UNDERSTANDING DIGITALLY PROGRAMMABLE HEARING AIDS

Other books of interest from the Longwood Division of Allyn and Bacon

Handbook of Auditory Evoked Responses
James W. Hall III
ISBN: 0-205-13566-8

Audiometric Interpretation: A Manual of Basic Audiometry, 2nd Edition
Harriet Kaplan, Vic S. Gladstone, and Lyle L. Lloyd
ISBN: 0-205-14753-4

Hearing Assessment, 2nd Edition
William F. Rintelmann
ISBN: 0-205-13537-4

Introduction to Aural Rehabilitation, 2nd Edition
Ronald L. Schow and Michael A. Nerbonne
ISBN: 0-205-13535-8

Acoustical Factors Affecting Hearing Aid Performance, 2nd Edition
Gerald A. Studebaker and Irving Hochberg
ISBN: 0-205-13778-4

UNDERSTANDING DIGITALLY PROGRAMMABLE HEARING AIDS

Edited by

ROBERT E. SANDLIN

Adjunct Professor
Department of Audiology
San Diego State University

ALLYN AND BACON

Boston   London   Sydney   Toronto

Copyright © 1994 by Allyn and Bacon
A Division of Simon & Schuster, Inc.
160 Gould Street
Needham Heights, MA 02194

Library of Congress Cataloging-in-Publication Data

Understanding digitally programmable hearing aids / edited by Robert E.
   Sandlin.
       p.   cm.
   Includes bibliographical references and index.
   ISBN 0-205-14845-X
   1. Hearing aids.   I. Sandlin, Robert E.
   [DNLM: 1. Hearing Aids   2. Software.   3. Signal Processing,
Computer-Assisted.   4. Speech Perception—physiology.   5. Hearing
Disorders—rehabilitation.   WV 274 U517 1993]
RF300.U53   1993
617.8'9—dc20   93-14194
                                                                CIP

Printed in the United States of America
10 9 8 7 6 5 4 3 2 1   97 96 95 94 93

This book is dedicated to those hearing health professionals who conscientiously endeavor to incorporate into their daily practice technological developments in hearing aid amplification in order to improve the communication abilities of those hearing-impaired individuals whom they serve.

Contents

PREFACE

The history of the development and utilization of electric hearing aid devices spans more than fifty years. During that half century plus, there have been many significant electroacoustic advances contributing to improved function for the hearing-impaired individual. Among the more important contributions have been improvement in transducer design and operation, efficient amplifiers providing less internal noise, transistor function, miniaturization of components without sacrificing performance, integrated circuitry, various forms of signal compression, and the application of automatic signal processing technology.

No development has been more significant, or has greater benefit potential, than the recent introduction of digitally controlled programmable hearing aid devices. The degrees of freedom afforded the hearing health professional in interfacing the electroacoustic response of the hearing aid with the magnitude and type of hearing loss are significant. The clinical utility of programming and reprogramming the output characteristics of a hearing aid is a great step forward. From a clinical point of view, the ability to change the response of the hearing aid without having to send it back to the manufacturer for modification represents conservation of time and improved efficiency. The ability to alter the acoustic response to meet changing amplification needs of the patient is most advantageous. The ability to adjust programmable hearing instruments to closely approximate recommended target gains has proven useful to clinicians embracing a specific fitting method, which prescribes frequency and gain values.

The primary intent of this book is to provide to the hearing health professional useful information about the development and application of digital technology applied to hearing aid devices. Although it is of considerable value to university and college students pursuing studies in audiology and hearing instrument dispensing, its primary value is for those professionals actively engaged in the selection and fitting of hearing aids. All readers will find valuable information about digitally controlled hearing aid systems and their contributions to effective use of amplification. The serious student will find this book of considerable interest, in that parts of it are given over to clinical evaluation of several commercially available digitally programmable hearing aids.

Even though digitally programmable hearing aids are commercially available, there has been no consensus among hearing health professionals regarding which instrument is most appropriate to meet acoustic demands of the hearing-impaired patient. Consensus is lacking regarding the superiority of a single-memory, digitally controlled, programmable hearing aid device over one having multiple memories, permitting the patient to select from a variety of electro-acoustic responses. Consensus is not to be found regarding methods of input/output function that should be incorporated into programmable hearing aid devices. For example, should the digitally controlled hearing aid provide automatic signal processing capabilities? If so, what should they be? Should the hearing aid have input or output compression (or both) to best compensate for the hearing deficit? Should there be a remote control transmission or other means of changing the hearing aid response to meet listening demands? The informed reader realizes that the same technical problems facing the designer of conventional analog hearing aid devices are those faced by engineers responsible for developing digitally controlled systems.

Digitally programmable systems represent a clinical and user convenience. Nonetheless, the convenience offered by these new hearing aid systems provides demonstrable advantage to hearing-impaired persons. Multiprogrammable systems, for example, have a number of specific acoustic responses from which to choose as background environmental conditions change in which listening is taking place. All that is required to create a more favorable acoustic response, as listening conditions change, is for the patient to select the appropriate acoustic output corresponding to need. The convenience of changing the response of the hearing aid on command has proven to be of considerable benefit to the user of the digitally multiprogrammable systems.

The argument remains, relative to the value of a *single programmable response* hearing aid compared to a *multiprogrammable* one. The proponents of single-response programmable systems feel that nothing additional is needed to maintain optimal function in any listening environment. The proponents of multi-programmable systems suggest that the acoustic response of the hearing aid should change as listening environments change. Both arguments are somewhat flawed, in that the electroacoustic behavior of a single programmable instrument and/or a multiprogrammable system is not uniform. There are single-response programmable units that provide significant change in electroacoustic response as the listening environment changes and, as such, are somewhat equivalent to multiprogrammable systems. The contrary opinion is that multiprogrammable systems offer greater change in electroacoustic behavior and, therefore, can provide the best acoustic correspondence as background environments change.

It is not our purpose in this book to answer these arguments. They will be resolved, eventually, through research, trial and error, modification of instrument performance, and individual preferences expressed by hearing-impaired individuals. If nothing else, we are at the early stage of this new technology. No one knows what performance characteristics are needed to best correspond with the presenting pathology. Nonetheless, evidence is mounting in support of the continued use of digitally controlled hearing aid devices.

Currently, only about 6% to 9% of hearing aids sold in the United States have some form of digital control application. Although disappointing, it is not surprising that many who dispense hearing aid devices are somewhat skeptical as to the clinical value of programmable instruments. Such hesitancy by hearing health professionals to adopt new and innovative approaches has been evident throughout the history of technological advance in hearing aid design and performance. One may hypothesize why it is that this *technology application* lag exists, but the conservative answer would include a number of possible reasons. Some of them are:

1. Programmable systems are no more electroacoustically advanced than current conventional systems.
2. The cost for the device is high and clinical value has not been demonstrated sufficiently to warrant the expenditure.
3. They are too complicated and one is not willing to invest the time to learn how to apply the new technology.
4. The dispenser is comfortable with his or her present selection and fitting procedures and chooses not to be bothered with this new hearing aid technology.

The best guess would be that there is a bit of truth in each of the attitudes expressed. My opinion is that much is to be gained by the hearing health professional and the patient to whom these new hearing aid devices are fitted.

This book is intended for those who have some knowledge base about the human auditory system and the application of hearing aid amplification. Although extensive academic or clinical backgrounds are not required, it is assumed that the reader has an active and professional interest in technological advances in hearing aid performance.

Let me mention here that only a relatively small number of digitally programmable hearing aids are reviewed in this book. Our intent was not to ignore or discount any contribution to digitally programmable hearing aid application. However, we have attempted to select hearing aid systems because they represent different approaches in the use of digital technology. We offer our apologies to those hearing aid manufacturing companies whose products are not mentioned here. There simply was not sufficient space to review all digitally controlled systems now available, or soon to be available to the hearing health professional. The primary purpose underlying the selection of those instruments discussed here was that each of them represented a unique utilization of digital technology in controlling the electroacoustic behavior of the hearing aids. Of the several companies manufacturing digitally programmable hearing aids, only seven are reviewed in depth. Of those seven, only the Phoenix, developed by Nicolet, represents a hearing aid system wherein the input signal is digitized, processed according to a specific algorithm, and reconverted to an analog signal. One may question the inclusion of this system in that it is no longer commercially available. The reason for so doing is rather straightforward. It was the first major effort of any company to use true digital technology in the design and function of a hearing aid system. Millions of dollars were spent in development, and technological advances were made because of that investment. Although the commercial success was less than needed to sustain production, the Phoenix true digital system demonstrated, clearly, that such technology is possible and that further research will improve upon its utility. The reader is advised to keep in mind that other commercial digitally programmable systems discussed do not alter the signal path. That is, the signal path in current digitally programmable hearing aids remains analog at all times.

Reviewed also is the utility of a specific cochlear implant system, which utilizes digitally programmable technology in establishing instrument performance. The Nucleus 22 developed by the Cochlear Corporation is an implantable hearing device selecting certain feature extractions of the input signal. Though radically different than a conventional hearing aid, it is nonetheless a hearing aid system employing digital technology. Through this form of cochlear implant, thousands of severe to profoundly deaf individuals have made significant gains in understanding and reacting to the acoustic world in which they live.

We are fortunate, indeed, to present the combined efforts of a number of well-qualified individuals who have contributed greatly to the several chapters presented here. Drs. Harry Levitt and Edward Cudahy tell us in Chapter 1 about the development of digital technology and its gradual application to hearing aid devices. Each of these gentlemen has attained national recognition as a researcher, and each evidences a keen interest in digital technology. Dr. Levitt, especially, has been in the forefront of its development. For some, the vocabulary found in this chapter may be new, but with sustained effort, the reader will find this to be a very necessary and useful chapter in understanding the subsequent contributions of others to this book.

Chapter 2 reviews the significant contributions that the ReSound Corporation has made to hearing aid technology and to the use of digitally programmable systems. Dr. Vincent Pluvinage, Director of Research and Development, carefully explores the rationale and development of the ReSound ITE and BTE devices. The underlying principle giving rise to this system is based on the recognition that loudness growth measured for the pathologic ear is significantly different than loudness growth measured for normal auditory systems. By measuring loudness growth by octave bands (LGOB), the hearing health professional can program into the hearing aid device input/output functions corresponding to the amplification needs of the impaired auditory system.

The Quattro multiprogrammable system discussed in Chapter 3 was developed by Widex in Copenhagen, Denmark. It is reviewed in a very competent and informative manner by Søren Westermann. Mr. Westermann is Research Manager for Widex. He points out that the most salient feature of the Quattro system is that of providing four separate hearing aid responses at the immediate command of the user. Each of these programs can be independently organized acoustically to correspond best to specific listening environments. That is, as the environment changes, the user of the system can select by remote control that electroacoustic response best suited for that specific listening condition. Although there is no general consensus as to the optimal number of programs that can be accessed, four would seem to represent a reasonable compromise. He ably discusses the rationale for the development of this digitally controlled, multiprogrammable system.

In Chapter 4, Pamela Burton of Siemens Hearing Instruments, Inc., presents a very competent analysis underlying the rationale for the Triton multichannel hearing aid and the PMC programming unit. Unlike most available digitally programmable systems, the Triton provides three channels of amplification, each of which can be independently programmed to interface with acoustic need. The value and limitations of such systems receive professional comment, much of which is supported by clinical research.

In Chapter 5, Dr. Thomas Powers expertly reviews the rationale and principles underlying the development of the PRIZM multiprogrammable hearing aid device. As Director of Sales for AudioScience, and with his strong background in clinical audiology, he offers to the reader unusual and pertinent insights into the contributions of the new Prizm system. He stresses the flexibility of this multiprogrammable unit and reviews in some detail its clinical application. The Prizm reflects much of the current state-of-the-art technology applied to digitally controlled, multiprogrammable systems. This is particularly apparent when discussing linear and nonlinear performance characteristics of the instrument.

Chapter 6 deals with the rationale and development of the technically sophisticated 3M Memory Mate system and its application to those with hearing impairment. It is ably written by Dr. Paul Stypulkowski, who is intimately familiar with all phases of research and development of this digitally programmable hearing aid device. Unlike most other programmable instruments, the 3M system provides eight separate and distinct programs to the user. Rationale is ably presented in defense of this number.

The Phoenix, a true digital hearing aid system developed by Nicolet, is discussed by Veronica Heide in Chapter 7. As mentioned previously, this is the only digitally programmable hearing aid system wherein the input signal is digitized. Ms. Heide does an excellent job in defining and justifying the rationale for its development, as well as the need for further research to refine its performance characteristics. It is the feeling of many that true digital technology will be commonplace among hearing aid devices in the not too distant future. Her frank and open discussion of problems associated with the development and utilization of the Phoenix is refreshing, indeed.

In Chapter 8, Judy Brimacombe, Director of Clinical Services for the Cochlear Corporation, describes in organized detail the contributions of cochlear implants, with particular reference to the Nucleus 22 device. Of the several implant systems commercially available, the Nucleus device uses coding strategies employing digital technology. Often we forget that cochlear implants are hearing aid devices. They differ significantly, however, from conventional programmable systems, in that they do not perform in the same conventional manner. That is, the stimulus to the auditory system is provided by means of implanted active electrodes.

In Chapter 9, Dr. Robert Sweetow takes a long and careful look at the clinical utility of programmable hearing aid systems. Penetrating questions dealing with selecting and fitting of programmable hearing instruments are asked and answers given. Dr. Sweetow is the first to admit that to attempt to select a system judged to be the best is impossible in that not every programmable system is suited for all hearing loss types and magnitudes. He is to be highly commended for a yeomen-like task. His comments should be of significant value to those contemplating the use of programmable hearing aid devices.

Dr. Michael Valente and his highly qualified colleagues at the Washington

University School of Medicine in St. Louis do an excellent job in presenting an overview of the several programmable systems. In Chapter 10, they review the advantages and limitations of several programmable hearing aids. Clinical observations are presented in a straightforward and clinically defensible manner, relative to the value of those systems discussed. In that all comments are based on clinical utility, this is a very important chapter to all who read this book.

Dr. Wayne Staab has a long and distinguished clinical background in essentially all aspects of hearing aid amplification. In Chapter 11, he takes a very careful look at the limitations imposed by today's programmable systems. Not only does he look at the technical and performance limitations, but he reviews currently held attitudes of hearing health professionals regarding the justification of digitally programmable hearing aid devices and their use. This was a difficult chapter to write, but Dr. Staab does an outstanding job in simplifying a very arduous task. He warns against a blanket adoption of digitally controlled hearing aid devices just because they are new. He strongly emphasizes that audiologists and dispensers need to understand the performance rationale and fitting protocol before proceeding with selection and fitting.

Finally, in Chapter 12, Dr. David Preves, Vice President of Engineering for the Argosy Corporation, takes a crystal ball gazer's look at what the future may hold for digitally controlled hearing aid devices. With his background in audiology and electrical engineering, one could not ask for a more qualified individual to review what may be in store for those who select and fit hearing instruments. As the reader may suspect, Dr. Preves feels strongly that technological advance will continue and improvements made will add to the success with which programmable hearing aids are utilized.

Unfortunately, as with most books dealing with technological advance, by the time of publication there undoubtedly will be other systems available incorporating advances in digital technology. Such is the lot of those who choose to write about currently available technology. However, in no way should such observations reduce the value of this book. One is deeply indebted to those professional men and women who have contributed to the successful conclusion of this collected work. The greatest reward that each could receive is to know that the information provided here was instrumental in directing attention to the value of applied technology and its benefit to the hearing impaired.

I wish to acknowledge the invaluable services of friends and colleagues who not only encouraged the completion of this book but offered cogent suggestions related to its content and construction. To mention them all would extend this acknowledgment beyond reasonable bounds. However, they know who they are. My sincerest thanks to each of them.

Robert E. Sandlin

CONTRIBUTING AUTHORS

Robert E. Sandlin, Ph.D., Robert E. Sandlin, Ph.D. & Associates, Inc., Alvarado Medical Center, 6505 Alvarado Road, Suite 107, San Diego, CA 92120. Dr. Sandlin is an adjunct Professor of Audiology at San Diego State University. He serves on the scientific advisory board of the American Tinnitus Association. Although retired from active audiological and dispensing practice, he has an active writing, research, and lecturing schedule.

Anne L. Beiter, M.S., Cochlear Corporation, 61 Inverness Drive East, Suite 200, Englewood, CO 80112. Ms. Beiter is the Clinical Services Manager for Cochlear Corporation and has participated in the clinical study of cochlear implants in children, adolescents, and adults since 1986. She is an instructor for cochlear implant training courses and has coauthored several studies on cochlear implants in children and adults.

Judith A. Brimacombe, M.A., Cochlear Corporation, 61 Inverness Drive East, Suite 200, Englewood, CO 80112. Ms. Brimacombe has been working in the field of cochlear implants since 1981, first with single-channel devices at the House Ear Institute, then with multichannel systems through Cochlear Corporation. Presently, she is Vice President of Clinical and Regulatory Affairs for Cochlear, the manufacturer of the 22-channel cochlear implant system.

Pamela L. Burton, M.A., Siemens Hearing Instruments, Inc., 13043 East 166th Street, Cerritos, CA 90701. Ms. Burton is the Programmable Product Specialist at Siemens. She has been with Siemens for the past six years. Ms. Burton has published several articles on programmable products and has spoken at numerous local, regional, and national seminars on this subject.

James M. Coticchia, M.D., Washington University School of Medicine, Box 8115, 517 South Euclid Avenue, St. Louis, MO 63110. Dr. Coticchia completed his undergraduate education at Ohio State University and graduated from the Ohio State University College of Medicine in 1986. He is currently a resident in the Department of Otolaryngology–Head and Neck Surgery at Washington University School of Medicine.

Edward Cudahy, Ph.D., Executive Director of the New York League for the Hard of Hearing, 71 West 23rd Street, New York, NY 10010. Dr. Cudahy's research interests include psychoacoustics and acoustic instrumentation, especially signal processing in hearing aids, and he has recently published a text on instrumentation in audiology and speech pathology. He has extensive experience in data acquisition, signal synthesis, and the use of computers in audiology.

Veronica H. Heide, M.S., Audible Difference, 5727 Pembroke Drive, Madison, WI 53711. Ms. Heide joined Project Phoenix in 1976 as a research audiologist and later provided applications support and customer training for the Audiodiagnostic and

Biomedical Divisions of Nicolet Instrument Corp. She has shared her knowledge of signal processing and enthusiasm for her work with hundreds of audiologists from all over the world. She is currently in private practice in Madison, WI, spreading the word about her business, Audible Difference™.

Gary Jenison, M.D., Ph.D., Washington University School of Medicine, Box 8115, 517 South Euclid Avenue, St. Louis, MO 63110. Dr. Jenison is a graduate of the University of California–San Diego, the University of Colorado Medical Center, and Louisiana State University Medical School. He has completed a postdoctoral fellowship at the Kresge Hearing Research Laboratory of the South and is currently an Otolaryngology–Head and Neck Surgery Resident of Washington University Medical Center.

Harry Levitt, Ph.D., City University of New York, Graduate School and University Center, 33 West 42nd Street, New York, NY 10036. Dr. Levitt is Director of the Digital Sensory Aids Laboratory at the Graduate School of the City University of New York with the rank of Distinguished Professor. His research interests include development and evaluation of sensory aids, including digital hearing aids, signal processing for noise reduction, digital processing of speech, computer-assisted testing, and the application of these techniques to audiology, speech training, and deaf education.

Vincent Pluvinage, Ph.D., Vice President of Research and International Operations, ReSound Corporation, 220 Saginaw Drive, Redwood City, CA 94063. Dr. Pluvinage graduated summa cum laude from the Université Catholique de Louvain in Belgium with a degree in Applied Physics Engineering, while concurrently attending three years of medical school course work. Elected Fellow of the Belgian American Educational Foundation in 1980, he went on to conduct four years of post-graduate research in ophthalmology at the University of Michigan (Ann Arbor), where he completed a Ph.D. in Bio-Engineering. In 1985, he joined the R & D staff of AT&T Bell Laboratories, to design digital signal processing hardware and software. In collaboration with Dr. Henry Levitt at City University of New York, the experimental digital sound processors, programmed for multiband dynamic range compression, were field tested, and the clinical results confirmed the laboratory findings of Edgar Villchur. Upon spin-off of the AT&T technology to ReSound in 1987, four members of the original development team continued the product design with about $15 million private and venture capital funding, until first commercialization in 1990. Dr. Pluvinage's current activities include directing research on electromagnetic hearing devices, as well as expanding ReSound's international sales activities to Japan and several European countries.

Lisa Gulledge Potts, M.S., Washington University School of Medicine, Box 8115, 517 South Euclid Avenue, St. Louis, MO 63110. Ms. Potts received her B.S. in communication disorders and sciences from Southern Illinois University and her M.S. in speech and hearing from Washington University. She is currently a Research Audiologist at Washington University School of Medicine, working with new developments in programmable and nonprogrammable hearing aids.

Thomas A. Powers, Ph.D., AudioScience, Inc., P.O. Box 225, Bound Brook, NJ 08805. Dr. Powers received his B.A. from SUNY at Geneseo and his M.S. and Ph.D. from Ohio University. Upon completion of his doctorate he entered a private practice in audiology, with an active hearing instrument dispensing program. He entered the hearing instrument industry over 13 years ago and has held various management positions. Dr. Powers is currently Vice President for Professional Relations for AudioScience, Inc.

David A. Preves, Ph.D., Vice President of Research and Development, Argosy® Electronics, Inc., 10300 West 70th Street, Eden Prairie, MN 55344. Dr. Preves has a bachelor of science and a master of science degree in electrical engineering from the University of Illinois and a doctorate in biomedical engineering from the University of Minnesota. He is adjunct Professor in the Department of Communication Disorders at the University of Minnesota. Dr. Preves is chair of the ANSI working group on hearing aid measurement standards and is a member of two other ANSI standards committees. He is a member of the executive committee of the American Auditory Society.

Margaret W. Skinner, Ph.D., Associate Professor and Director of Audiology, Box 8115, 517 South Euclid Avenue, St. Louis, MO 63110. Dr. Skinnner's clinical research has focused on the selection of hearing aid and cochlear implant parameters that will optimize speech recognition and benefit in everyday life for individuals with hearing impairment.

Wayne J. Staab, Ph.D., President, Dr. Wayne J. Staab and Associates, 512 East Canterbury Lane, Phoenix, AZ 85022. Dr. Staab is an internationally recognized author, lecturer, marketer, and expert on hearing aids. His continued involvement in innovate hearing aid ideas puts him in the forefront of new technology issues. He is a past President of the American Auditory Society, Fellow of the International Collegium of Rehabilitative Audiology, and is active in other organizations.

Paul H. Stypulkowski, Ph.D., Hearing Health, 3M Life Sciences Sector, 3M Center, St. Paul, MN 55144. Dr. Stypulkowski holds his Ph.D. in Auditory Physiology from the University of Connecticut and has been involved in basic and clinical research in the hearing health care field at 3M Company since 1979. He has published in the areas of auditory electrophysiology, ototoxicity, evoked potentials, cochlear implants, and programmable hearing aids, and is currently a senior technical specialist with the Hearing Health Program at 3M.

Robert W. Sweetow, Ph.D., University of California, San Francisco, 400 Parnassus Avenue, A-705, San Francisco, CA 94143. Dr. Sweetow is currently the Director of Audiology and Associate Clinical Professor in the Department of Otolaryngology at the Medical Center of the University of California, San Francisco. He received his Ph.D. from Northwestern University in 1977 and also holds an M.A. from the University of Southern California and a B.S. from the University of Iowa. He is a popular lecturer and the author of numerous textbook chapters and scientific articles on tinnitus and amplification for the hearing impaired.

L. Maureen Valente, M.S., Department of Communication Disorders, St. Louis University, 3733 West Pine Boulevard, St. Louis, MO 63108. Ms. Valente received her Bachelor's and Master's degrees from the University of Illinois in Champaign-Urbana. Past clinical experiences have included a variety of hospital and private practice settings. She is currently a lecturer and clinical supervisor with St. Louis University's Department of Communication Disorders. Areas of interest include pediatric audiology and aural rehabilitation.

Michael Valente, Ph.D., Washington University School of Medicine, Box 8115, 517 South Euclid Avenue, St. Louis, MO 63110. Dr. Valente received his Ph.D. from the University of Illinois in 1975. He is currently Director of Adult Audiology at Washington University School of Medicine. He has published extensively on hearing aid fitting and selection.

Søren Westermann, M.S., Widex ApS, Ny Vestergaard Vej 25, DK 3500, Vaerloese, Denmark. Mr. Westermann received his General Certificate of Education in Mathematics and Physics in 1972 and his Master of Science degree in Electronics in 1980 from the Technical University of Denmark. As Manager of the Research and Computer Department, he participates in the development of hearing aid technology and its application to the hearing impaired. He has contributed to the hearing aid science literature in this country and in Europe.

CHAPTER 1

DIGITAL HEARING AIDS: A HISTORICAL PERSPECTIVE

Edward Cudahy and Harry Levitt

Analog hearing aids have improved considerably over the last decade. However, the introduction of digital technology at a reasonable cost is significantly impacting the development of new hearing aids. Another important factor is the continuing miniaturization and integration of more and more complex components, as evidenced by the evolution of the digital technology for the personal computer. Ten years ago, large desktop computers with limited memory and processing power were being introduced. Notebook computers, about one-tenth the size of these desktop machines, with large amounts of memory, high-capacity disk drives, and far more processing power than the original desktop units are currently available, with sub-notebook computers expected to be widely available by 1993. Software, which determines the utility of all this computer power, has made a similar evolution in sophistication and ease of use. The concept of a sophisticated computer that you carry much like you would a pad of paper and that is easy to use is well on its way to reality at a pace that would have been inconceivable even five years ago.

The same pace of development is evidenced in the hearing aid marketplace. While programmable (quasi-digital and digital) hearing aids constituted only 7% of the hearing aid market in 1990, in early 1991, 40% of dispensers indicated that they planned to dispense programmable instruments in the near future (Cranmer, 1991). This development has been predicted for quite a while (see Levitt, Neuman, and Toraskar, 1987), but it is only within the last couple of years that a wearable digital hearing aid has been introduced to the market. The continuing reduction in component size for digital technology and especially some of the exciting developments in the management of power for these components make it reasonable to predict that digital technology for in-the-ear instruments is very close to being available. A completely digital behind-the ear hearing aid has already been developed, although it has not been marketed.

Digital technology has made its way into hearing aids in such a variety of ways that the current state of affairs regarding digital technology and hearing aids can be very confusing. It has become especially difficult to understand exactly what constitutes a "digital" hearing aid. This chapter will examine digital technology and some of the ways in which it is used in hearing aids. Future applications of digital technology to hearing aids will also be discussed.

ADVANTAGES OF DIGITAL HEARING AIDS

Digital hearing aids promise many advantages over completely analog hearing aids. Potential features include:

1. Programmability
2. Much greater precision in adjusting electro-acoustic parameters
3. Self-monitoring capabilities, including self-calibration
4. Control of acoustic feedback (a serious practical problem with high-gain hearing aids)
5. The use of advanced digital signal processing techniques for noise reduction
6. Automatic control of signal levels
7. Self-adaptive adjustment to changing acoustic environments

A few of these features are available in the current generation of digital hearing aids, but some have not been implemented because of the constraints on chip size and power consumption. All of the above-mentioned features have already been demonstrated in a master digital hearing aid (Levitt, 1982; Levitt et al., 1986), and with the development of more advanced signal processing chips, an increasing number of these attractive features are being incorporated into wearable digital hearing aids.

The many advantages offered by digital hearing aids can be subdivided into three broad groups:

1. Signal processing capabilities that are analogous to, but superior to, those offered by conventional analog hearing aids
2. Signal processing capabilities that are unique to digital systems and that cannot be implemented in conventional analog hearing aids
3. Methods of processing and controlling signals that change our way of thinking about how hearing aids should be designed, prescribed, and fitted

The first two groups are fairly obvious. The first includes the ability to tune more finely the same electroacoustic parameters that would be adjusted in an analog hearing aid. The second includes sophisticated noise and feedback reduction techniques requiring storage of the signal for processing.

The third type of advantage is the most subtle and involves the greater flexibility provided by digital technology. For example, a digital hearing aid can be programmed not only to amplify audio signals input into the hearing aid, but also to generate audio signals. As such, the instrument can be programmed to serve as an audiometer in order to facilitate the measurement of audiological characteristics relevant to the prescriptive fitting of hearing aids (Levitt et al., 1986; Levitt, Sullivan, and Hwang, 1986). Although similar in concept to the real-ear measurement system in dealing with the very difficult problem of correcting for the frequency-dependent differences in sound level between the traditional audiometer headphone and the patient's own hearing aid receiver, the use of the hearing aid as audiometer has the advantage of using the same sound processing system that the person will be using every day. This idea is a logical extension of the observation that today's digital audiometers and a digital hearing aid use the same hardware for signal generation and the major difference between the two devices is software.

An important part of the research and development effort surrounding digital hearing aids has been the use of computer simulation. As noted at the beginning of this chapter, the development of digital technology for computers has closely paralleled such development for hearing aids. In fact, the first working digital hearing aid was achieved using real-time computer simulation (Levitt, 1982; Levitt et al., 1986), thereby providing a glimpse of the many possible features that could be incorporated in the digital hearing aids of the future.

The results currently being obtained using computer simulation techniques are having a profound effect on our thinking with respect to which features should or should not be included in a modern hearing aid. Whereas, in the past, investigation of signal processing and control features that would lead to more effective hearing aids was limited primarily by what could be achieved technologically, the present situation, with the help of computer simulation and the realization of practical digital hearing aids, is one in which progress is limited primarily by our own lack of understanding of what is important in processing signals for hearing impairment.

A BRIEF HISTORY OF DIGITAL HEARING AIDS

Early Applications of Digital Techniques

A description of the early developments in signal processing theory and technology, especially as they relate to hearing aids, is provided in Levitt, Neuman, and Toraskar (1987). As is frequently the case in technological development, many of the same issues discussed there, such as the need for digital-to-analog (D/A) and analog-to-digital (A/D) converters of sufficient speed, accuracy, and power consumption, are still current. The use of computer simulation, as indicated earlier, has continued to play a big role in the development of hearing aid fitting techniques for digital hearing aids, as well as for hardware development.

The introduction of personal computers, and especially portable computers, has accelerated this trend. A recent development is signal processing boards incorporating virtually all the components required for processing audio signals and fitting neatly inside a personal computer. Such integrated systems are currently used extensively in experiments on acoustic amplification and signal processing for hearing impairment. The portable system in particular has permitted the field testing of new signal processing features,

something not possible with the older laboratory systems and a feature that should lead to improved transfer of proof of concept from the laboratory to everyday use in hearing aids.

A closely related application of computers in this context is that in which a personal computer is used as an audiometer and prescriptive tool. A system of this type has been developed (Popelka and Engebretson, 1983; Engebretson, Morley, and Popelka, 1987) in which the computer is used to facilitate the measurement, display, and interpretation of audiological data in order to prescribe a hearing aid more efficiently. The computer can also be used to search for the best hearing aid for a given patient from a data base containing detailed electroacoustic specifications of available hearing aids (Hertzano, Levitt, and Slosberg, 1979). A number of companies have developed similar computerized hearing aid fitting systems (Johnson and Schnier, 1988; Mangold and Leijon, 1979; Pluvinage and Benson, 1988; Widin and Mangold, 1988).

"Digital" hearing aids actually are represented by two classes of instrument: the quasi-digital (sometimes referred to as hybrid) hearing aid and the all-digital hearing aid. Both are frequently referred to as digital hearing aids. While similar in many ways, there are also significant differences in the nature of the signal processing, which has implications for their potential applications.

Quasi-Digital Hearing Aids

In a quasi-digital hearing aid, conventional analog amplifiers and filters are controlled by digital means. A simple, practical realization of this approach is to use a computer for programming the hearing aid. Once programmed, the hearing aid is disconnected from the computer and is then used in essentially the same way as a conventional hearing aid.

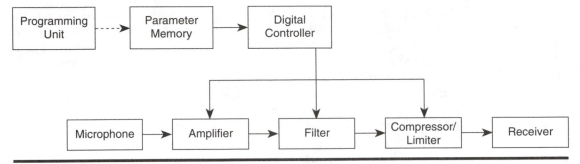

FIGURE 1.1.   A block diagram of a quasi-digital hearing aid. The programming unit is shown as temporarily connected. The digital controller is shown as controlling an analog amplifier, filter, and compressor/limiter.

The next step in the development of a practical quasi-digital hearing aid is that in which both the analog components and the digital controller are combined in a single wearable unit. The basic architecture of such a hearing aid is shown in Figure 1.1. Note that the digital controller not only controls or programs the operation of the analog components (amplifiers, filter, and compressor/limiter), but is itself programmed by an external computer (programming unit) using a temporary connection. The external programming and control are performed in the clinic or hearing aid dispensary when the unit is first prescribed and fitted. The control data is then stored in a memory bank tied to the controller in the hearing aid.

The concept of a digitally controlled analog hearing aid is very attractive from a practical perspective because of the low power consumption involved. The technology of low-power analog amplifiers and filters is well advanced, whereas the present generation of chips for digital signal processing draws relatively large amounts of power. The possibility of combining the low power consumption of analog components with the greater signal processing capability of digital components now appears to be a viable option. For example, Graupe, Grosspietsch, and Basseas (1987) have developed an adaptive

noise-reducing filter on a single chip using a quasi-digital approach. This chip is small enough and of sufficiently low power consumption to fit in a conventional behind-the-ear or in-the-ear hearing aid.

Quasi-digital technology is currently the approach taken for all programmable hearing aids (see Bentler, 1991, for a list of programmable hearing aid manufacturers). This approach has the advantage that the programmer (computer) is essentially sending lists of parameters to the hearing aid, which are then stored and used to drive the digital controller in the hearing aid. The difficulty in the present situation is that many hearing aid manufacturers use a unique way of handling the control information, requiring separate programmers for each hearing aid. Since the control information is just data, it should be possible for companies to agree on a common interface standard. What data are sent can be handled by software, thus helping protect proprietary knowledge regarding the inner workings of the hearing aid. There has been an attempt to set up just such a situation by getting a consortium of companies to agree on a common interface standard and programmer, with individual software control modules produced by each company (Branderbit, 1991).

Another form of quasi-digital hearing aid (which may have been used in the applications cited above) is that of a sampled-data system in which the audio signal is sampled at discrete intervals in time, but the samples are kept in analog form during processing. Such a system can be implemented fairly easily in practice using switched-capacitance techniques. Consider, for example, a sequence of capacitors with each capacitor containing a charge representing a single sample in a sampled-data sequence. At each sampling instant, the charge on each capacitor is switched to the next capacitor in the sequence. The value of the charge on each capacitance is multiplied by a coefficient. The sum of these products is the output of the filter. (For further discussion of the technical characteristics of such a filter, see Oppenheim and Schafer, 1975; Levitt, Neuman, and Toraskar, 1987.)

The characteristics of this filter are determined by the choice of the coefficients. In a programmable version of the filter, the coefficients are adjusted by a digital controller. Note that although the incoming audio waveform is sampled discretely in time (which requires anti-aliasing and anti-imaging filters), the samples themselves remain in analog form throughout processing. In an all-digital version of the above filter, the samples would be converted to binary form prior to processing.

The use of quasi-digital methods has the important advantage that digital signal processing techniques can be used without the need for A/D or D/A converters. The power consumed by an A/D converter increases rapidly with degree of quantization. The development of high-resolution A/D converters of small size and low power consumption, suitable for use in a practical hearing aid, is still a difficult technical problem.

All-Digital Hearing Aids

In an all-digital hearing aid, both the processing of the audio signals and the control for the processing are done by digital means. Analog signals transduced by the microphone are sampled and converted to binary form for processing and then converted back to analog form after processing to drive the earphone. Figure 1.2 shows a block diagram for an all-digital hearing aid. Note that it is very similar to a quasi-digital hearing aid, except that all analog circuitry between the microphone and receiver has been replaced by the signal processor with A/D and D/A converters. Graupe and Causey (1975) appear to have been the first to implement such a system using an 8080 microprocessor. The approach used was conceptually similar to that of the digitally

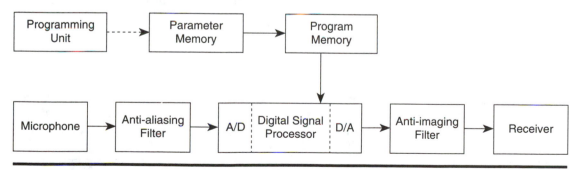

FIGURE 1.2.   A block diagram of an all-digital hearing aid. This figure is the same as Figure 1.1, except that the analog amplifier, filter, and compressor/limiter have been replaced with a digital signal processor controlled by the programs in program memory.

controlled analog system shown in Figure 1.1, except that the filter, limiter, and amplifier were replaced by equivalent digital components. Further, because of the great flexibility of control afforded by the microprocessor, it was possible to program the system to be self-adaptive, thereby opening the door to the use of advanced signal processing techniques for noise reduction and intelligibility enhancement. Although the 8080 microprocessor used by Graupe was both slow and relatively large in size, he clearly anticipated the day when microprocessors would be fast enough and small enough for use in a practical hearing aid.

At about this time (the late 1970s) the concept of an all-digital programmable hearing aid was also being developed in Germany (Moser, 1980), as well as at the Institute for Hearing Research in Nottingham, England (personal communication between M. Haggard and Levitt). The approach followed by the latter group was that of using a self-standing digital filter controlled by a standard microcomputer, a technique that was to be adopted later by several other research laboratories (Levitt et al., 1986; Studebaker, Sherbecoe, and Matesich, 1987).

Although the concept of a digital hearing aid was anticipated at an early date, two major technical problems had to be resolved before anyone could develop a practical all-digital instrument. The first was the development of a digital signal processor fast enough to operate in real time. The second, more difficult problem is that of developing digital circuitry that is small enough and sufficiently low in power consumption for practical use in a small, wearable unit. Although the technology is currently advanced sufficiently that a behind-the-ear all-digital hearing aid can be produced, the cost is still high and, given the popularity of in-the-ear devices, it is very difficult to market.

The first breakthrough regarding real-time signal processors came with the development of the array processor, in which an array of numbers is processed simultaneously, instead of only one number at a time as in a conventional digital computer. The saving in processing time resulting from the use of this technique is sufficient to allow for real-time processing of audio signals. High-speed array processors were introduced toward the end of the 1970s, and shortly afterwards an all-digital hearing aid was developed configured around one of these units (Levitt, 1982). Although still too large to be wearable, that instrument has been used effectively as a master hearing aid in a series of experimental investigations on the prescriptive fitting and evaluation of digital hearing aids (Levitt et al., 1986; Levitt, Neuman, and Toraskar, 1987; Neuman et al., 1987).

Another important development was the introduction of a family of high-speed digital signal processing (DSP) chips in 1982. Although not as fast as an array processor, these chips are currently fast enough for extensive real-time processing of speech signals. These chips have been used as the central component for personal computer-based signal processing boards with all of the other circuitry needed for audio signal processing, such as A/D and D/A conversion and anti-aliasing and anti-imaging filters, plus large amounts of memory for program and data storage built into the board.

A recent computer simulation of a hearing aid, using a personal computer with a signal processing board, was a two-channel compression hearing aid with a programmable filter before and after compression in each channel. This system allows for simulation of a wide array of hearing aid configurations, especially compression, as implemented in current and future hearing aids (Fabry, 1991) with a view to finding parameter sets that are most beneficial in particular situations.

A significant advantage of these chips is

that because audio signal processing is only one of the applications for such chips, the economy of scale has made their cost decrease considerably. As in the beginning history of analog hearing aids, the major industry driving this cost reduction is the audio entertainment industry. Furthermore, their small size permits packaging in a unit small enough to be wearable. Experimental body-worn digital hearing aids were developed soon after such high-speed DSP chips became available (Cummins and Hecox, 1987).

The second major problem, that of reducing power consumption and physical size so that the digital chips are small enough to fit in an in-the-ear hearing aid, has yet to be resolved. Under normal operation, the various DSP chips on the market in 1991 are too large and draw far too much current for a practical in-the-ear unit. The current generation of chips is small enough and of sufficiently low power consumption that a small (about half the size of a pack of cigarettes), body-worn, all-digital hearing aid was developed and marketed (Sammeth, 1990). Unfortunately, as often happens with the first generation of an advanced technological device, it was expensive and was not a financial success. The same company did design and make a BTE all-digital unit (Hecox, personal communication), but it was never marketed.

HOW DOES DIGITAL SIGNAL PROCESSING WORK?

Analog-to-Digital Conversion

The key element in a digital hearing aid is its use of sound signals that have been sampled discretely in time so that they have become represented by a series of data points instead of by a continuously varying value analogous to the waveform itself. Figure 1.3 illustrates the process whereby an analog signal is converted to digital form. The uppermost section

of the diagram shows a continuous waveform; in this example, voltage as a function of time is shown for a single cycle of a sine wave.

The middle section of the diagram shows the sampled data at three sample rates. Note that the signal is no longer continuous but consists of a series of discrete steps. The height of each step is equal to the conversion value of the continuous waveform at the sampling instant. At this stage of the conversion process, the step heights are specified in numerical form—that is, the value of each sample is recorded at its decimal equivalent of the binary level within the range of the signal's continuous variation. For the purpose of this example, eight arbitrary levels of quantization are shown. Each of the analog samples shown in the top section of the diagram has been approximated by a sample with a height equal to one of these eight levels of quantization. Each of the three binary waveforms represents a different sample rate.

Two potential types of A/D conversion are available today, linear and logarithmic. A linear converter uses a linear scale with a resolution determined by the power of 2 represented by the number of binary digits (bits) in the converter. For example, a 16-bit converter will have a resolution of one part in 65,536, with each step being equal in size. (For a more detailed discussion of linear analog-to-digital converters, see Cudahy, 1990). A logarithmic or floating-point converter uses a logarithmic scale. The value of the logarithmic converter is that the highest resolution will be with the smallest signals, yielding good signal-to-noise ratios for these signals. (For a more detailed discussion of floating-point A/D conversion, see Harris et al., 1991.) Harris et al. (1991) reported that to reproduce speech without affecting intelligibility required a 5-bit floating-point conversion or a 12-bit integer conversion, but although the floating-point conversion is more efficient, it requires greater processing power.

Original Sine Wave

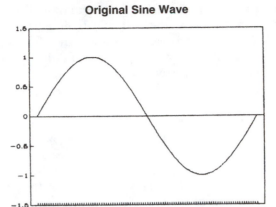

Time

Digitization as a Function of Sample Rate

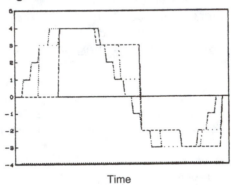

Time

Relation Between Signal Frequency and Sample Rate

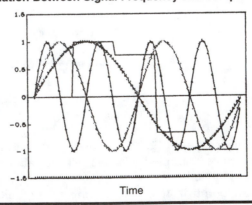

Time

FIGURE 1.3.   Conversion of an analog signal to digital format. The top panel shows a typical analog waveform. The middle panel shows the digitized samples derived from that waveform at three sample rates. The bottom panel shows three analog waveforms at different frequencies that could be generated using the lowest-frequency digitized waveform from the middle panel.

Potential Problems in Digital Signal Processing: Quantization

Regardless of the type of converter, the process of converting an analog sample to digital form involves a sequence of binary "decisions." In the example shown in the middle panel of Figure 1.3, three binary decisions were used leading to a binary representation consisting of three binary digits or bits. Therefore, the binary representation is said to have "an accuracy of 3 bits."

Referring once again to the middle section of Figure 1.3, it can be seen that all binary samples do not lie directly on the original waveform. The waveform to be digitized for the example shown is from –1 to +1. Since there are eight steps, the distance between steps (quantization levels) in this example is 0.25. The largest error that can occur is half a quantization step, which in this case is 0.125. In general, an N-bit A/D converter will have 2^N quantization levels, and the error of quantization will not exceed 1/2 of $1/2^N$, or $1/(2^{N+1})$, of the range of the A/D converter. In the above example, N = 3 and the range of quantization was 2; the number of quantization levels was thus 8 (2^3) and the precision of quantization was $1/(2^4)$ or 1/16 of the range, which is 2/16 (=0.125).

Since the timing of the error is usually random (sample rate issues are discussed later), quantization error generates a broadband noise. The advent of digital processing in hearing aids has led to research into the perceptual consequences of digital conversion (Harris et al., 1991; Cudahy and Kates, 1993). This research will provide guidance regarding the kind and amount of digital conversion required for adequate sound quality.

Potential Problems in Digital Signal Processing: Aliasing

Another potential problem in the digitization of analog signals is the risk of "aliasing." The lowest section of Figure 1.3 shows three analog waveforms, each of which would yield the same sequence of samples shown in the figure along with the waveforms. Two of the waveforms shown are valid waveforms—that is, they represent the waveforms that were originally sampled. The third is an alias of the true waveform. (It can be shown that there are an infinite number of possible aliases of the true waveform.) If sampling is to be used as a means of preparing continuous signals for digital signal processing, it is essential that there be no ambiguity as to which waveform the sample waveform represents.

A Rule for Avoiding Aliasing. The analog waveforms in the lowest section of the diagram differ in frequency. The highest-frequency waveform differs from the other waveforms in one important respect: It is represented by less than two samples per period. The two lower-frequency waveforms are sampled at a rate of more than two samples per period. For example, there are five samples for four periods of the highest-frequency waveform; the rate of samples is thus less than two samples per period. This is true of any other alias corresponding to the sample waveform shown. A simple rule is thus to assume that a true waveform is one sampled at more than two samples per period. In order for this rule to hold, it is essential that the sampling rate always be greater than twice the highest frequency of the waveform being sampled. Stated another way, if it is known that the highest frequency in the signal does not exceed half the sampling rate (i.e., there are at least two samples per period of the highest-frequency component in the signal), then there can be no aliasing errors.

In order to ensure that there are no aliasing errors, it is common practice to use an anti-aliasing filter prior to the sampling operation. An anti-aliasing filter is typically a low-pass filter with a very high rate of attenuation above the cutoff frequency, fc, where fc < 1/2 sampling rate. Due to the fact that filters do not eliminate energy completely at frequencies above fc, a typical rule is to use 40% of the sampling rate. Similarly, in order to avoid the generation of spurious waveforms when a sample waveform is converted back to analog form, it is common practice to use an anti-imaging filter after the D/A converter. It is usual for the anti-imaging filter to have the same low-pass characteristics as the anti-aliasing filter.

ELEMENTS OF A DIGITAL HEARING AID

The basic operations performed by a hearing aid are amplification, filtering, and output limiting using the numerical information provided by the conversion techniques described earlier. Amplification in a digital system is achieved by simply multiplying the samples representing the audio signal by a constant A. The magnitude of A determines the amount of amplification. Amplitude limiting is also achieved fairly simply by setting a maximum allowable value for the samples contained in the digital representation. An alternative method of output limiting is to adjust the amplification constant A in inverse proportion to the short-term energy of the signal (represented by an amplitude average of the number of samples corresponding to some time constant), thereby reducing the gain as signal level is increased. The first of these two methods is the digital equivalent of peak clipping (a technique commonly used in older conventional hearing aids); the second method is the digital equivalent of amplitude compression (a technique used regularly in modern conventional hearing aids). Considerable control of the temporal characteristics of compression is given by the ability to manipulate the time constant easily in response to a parameter of the audio signal, for example, the instantaneous amplitude.

In contrast to the above operations, the process of filtering audio signals represents a particularly interesting and innovative application of digital techniques. Unfortunately, digital filters are difficult to describe without some use of mathematics. Levitt, Neuman, and Toraskar (1987) provide some mathematical background to the key concepts underlying digital filtering.

Digital filters operate on sample waveforms in much the same way (but not in exactly the same way) as an electronic filter operates on an electrical waveform. It may be noted that this filtering operation is also analogous to taking a running arithmetic average of the data sequence.

An important advantage of digital filtering over conventional electronic filtering is the potential for increased precision, which may be several orders of magnitude greater than can be achieved in practice using conventional electronic (analog) components. For example, it is not difficult to create a digital filter with a very steep rate of attenuation (e.g., over 1000 dB/octave). This is a major difference between quasi-digital and all-digital hearing aids. The all-digital instrument can perform manipulations of the frequency gain characteristic that a quasi-digital instrument would find impossible because it is impossible to design and build such a filter from analog components that would fit in a hearing aid.

A second important advantage is that the digital filter can be reprogrammed to have vastly different characteristics without any change in hardware—that is, the same piece of equipment is used. This change can be made to take place in a fraction of a second. The same would be true for other aspects of the hearing aid, such as designing two different forms of compression in the same hearing aid. For an all-digital instrument it is simply a matter of software, and a switch between the two would be virtually instantaneous. A quasi-digital instrument would not be able to contain all the necessary analog components.

A third fundamental advantage of the digital filter is that it can be programmed to include logical operations, such as switching itself off or changing its characteristics in response to preselected events in the signal. These features could be used for feedback control (Kates, 1991) or sophisticated noise reduction (Weiss, 1987; Preves, 1990).

Programmable Hearing Aids

Many of the features described above depend on the fact that the hearing aid is programmable in the same manner as a computer. This programmability has several implications for the flexibility, limitations, and everyday use of a hearing aid.

The ability of the digital hearing aid to change almost instantaneously its characteristics significantly applies equally to quasi-digital and fully digital hearing aids because all that is required is sufficient memory to store different sets of parameter information. The degree of change possible, however, is greater with the all-digital instrument than with the quasi-digital instrument because of limitations in the degree of variation permitted by the analog circuitry.

Easy and flexible manipulation of hearing aid parameters has also led to extensive use of prescriptive techniques as described by Skinner (1988). Although such techniques have been available for a long time, the advent of the programmable hearing aid made it easy to use the techniques because the programming unit (computer) does all the necessary calculations and then sets up the hearing aid parameters accordingly.

Some quasi-digital hearing aids have sufficient memory for storing several sets of parameters. This improves the flexibility of the hearing aid by permitting the person fitting the hearing aid to "fine-tune" the hearing aid with several sets of characteristics. Although this does not avoid the limitation given above, it does allow the user to alter his/her hearing aid by selecting the parameter set that he/she feels best fits the current communication situation. Johnson et al. (1988) report that users will restrict a majority of their parameter set selections to two or three, even though as many as seven may be available. Based on this information, the most common situation is for a programmable hearing aid to have three to four parameter sets available.

PERSPECTIVE

Hearing aid development has been as tumultuous as the development of digital technology itself, and great progress has been made. There are some issues that remain for hearing aid manufacturers to solve before cosmetically acceptable hearing aids incorporating the full range of digital technology can be produced and marketed. There are also issues that must be addressed by the researchers in order for such technology to be truly usable and useful.

The manufacturers still must contend with the size and power issues. The size issue will probably resolve itself within the next two to three years. The power issue is more recalcitrant and involves both battery and hearing aid manufacturers. Some exciting developments in the computer field may presage a solution to these problems on a long-term basis. Faced with the same power issue in making extremely small portable computers, the manufacturers have resorted to software solutions. The software employed monitors power usage by the machine and adjusts the power requirements placed on the battery power supply so that maximum usage is made of available power. Significant gains, on the order of two to three times, have been made. It may be that a similar approach will hold promise for the hearing aid manufacturers.

Another issue facing the manufacturers as a group is the determination of a standard programming interface. The most intrusive aspect of current programmable hearing aids is the need for a separate programming unit for each manufacturer's hearing aid. This impacts acceptance both by the clinical community, because of cost and lack of ease of use, and by the user community, because the cost is passed to the consumer. An approach was described earlier for a small group of manufacturers. This effort must be taken up by standards committees and handled expeditiously to promote development of new types of hearing aids and remove the onus of developing independent interfaces. A standard interface will have considerable benefits, including economy of scale, because all manufacturers would be using the same interface, thereby driving down costs. The telecommunications industry is benefitting from its standards by permitting a large variety of services and software to be utilized through standard communications channels and criteria.

There is also considerable need for research to determine how to use this exciting technology. The current state of affairs, as referred to at the beginning of this chapter, is that our technology, certainly in terms of what can be implemented in a computer simulation, exceeds our knowledge of how to guide the selection of hearing aid parameters in the most beneficial way for hearing aid users. Issues include how to implement noise reduction and feedback control; how to specify the variety of compression parameters available, involving both type of compression as well as factors such as attack and release times; minimal specifications for acceptable sound quality in a digital hearing aid in terms of type and resolution of the converters or in terms of some degradations of the signal that occur during signal processing; and finally, how can the user options, such as control over the hearing parameter set, be designed so that the user gets optimal benefit from the hearing aid. There is, of course, always the question that has plagued hearing aid researchers since hearing aids were first invented, namely, how to predict the optimal fit for a hearing aid. If we have learned anything from our experience with programmable hearing aids, it is probably that there is no single optimal fit for an individual, but rather several fits that together provide the flexibility required to deal with the particular communication situations for the user.

REFERENCES

Bentler, R.A. (1991). Programmable hearing aid review. *American Journal of Audiology: A Journal of Clinical Practice* 1(1): 25–28.

Branderbit, P.L. (1991). A standardized programming system and three-channel compression hearing instrument technology. *Hearing Instruments* 42(1): 28–30.

Cranmer, K.S. (1991). Hearing instrument dispensing–1991. *Hearing Instruments* 42(6): 6–13.

Cudahy, E.A. (1988). Instrumentation for signal acquisition, generation, and analysis. In: J. Butler (ed.), *Introduction to Instrumentation in Speech and Hearing* (pp. 211–241). Baltimore: Williams & Wilkins.

Cudahy, E.A., and Kates, J. (1993). Measuring the performance of modern hearing aids. In: G. Studebaker and I. Hochberg (eds.), *Acoustical Factors Affecting Hearing Aid Performance*, 2nd ed. Boston: Allyn and Bacon.

Cummins, K.L., and Hecox, K. (1987). Ambulatory testing of digital hearing aid algorithms. *Proceedings of the 10th Annual Conference on Rehabilitation Technology (RESNA '87)* (pp. 398–400). Washington, DC: Association for the Advancement of Rehabilitation Technology.

Engebretson, A.M., Morley, F.F., and Popelka, G.R. (1987). Development of an ear-level digital hearing aid and computer-assisted fitting procedure: An interim report. *Journal of Rehabilitation Research and Development* 24(4): 55–64.

Fabry, D.A. (1991). Hearing aid compression. *American Journal of Audiology: A Journal of Clinical Practice* 1(1): 11–13.

Graupe, D., and Causey, G.D. (1975). Development of a hearing aid system with independently adjustable subranges of its spectrum using microprocessor hardware. *Bulletin of Prosthetic Research* 12: 241–242.

Graupe, D., Grosspietsch, J.K., and Basseas, S.P. (1987). A single-microphone-based self-adaptive filter of noise from speech and its performance evaluation. *Journal of Rehabilitation Research and Development* 24(4): 119–126.

Harris, R.W., Brey, R.H., Chang, Y.S., Soria, B.D., and Hilton, L.M. (1991). The effects of digital quantization error on speech intelligibility and perceived speech quality. *Journal of Speech and Hearing Research* 34(1): 189–196.

Hertzano, T., Levitt, H., and Slosberg, R. (1979). Computer-assisted hearing aid selection. *Speech Communication Papers, 97th Meeting of the Acoustical Society of America*. Boston: Acoustical Society of America.

Johnson, J.S., and Schnier, W.R. (1988). An expert system for programming a digitally controlled hearing instrument. *Hearing Instruments* 39(4).

Johnson, J.S., Kirby, V.M., Hodgson, W.A., and Johnson, L.J. (1988). Clinical study of a programmable, multiple memory hearing instrument. *Hearing Instruments* 39(11).

Kates, J.M. (1991). Feedback cancellation in hearing aids: Results from a computer simulation. *IEEE Transactions on Signal Processing* 39(3): 553–562.

Levitt, H. (1982). An array-processor, computer hearing aid. Annual Convention of the American Speech-Language-Hearing Association, Toronto. See also *ASHA* 24, 805.

Levitt, H., Neuman, A., and Toraskar, J. (1987). Orthogonal polynomial compression amplification for the hearing-impaired. *Proceedings of the 10th Annual Conference on Rehabilitation Technology (RESNA '87)* (pp. 410–412). Washington, DC: Association for the Advancement of Rehabilitation Technology

Levitt, H., Neuman, A., Mills, R., and Schwander, T. (1986). A digital master hearing aid. *Journal of Rehabilitation Research and Development* 23(1): 79–87.

Levitt, H., Sullivan, J., and Hwang, J.Y. (1986). A computerized hearing aid measurement/simulation system. *Hearing Instruments* 37(2).

Mangold, S., and Leijon, A. (1979). A programmable hearing aid with multi-channel compression. *Scandinavian Audiology* 8: 121–126.

Megahed, S., and Dopp, R. (1990). Batteries for present and future hearing aids. *ASHA* June/July: 52–54.

Moser, I.M. (1980). Hearing aid with digital processing for: Correlation of signals from plural microphones, dynamic range control, or filtering using an erasable memory. U.S. Patent #4,187,413, February 5, 1980.

Neuman, A., Levitt, H., Mills, R., and Schwander, T. (1987). An evaluation of three adaptive hearing aid selection strategies. *Journal of the Acoustical Society of America* 82(6): 1967–1976.

Oppenheim, A.V., and Schafer, R.W. (1975). *Digital Signal Processing*. Englewood Cliffs, NJ: Prentice-Hall.

Pluvinage, V., and Benson, D. (1988). New dimensions in diagnostics and fitting. *Hearing Instruments* 39(8).

Popelka, F., and Engebretson, A.M. (1983). A computer-based system for hearing aid assessment. *Hearing Instruments* 34(7).

Preves, D. (1990). Approaches to noise reduction in analog, digital, and hybrid hearing aids. *Seminars in Hearing* 11(1): 39–67.

Sammeth, C.A. (1990). Current availability of digital and hybrid hearing aids. *Seminars in Hearing* 11(1): 91–100.

Skinner, M.W. (1988). *Hearing Aid Evaluation*. Englewood Cliffs, NJ: Prentice-Hall.

Studebaker, G.A., Sherbecoe, R.L., and Matesich, J.S. (1987). Spectrum shaping with a hardware digital filter. *Journal of Rehabilitation Research and Development* 24(4): 21–28.

Widin, G.P., and Mangold, S. (1988). Fitting a programmable hearing instrument. *Hearing Instruments* 39(6).

CHAPTER 2

RATIONALE AND DEVELOPMENT OF THE RESOUND SYSTEM

Vincent Pluvinage

ReSound's hearing devices incorporate technology initially designed at AT&T Bell Laboratories. The unique sound processing is called "Multiband Full Dynamic Range Compression" (MBFDRC). After a front-end AGC, sounds are split into two bands, each processed by a syllabic compressor. The design of these compressors is unique in three important aspects: The thresholds are low (45 dB SPL); the dynamic range compression operates over a wide range (40 dB: from 45 to 85 dB SPL); and the compression ratio is programmable in eleven steps, from linear to 3:1 compression. This design allows the frequency response to adjust itself automatically in response to changes in both bass and treble sound intensities. The processing can be programmed to match the patient's loudness contours. The resulting benefit is improved comfort and speech intelligibility, as shown scientifically by Villchur (1973) and Moore et al. (1992).

The P³ fitting system is hand held, battery operated, and performs three functions. First, it automatically computes the initial fitting based on the audiogram and/or the results of an automated loudness test. The fitting algorithm was progressively refined over several years of field testing and statistical analysis of over a thousand fittings. Second, it supports paired-comparison fine-tuning. Third, it programs the nonvolatile memories of both the remote control and the hearing device. The latter preserves all patient information (fitting, name, audiogram, dates, etc.) even when the battery is removed, thus allowing for optional use of the remote. The P³ fitting system is designed also to function as a "slave" interface of a personal computer.

Two models of hearing device are available: an ITE and a BTE. Both can be operated with an optional remote control that allows volume adjustments and selection of two programs for each ear—that is, four programs in the case of a binaural fitting. If necessary, the hearing device memories and the remote control can be programmed with different fittings. In such a case, the patient can access one program simply by closing the battery door and two additional programs by transmitting from the remote (for a total of three choices per ear). The crossover frequency between the two bands can be selected from .4 kHz to 4.7 kHz, in half-octave steps. The gain for weak sounds (50 dB SPL input) can be selected in each band from 2 dB to 54 dB, in 2 dB steps. For intense sounds (80 dB SPL input), the gain range is 2 dB to 34 dB.

Products are developed to satisfy specific customer needs. Thus, a natural way to describe new, high-technology products is to first describe those needs and the rationales underlying the product design. This approach allows the practitioner to judge whether, *in principle*, the technology is based on solid foundations. Following a brief product description, we will then review the scientific and clinical data available and evaluate how the *actual*, *measured* benefits compare with the design goals.

DEVELOPMENTAL HISTORY

The origin of ReSound's technology lies with research conducted in the early 1970s by Edgar Villchur. Following the extraordinary growth of Acoustic Research, the company he founded to commercialize his invention (the acoustic suspension used in modern loudspeakers), Villchur designed sound processing laboratory equipment to conduct experiments with patients suffering from sensorineural hearing losses. In 1973, he published the results in the *Journal of the Acoustical Society of America*, showing significant improvement in speech recognition in background noise when sounds are processed by multiband full dynamic range compression electronics (Villchur, 1973). In the 1980s, Moore and his colleagues published similar results using a slightly different multiband compression design (Laurence, Moore, and Glasberg, 1983; Moore et al., 1986; Moore, 1987).

In both cases, tests were conducted using multitalker speech interfering noises and "target" speech level varying over a dynamic range similar to that found in real-life situations. To date, *no commercially available sound processing* other than ReSound's (see Moore et al., 1992) has been shown in the scientific literature to yield similar results. Despite such outstanding research achievements, successful commercialization of multiband dynamic range compression would have to wait over a decade.

During the early 1980s, Fred Waldhauer, then at AT&T Bell Laboratories, became increasingly interested in Villchur's findings. Their friendship and the breakup of the Bell system offered the opportunity to design products based on Villchur's idea. In 1984, AT&T formed an internal venture organization to fund projects that could lead to new markets previously closed to AT&T by the antitrust laws. Citing examples ranging from Alexander Graham Bell's work with the deaf to Bell Laboratories' invention of the audiometer and the expertise of the Acoustic Research laboratory, Waldhauer convinced AT&T's management to form a team that could develop the world's best hearing aids.

In 1985, the author joined Waldhauer's efforts and, over a two-year period, the team grew to twenty people. Following a restructuring, several internal "medical" ventures of AT&T were canceled at the end of 1986. Three months later, three Silicon Valley entrepreneurs, Drs. Rodney Perkins, Eugene Kleiner, and Richard Goode, founders of ReSound, a Hearing Health Care Corporation, acquired the rights to the AT&T technology and hired four members of the AT&T team.

Three years of intense product development, fueled by over $15M of equity financing, led to the commercial launch in early 1990 of a programmable in-the-ear hearing device incorporating sound processing based on Villchur's ideas, together with an ultrasonic remote control and a custom computer fitting system (Pluvinage and Benson, 1988). In early 1992, a second-generation hand-held fitting system, an ITE with nonvolatile memory, and a small BTE incorporating the same multiband dynamic range compression sound processing were introduced.

DESIGN RATIONALE

The philosophy behind ReSound's products is based on a few key postulates:

1. The most important goal of a hearing device is to improve social interactions of the communication-handicapped patients with sensorineural hearing loss. Thus, the ability to follow conversation in the presence of competing noises found in social and professional gatherings is a key measure of performance.

2. The brain is by far the most effective information processor, the only one able to extract a desired speech signal from a loud background of competing noises. To perform this task, both signal and noise must be "heard" by the nervous system with the least amount of distortion and loss of cues. Distortion and information loss produced by the acoustic transducers, the electronic processing, the middle ear, and the cochlea must be minimized.

3. The process of fitting (or fine-tuning) a given sound processing system to the specific needs of a patient is crucial and requires a methodical but not lengthy approach. Two steps are mandatory for proper adjustment of a complex sound processor: initial "computation" of the likely settings based on available audiological data and fine-tuning based on aided psychoacoustic patient responses. A fitting algorithm must be developed for the specific sound processing being prescribed in order to provide a reliable starting point for the fine-tuning.

During a conversation, a listener must correctly identify a minimum percentage of the words in order to carry on a meaningful dialogue. In noisy situations, *normal-hearing* people adjust the level of their voices so as to allow just enough words to be recognized by a *normal-hearing* interlocutor. As shown in Figure 2.1, the speech level is automatically adjusted near the noise level, maintaining a signal-to-noise ratio within the range of –5 dB to +5 dB. For this signal-to-noise range, a normal listener will recognize slightly more than 50% of the words,

enough to follow the conversation; there is no need for the interlocutor to raise his/her voice further. Hearing-impaired listeners frequently recognize a smaller percentage of words in those conditions and thus are unable to participate effectively in the social interaction. The consequence is progressive social isolation.

Thus, a prosthetic sound processing system must allow at least 50% word recognition at signal-to-noise ratio of 5 dB or worse in order for a user to converse easily in noisy social gatherings and not be confined to communication in quiet environments. Unfortunately, this goal is not met by most hearing devices on the market today.

RATIONALE FOR MULTIBAND FULL DYNAMIC RANGE COMPRESSION (MBFDRC)

The name used to describe ReSound's sound processing (MBFDRC), although correct, is unfortunate in that it wrongly suggests similarities with traditional "compression limiting" (threshold higher than 60 dB SPL, fixed compression ratio). There are multiple ways to describe MBFDRC and, taken together, the correct perspective is easily reached.

Recruitment Compensation

Figure 2.2 illustrates the relationship between loudness and intensity of a narrowband sound stimulus centered at a given frequency. One curve describes "normal" loudness growth, the other describes abnormal loudness growth typically found in sensorineural hearing losses. At point A, an intensity of about 15 dB SPL evokes, in a normal-hearing listener, a "very soft" sensation. Sounds of increasing intensities are heard as progressively louder until discomfort is reached, at point B. For a patient with a pure

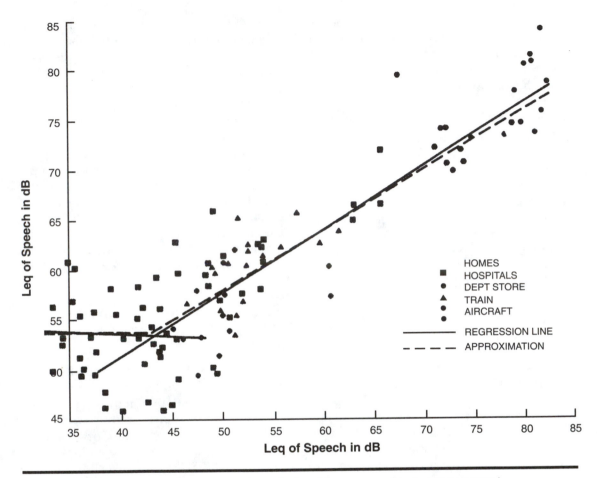

FIGURE 2.1.   Measured speech intensity level for conversation between normal-hearing people, as a function of the level of background noise in various environments. Reprinted with permission from Pearsons, Bennett, and Fidell (Cambridge, MA: Bolt, Beranek and Newman, 1976).

tone threshold of 60 dB SPL, the stimulus will not be heard until it reaches a much higher intensity, as shown by point C. Thereafter, loudness grows quickly with intensity until point D, where normal loudness perception occurs. Recruitment, or abnormally steep loudness growth, is exhibited by *all* sensorineural hearing-impaired patients*. The abnormal loudness growth is typically much steeper than normal for

*This is simply a correlate of the following statement: In cochlear losses, the loudness discomfort level (LDL) is not increased by the amount of threshold loss (HTL). Therefore, the dynamic range between HTL and LDC is reduced somewhat, and the loudness function *must* be steeper than normal.

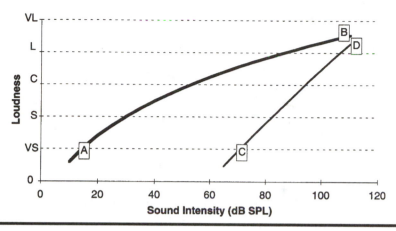

FIGURE 2.2.   Relationship between the loudness and the intensity of a narrowband signal for a normal (curve A-B) and for a hearing-impaired (curve C-D) listener.

high-frequency sounds just above the impaired threshold. (Note: dynamic range compression is thus *most* needed at *soft* levels and *less* needed at *high* levels; see Killion, 1979). Thus, relatively small modulations in intensity typical of consonants are perceived with exaggerated loudness fluctuations. This "jumbling" of the consonants is the signature of cochlear recruitment distortion. A frequent misconception is that recruitment refers only to the less-frequent cases of hypersensitivity to high-intensity sounds.

Figure 2.3(a) illustrates the effect of linear amplification with a constant gain of 30 dB (the length of the horizontal arrow). The dark gray line corresponds to the aided loudness perception: Each loudness level is reached for an incoming intensity 30 dB lower than in the unaided condition. At mid-intensities, a "comfortable" sensation is evoked at normal intensity levels. However, below that level, sounds are softer than for normal listeners, and above that level, they are louder. This last discrepancy usually is corrected by adding a high-level AGC (or compression limiting) to

decrease the gain provided at high-intensity input levels [see Figure 2.3(b)]. Unfortunately, soft speech cues, especially weak consonants precious to speech intelligibility, are left under-amplified by this type of processing.

Full dynamic range compression refers to sound processing that provides maximum gain for the softest speech components and *progressively* less gain for higher-intensity sounds [Figure 2.3(c)]. Thus, sound intensity variations lead to an automatic adjustment of the gain. For weaker sounds, the gain is increased. For stronger ones, the gain is decreased. To ensure proper loudness for all speech sounds, three conditions must be met. First, very weak consonants must be amplified more than stronger speech sounds. This requires a low compression threshold, around 40 dB SPL. Second, while the weakest speech cues must be made audible, the strongest speech sounds should be perceived as loud, but not too loud. This requires that the amount of gain adjustment be tailored to the patient's dynamic range of hearing. In other words, the compression ratio of the amplifier must be ad-

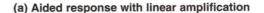

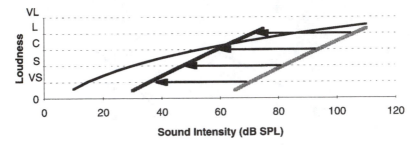

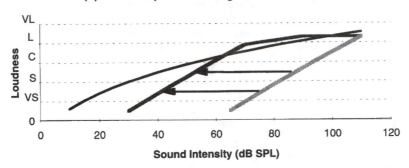

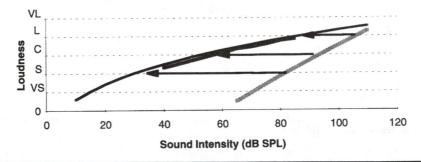

FIGURE 2.3. (a) Effect of linear amplification on loudness perception. The dark gray line, describing the aided loudness/intensity relationship, is parallel to the light gray line, describing the unaided relationship. The horizontal shift is the functional gain. In this case, it does not vary with input intensity. (b) Effect of linear amplification with compression limiting. High-intensity sounds are prevented from exceeding their normal loudness. (c) Effect of full dynamic range on loudness perception. The functional gain is level dependent: It is maximum at low level and minimum at high level. Abnormal loudness growth can be substantially corrected over the speech intensity range.

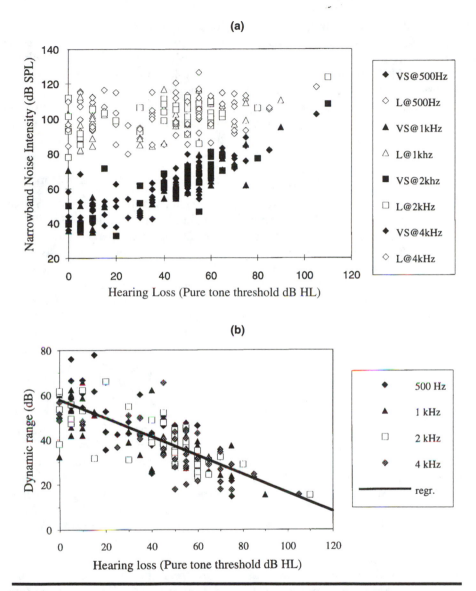

FIGURE 2.4.   (a) Average intensity of narrowband noises perceived as very soft and loud by fifty hearing-impaired subjects, as a function of their pure tone threshold. The various symbols are for frequencies of 500, 1000, 2000, and 4000 Hz, measured using the LGOB test. (b) Dynamic ranges for the data shown in part (a), computed as the difference between loud and very soft intensities.

justable. Third, since recruitment is typically more severe in the frequency range of greater hearing loss, different compression ratios are required at low and high frequencies.

To cover the range of recruitment typically found in mild to severe sensorineural losses, the ReSound compressors are designed to operate from a low threshold of 45 dB SPL to a high level of 85 dB SPL. Above 85 dB SPL input level, a front-end, wideband AGC is responsible for preventing circuit overload. To accommodate the range of recruitment found in sensorineural patients with losses from mild to severe, compression ratios are independently adjustable in each band from 1:1 (linear) to 3:1. The dynamic range between very soft and loud sounds decreases from about 60 dB in a normal listener to an average of 20 dB for severe hearing losses (Figure 2.4).

An adjustable compression ratio is clearly necessary to allow for correction of abnormal loudness growth, as shown in Figure 2.5. Just as the audiogram measures the hearing loss at threshold, one can define a similar "sensitivity loss" at specific suprathreshold levels. For each stimulus intensity, one can measure the intensity increase (in dB) necessary to elicit a normal loudness sensation. On a loudness growth plot [i.e., Figure 2.3(a), (b), and (c) and Figure 2.5], this is simply the horizontal distance between the normal and the abnormal loudness functions. The lower the reference intensity, the larger the "sensitivity loss": In Figure 2.2, the intensity corresponding to point A must be raised to that of point C to allow the patient to hear the stimulus at the normal loudness level. Thus, the sensitivity loss is the "distance" (in dB) between A and C. At higher intensities, the loudness functions typically converge toward the normal curve. Thus, the "sensitivity loss" decreases toward "zero" (a complicated way to say that sensorineural patients perceive intense sounds more or less normally).

Figure 2.5(b) shows the "sensitivity loss"

for various degrees of recruitment. Note that the slopes vary. By providing a gain equal to the sensitivity loss over the speech intensities, proper loudness of all speech components can be achieved. As is apparent in Figure 2.5(c), this goal requires a programmable compression ratio, allowing the gain to match the "slope" of the sensitivity loss.

Level-Dependent Equalization

A different approach (Figure 2.6) may help in visualizing the need for MBFDRC. To restore normal loudness perception for very weak stimuli, the frequency response of a linear amplifier must be adjusted to match a significant fraction of the hearing loss; for example, a gain at each frequency equal to 4/5 of the threshold hearing level (often referred to as "mirroring the audiogram"). On the other hand, strong sound stimuli require a much smaller amount of amplification in order to be heard as comfortably loud, typically 1/5 of the threshold loss. Notably, the real world rarely presents only very weak or only strong sounds. For this reason, dispensers of "linear" hearing devices must compromise and usually follow some intermediate "gain rule," for example, the "half gain rule," to select the appropriate frequency response. However, as shown by many investigators (see, for example, Skinner, 1976, and Zurek et al., 1990), the optimum preferred frequency response depends on the level of the speech stimulus. For high-frequency losses, more treble boost is needed for soft sounds, and progressively less for louder ones.

In summary, another way to describe ReSound's MBFDRC is to point out that it automatically adjusts the "frequency equalization" with signal level. It is an "adaptive, multiple gain rule" amplifier. The decrease in gain for high-level, low-frequency sounds and the extra boost to low-level, high-frequency sounds both contribute to the release from upward spread of masking. Thus, it is possible for the

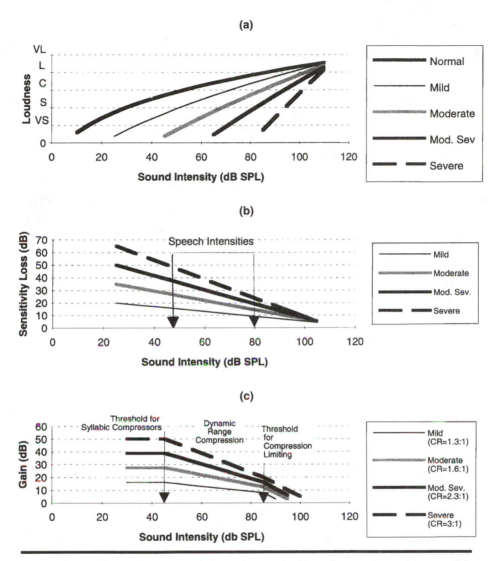

FIGURE 2.5. (a) Loudness growth for various severities of sensorineural losses. (b) Sensitivity loss as a function of sound intensity. These curves are derived from part (a): Loss is the horizontal distance between impaired and normal loudness curves. (c) Gain provided by ReSound's sound processing. Note that it matches the sensitivity loss over the speech intensities.

frequency response simultaneously to follow a 1/5 gain rule in the low band and 4/5 gain rule in the high band. Moments later, as conditions change, some loud high-frequency kitchen noises can reduce the high-frequency

gain according to a 1/5 gain rule, while a very soft vowel is boosted by a gain equal to 4/5 of the low-frequency loss.

As an example, Figure 2.7 shows the output sound pressure of various hearing de-

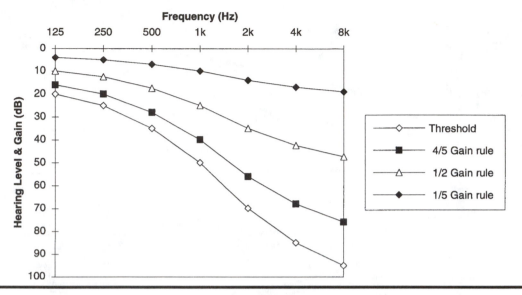

FIGURE 2.6. High-frequency loss audiogram with three different gain rules: 1/5 for loud sounds (very little gain); 1/2 for comfortable ones (also indicative of the linear compromise according to Pogo, NAL, etc.), and 4/5 for very soft sound (called almost "mirroring" the audiogram).

vices when the input is a single frequency of increasing intensity. In Figure 2.7(a), the output is simply the input multiplied by a constant factor. In other words, the gain is constant, regardless of the input intensity. As the input amplitude increases, so does the output. In Figure 2.7(b), peak clipping is added. As a result, high-intensity output signals are "chopped off." In Figure 2.7(c), compression limiting achieves the same goal by reducing the gain when the signal is above compression threshold. The advantage over peak clipping is less distortion, as can be seen by inspecting the waveform. Finally, in Figure 2.7(d), the effect of full dynamic range compression is shown: For small input signals, the gain is greater than for either PC or AGC limiting. This is possible, without overamplifying louder sounds, because the gain is progressively reduced as the input increases. At high intensities, the gain progressively decreases.

Dynamic Range Compression

The loss of hearing in a specific frequency range (most commonly high frequencies) is the obvious justification for frequency shaping in hearing aids. Yet, the loss of dynamic range is often left uncorrected. As depicted in Figure 2.8, the elevation of hearing threshold leads to a "squeezing" of the equal loudness contours. In this highly schematic figure, the equal loudness contours are depicted by horizontal lines of various styles. In Figure 2.8(b) the lower ("softer") loudness contours are most affected by the hearing loss, while higher ("louder") loudness contours are closer to normal.

With compression limiting [Figure 2.8(c)], the gain (vertical arrows) is matched to the distance between abnormal and normal "comfortable" loudness contours. At higher levels, the gain is reduced (shorter arrows). However, below the comfortable level, the

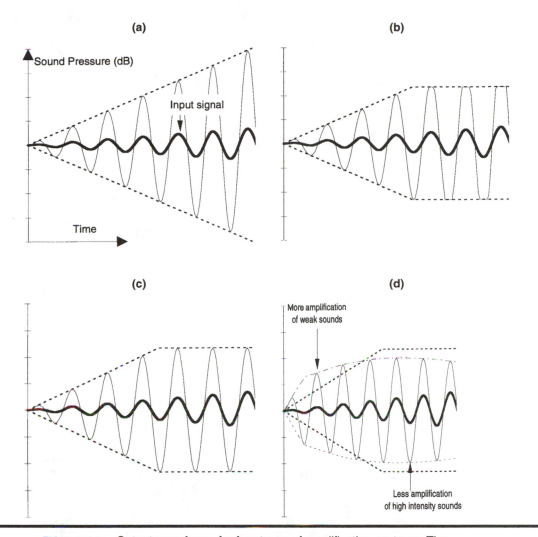

FIGURE 2.7.   Output waveforms for four types of amplification systems. The input signal is a fixed frequency tone that increases in intensity at a constant rate (dB/second). For example, this signal could be the whistle of an approaching locomotive. (a) Linear amplification. (b) Peak clipping. (c) AGC limiting. (d) Full dynamic range compression.

gain is *not* increased to close the gap between normal and abnormal contours (the arrow's length is not increased). This is simply because, below compression threshold, the gain does not change with stimulus intensity. In Figure 2.8(d), the gain is systematically matched across two dimensions: frequency

and intensity. Thus, all loudness contours are properly restored by MBFDRC.

In the absence of adequate dynamic range correction, fluctuations in sound intensity inevitably produce exaggerated fluctuation in loudness, *regardless* of the frequency shaping selected. Devices with multiband AGC com-

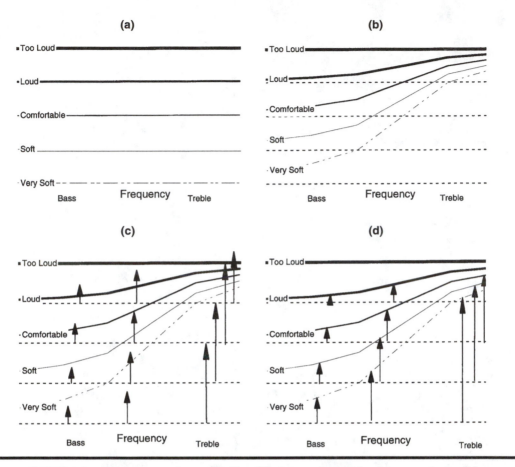

FIGURE 2.8. Loudness contours. (a) Simplified normal equal loudness contours. (b) Impaired loudness contours for a high-frequency sensorineural loss. (c) Gains provided by linear amplification with compression limiting (arrows). (d) Gains provided by ReSound's sound processing (arrows). Note that in each frequency range, the gain is level dependent and matches the appropriate loudness contours.

pression limiting only (defined here as those with a threshold of 60 dB SPL or higher) can reduce the dynamic range of incoming sounds. However, compression is provided only for the stronger sounds, for which the patient's loudness growth is typically close to normal. All weak sounds, including the consonants, are processed linearly and thus are perceived with the wrong loudness relative to other speech sounds. Unfortunately, this handicap cannot be compensated for by manual volume adjustments or manual selection of an alternative fitting program. This is because adjustments must be made at syllabic rate, much too fast for any user.

Linear amplification of weak sounds (found in all hearing devices, except Killion's K-amp and ReSound's processing) fails to correct the exaggerated loudness growth near threshold. Speech remains "perceptually" distorted, thereby compromising the brain's ability to extract information from noise. Proper correction requires a nonlinear gain function matched to the level-dependent "sensitivity loss" (as shown in Figure 2.5). This is analogous to the Dolby processing found on most hi-fi tape players: The music is compressed before recording so as to record soft sounds at a level above the tape's own low-level background noise while at the same time preventing distortion of loud sounds due to tape magnetic saturation. Upon playback, the signal read from the tape is expanded back to its original dynamic range, which could be called, in simplistic ways, an electronic "recruitment" mechanism (in the case of sensorineural hearing-impaired patients, the impaired cochlea fails to provide its normal compression function, and the loudness growth is therefore accelerated). Pre- and post-recording processing must be complementary in order to avoid audible distortion. Similarly, the amount of dynamic range compression must be matched to cochlear recruitment.

Dynamic range compression actually "expands" the patient's listening range. The word "compression" is selected by engineers. Psychoacousticians would probably prefer the words "listening range expanders," looking at it from the patient's perspective rather than from the electronic point of view. For example, with a 3:1 compression ratio, lowering the compression threshold from 65 dB SPL to 45 dB SPL lowers the aided threshold (thus increasing the patient's hearing range) by 6.6 dB. Assuming a typical loudness growth for a severe sensorineural loss, these 6.6 extra decibels can cover a sensation range equivalent to 20 dB in a normal-hearing person.

Specific values for compression ratios are meaningless if the range of compression is not specified. When the compression threshold is low and the nonlinear amplification covers a large range (over 40 dB) of incoming intensities, small compression ratios translate into substantial differences in gain provided to low- and high-intensity sounds. For ex-

ample, a compression ratio of 3:1 over an input range of 40 dB produces an amplification of low-intensity sounds that exceeds the amplification of high-level sounds by 26 dB. Furthermore, it should be noted that this "differential amplification" of low- and high-level sounds increases nonlinearly with compression ratio. For example, with a full dynamic range compressor, an increase in compression ratio from 1.2:1 to 1.5:1 provides an extra "boost" of 6.6 dB to soft sounds. For the same compressor, an increase in compression ratio from 2:1 to 3:1 provides the same amount of "boost." The relationship between these variables is mathematically described by the following formulas:

Compressor output dynamic range
$$= \frac{\text{Compressor input dynamic range}}{\text{Compression ratio}}$$

Low-level extra boost
$$= \text{Gain at compressor's threshold} - \text{Gain at high level}$$

Maximum low-level extra boost
$$= (\text{Compressor dynamic range}) \times (1 - 1/\text{Compression ratio})$$

ReSound's compressors have a 40 dB input range and a maximum of 3:1 compression ratio. Thus, if the high-level gain is adjusted to match that of a linear aid, the patient's ability to hear soft sounds can be increased up to $40 \times (1 - 1/3) = 26$ dB.

Full dynamic range compression increases amplification of all soft sounds: soft speech cues as well as soft noises. However, if the compression ratio is selected appropriately, the soft noises are perceived at their "normal" loudness. Typically, this requires different compression ratios at the low and high frequencies and thus cannot be accomplished with a single, wideband compression system. Excessive amounts of dynamic compression can lead patients to complain about hearing too many soft sounds. Fitting algorithm accuracy and careful fine-tuning are essential to producing the correct balance.

Time-Varying Aspects

Compressors react to changes in input intensity by adjusting the gain accordingly. How fast the adjustment should be made is a tricky question. Typically, reaction times to sudden increases in signal intensity (attack time constant) must be fast (<a few msec) in order to prevent discomfort due to overamplification of high-level sounds. Reaction time to sudden decreases (release time constant) must be slow enough to avoid audible distortion, yet fast enough to prevent soft sounds to be "attenuated" by preceding loud ones. Reaction times comparable to the duration of typical syllables ("syllabic compressors") are achievable when separate compressors independently process the low and high frequencies. Indeed, loud vowels presented in rapid alternation with soft consonants can produce a *simultaneous* decrease in low-frequency gain and increase in high-frequency gain. Thus, a release from upward spread of masking can be achieved.

Furthermore, when a loud noise and a soft signal are in different frequency bands, a dual-band compression system will effectively *increase* the signal-to-noise ratio. By comparison, linear amplification will keep this ratio constant while a wideband compressor will *decrease* the signal-to-noise ratio.

Nonlinear sound processing, by definition, always introduces some degree of signal distortion, so great care is required to ensure that nondesirable effects are inaudible. Over a year of listening tests and design modifications were required to achieve this objective in the ReSound sound processing integrated circuit.

Electronic Design

The ReSound electronics consist of three integrated circuits: a bipolar sound processing circuit, a CMOS digital circuit, and a nonvolatile memory (EEPROM). Traditional transducers and battery are used. In addition, an ultrasonic remote control allows volume changes and user-controlled selection of alternative sound processing programs. Specifications are summarized in Table 2.1.

Figure 2.9 shows the signal path block diagram. A front-end preamplifier is followed by a high-threshold (85 dB SPL) wideband AGC protecting the rest of the circuitry from overload. Next, a split-band filter separates the low and high frequencies. The separation frequency between bands (crossover frequency) is adjustable in half-octave steps, from .4 kHz up to 4.7 kHz. Each of the two dynamic range compressors has a low threshold around 45 dB SPL and is capable of adjusting the gain over an input range of about 40 dB or more. Attack time constants are fast (<1 msec), while the release time constants of the compressors are compression ratio dependent and vary from about 70 msec to 90 msec (per ANSI definition).

Each dynamic range compressor has two programmable degrees of freedom. In each band, these two adjustments allow independent setting of gain for low-level (50 dB SPL input) and for high-level (80 dB SPL input) sounds. An alternative, and strictly equivalent, programming selection consists in specifying only one of these two gains and specifying the desired compression ratio [a straight-line input/output line can be uniquely specified by two points or one point and a slope (see Figure 2.10)]. The low-level gains (G50) can be programmed from 2 dB to 44 dB (in 2 dB steps), while the high-level gains (G80) can be set from 2 dB to 24 dB. Another 8 dB to 10 dB can be added in the input and output stages, but at the sacrifice of volume control "headroom." A total of 11 compression ratios are available, ranging from 1:1 (linear) to 3:1. As an example, if a gain G50 equal to 40 dB and a gain G80 of 20 dB are specified, 50 dB SPL sounds will produce a (50 + 40) 90 dB SPL

TABLE 2.1. Final Specifications: ReSound Personal Hearing System ED3

MULTIBAND FULL DYNAMIC COMPRESSION

Filters

Programmable High Band/Low Band Crossover Frequency (fc):	400 to 4700 Hz
Programming Step Size:	1/2 Octave
High Band Filter Slope:	−18 dB/Octave
Low Band Filter Slope:	−12 dB/Octave

Independent High Band and Low Band Compressors

Programmable Compression Ratios:	1.0, 1.1, 1.2, 1.3, 1.4, 1.5, 1.7, 1.9, 2.1, 2.5, 3.0*
Compression Input Threshold:	45 dB SPL (At Maximum Compression)
Attack Time:	1 msec
Release Time (per ANSI):	70 to 140 ms Depending on Program
Gain Control RC Time Constant:	40 msec

*Compression Ratio = 30/(30-G50 + G80)

Programmable Gains Provided With Nominal Volume Control Setting and fc = 1.3 kHz

High Band

For 50 dB SPL Input (G50):	4 to 46 dB @ 2000 Hz*
For 80 dB SPL Input (G80):	6 to 30 dB @ 2000 Hz*

Low Band

For 50 dB SPL (G50):	2 to 40 dB @ 500 Hz*
For 80 dB SPL (G80):	2 to 24 dB @ 500 Hz*
Programming Step Size:	2 dB

*Add up to 8 dB for Maximum Volume Control Setting

Frequency Equalization (Gain Difference Between Compressors)

For 50 dB SPL (G50):	0 to 44 dB
For 80 dB SPL (G80):	0 to 28 dB

DIGITAL VOLUME CONTROL

Range:	Up to 30 dB (−22 to +8 dB relative to Nominal)
Programming Step Size:	2 dB
Functional Placement:	40% Before Compressors (Output Compression)
	60% After Compressors (Input Compression)

INPUT AGC

Threshold (Referred to Input):	85 dB SPL*
Release Time:	40 msec

*For nominal volume control setting

continues

TABLE 2.1.   Continued.

BATTERY INFORMATION

Battery Size:	13 to 312
Typical Current Drain:	2.3 mA
Typical Battery Life:	100 Hours (With Size 13 battery)

ANSI S3.22 1987 DATA

HFA Full-On Gain:	52 dB
Peak Gain:	57 dB
Maximum Output (SSPL 90):	118 dB SPL
HF Average (SSPL 90):	115 dB SPL
Typical Frequency Range:	200 to 6000 Hz
Maximum Equivalent Input Noise:	28 dB SPL*

*With Device Programmed for Maximum Linear Gain

output, and 80 dB SPL sounds will produce an (80 + 20) 100 dB output. Thus, the 30 dB range between the incoming sounds (80 − 50) will be compressed into a 10 dB output dynamic range (100 − 90). The resulting compression ratio is then 30/10 = 3:1. Similarly, other cases can be computed using the following formula:

$$CR = \frac{30}{30 - (G50 - G80)}$$

Because of the wide input intensity range of the compressors, compression ratios ranging from 1:1 to 3:1 were found to be adequate for most cases up to and including severe losses. Most well-fitted patients rarely need to make volume adjustments. The volume control can nevertheless provide additional, user-controllable fine-tuning that is often crucial during the first few weeks after the initial fitting. For each volume control step (up or down) of 2.5 dB, 40% of the gain adjustment is made before the front-end AGC, and the

other 60% takes place after the compressors. Increase in volume setting beyond the nominal level produces a lowering of the threshold of syllabic compression (and vice versa). The output gain adjustment affects the maximum power output (MPO). Thus, volume adjustments allow the patient to fine-tune two critical parameters.

The CMOS digital control circuit is shown, in block diagram form, in Figure 2.11. It has three functions: decoding of ultrasonic transmission; communication with the nonvolatile memory; and digital control of the bipolar sound processing circuit. The ultrasound signals control the following: up and down volume adjustments; turning off the amplification; and "reprogramming" of the sound processing. To increase the reliability of ultrasonic transmission, special "bits" of information control are added to the "digital fitting parameters" sent from the remote control to the hearing device(s). A group of bits is programmed to match the last digit of

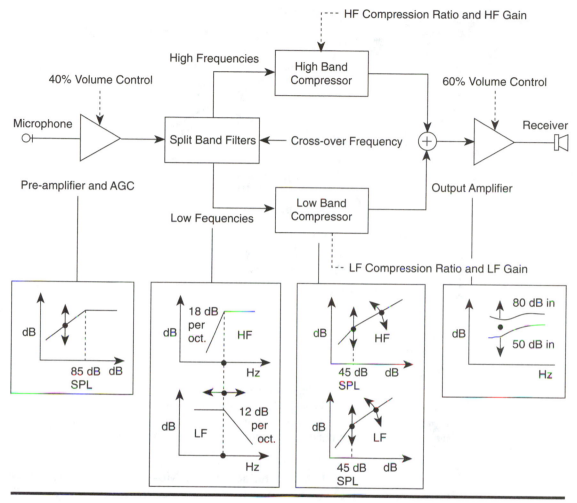

FIGURE 2.9.   Block diagram of ReSound's sound processing. The arrows in the bottom half of the figure indicate the programmable parameters.

the device serial number (this avoids controlling someone else's device), and seven "parity bits" provide redundancy used by the hearing device to verify that the transmission was not scrambled. This coding scheme allows reliable communication from the remote control to the hearing device(s). When a binaural user selects a program on the remote control, both left and right ear prescriptions are sent at once, and each de-

vice is capable of recovering the appropriate information.

The nonvolatile (information is not lost when the battery is removed) memory stores the fitting prescription, as well as other information such as audiogram, patient name, and so on, (a total of 1024 bits). Thus, the complete patient file is stored in the device and can be retrieved by any ReSound dispenser using the Portable Prescriptive Programming Sys-

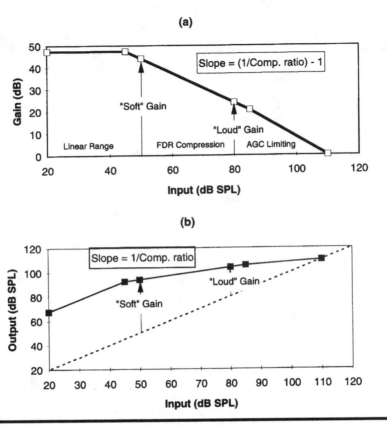

FIGURE 2.10. (a) Gain. The slope and vertical position of the curve are programmable. (b) Output. Each band can be programmed independently.

tem (P^3). This is especially useful for patient follow-up in multi-office practices. If the user prefers to leave the remote control at home, the prescription is automatically loaded from this memory when the battery is replaced. The pen-like remote control (Figure 2.12) is operated at arm's length.

SELECTION AND FITTING RATIONALE

Selecting the proper program for a specific patient presents three challenging steps:

1. *Collecting the necessary audiological information.* Threshold audiograms alone allow only a guess at the suprathreshold hearing

characteristics. Most other tests are either non-frequency specific or nonstandardized. To remedy that situation, ReSound developed an automatic procedure that measures loudness growth at four octave frequencies (the LGOB test; see Pluvinage, 1989, and Allen and Jeng, 1990, for a complete description of this test). Undoubtedly, advanced sound processing will bring increasing pressure for developing standardized and automated tests and integrating them into the fitting process. After all, what would the performance of the Ferrari be without electronic test equipment and a precise, methodical tune-up manual? Because of the length of time required by the LGOB test (10

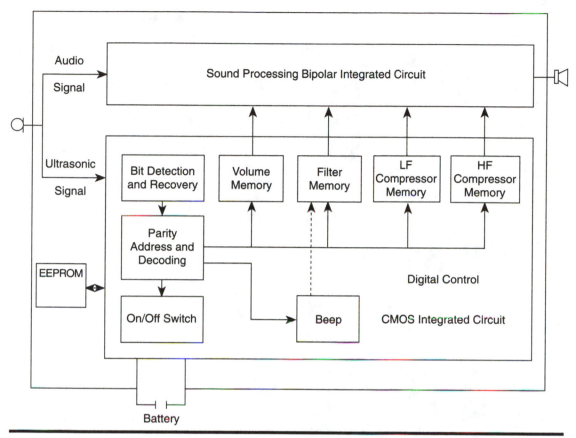

FIGURE 2.11.   Block diagram of the digital integrated circuit. It has four functions: ultrasonic communication; hardwired communication via a battery pill connection; control of the sound processing according to the prescribed parameters; and EEPROM communication.

to 15 minutes per ear), it sometimes must be omitted. In this case, the software of the P³ system calculates the statistically most likely suprathreshold contours based on the audiogram.

2. *Computing the appropriate programmable parameters.* Automatic computation of a reasonable fitting is a mandatory starting point: The task of fine-tuning a nonlinear sound processing with five or six interrelated degrees of freedom is a complex one, and the risk of getting lost (diverging instead of converging) must be minimized. The original programming system

software, shipped in 1990, incorporated experience learned during months of clinical testing. However, this was insufficient and many of the early ReSound dispensers either learned to modify effectively the automatic computations or struggled with the frustration of having some patients raving about the sound processing while others were less enthusiastic. This lesson led to a systematic analysis of thousands of fittings. For a period of several months, audiological data, fitting parameters, and patient's responses to a three-page questionnaire were collected and analyzed.

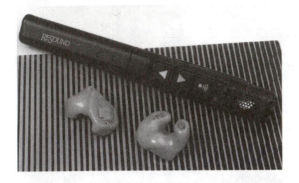

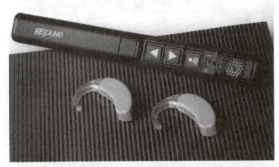

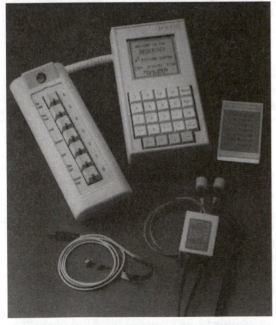

FIGURE 2.12. Remote control and the ITE Model ED3 (top) and the BTE Model BT2 (middle) and P³ fitting systems (bottom).

The resulting fitting algorithms have been incorporated into the P³ fitting system, resulting in a much more appropriate starting point for initial fittings.

3. *Fine-tuning the computed program.* After the initial fitting computation, the dispenser typically adjusts the overall level as required (increasing or decreasing all four prescribed gains simultaneously). While no other adjustments are recommended at this time for the first program (indicated as Program I on the remote control), the second program (Program II) may be set with parameters modified to match the patient's preference. The patient is then encouraged to use both Programs I and II in various real-life situations and to note specific differences. Upon return a week or two later, these paired comparisons are a precious source of information to complete the fine-tuning process. A concise fitting guide is provided to help with specific fitting modifications required by occlusion, feedback, fluctuating hearing loss, telephone use, and so on.

In summary, the P³ fitting system allows:

1. Automated suprathreshold testing
2. Audiogram entry
3. Automated fitting computation based on (1) or (2) or both
4. Paired comparison via ultra sonic programming or hard-wired programming
5. Remote control and device programming
6. Storage of patient file in the hearing device EEPROM memory
7. Hand-held operation
8. PC-based operations, with the P³ acting as an interface
9. Foreign languages, new devices support; easy algorithm upgrade via programming cards sent by mail

More systematic fine-tuning techniques are being developed to simplify further the dispenser's task and increase the patient's satisfaction with the product. Overall, the development of practical effective fitting algorithms and techniques has proven to be a formidable but mandatory task. It is not an exaggeration to point out that the psychoacoustic strategies for selection of sound processing parameters and the design of the fitting tools were as demanding and perhaps even more challenging than the electronic and software design.

THE CLINICAL RESULTS

Clinical and real-life verification of the performance of ReSound's sound processing scheme and of the fitting technique were obtained in a series of clinical and laboratory evaluations. An extensive investigation by Moore et al. (1992) went beyond most earlier studies of multiband compression systems by employing wearable in-the-ear hearing devices and by allowing the subjects to wear the aids in a variety of everyday situations for some time before being tested . Twenty experienced and reasonably well-satisfied hearing aid users with moderate sensorineural hearing losses were tested using ReSound in-the-ear devices programmed as linear amplifiers and as two-band compressors. Subjects also

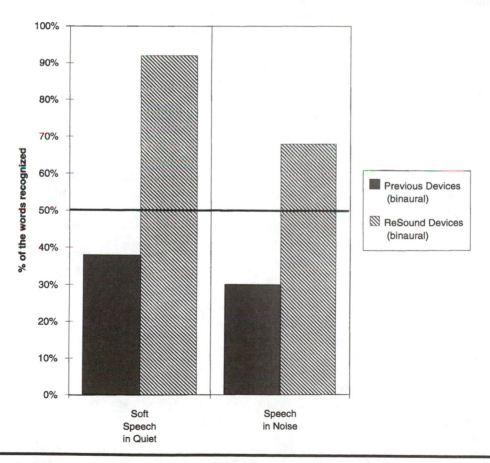

FIGURE 2.13.   ReSound vs. traditional hearing devices: improvements in speech recognition in quiet and in noise. Data from Moore et al.

were tested unaided and using their own hearing devices. Speech recognition was measured in quiet at three intensity levels, 50, 65, and 80 dB SPL, and in 12-talker babble under a variety of monaurally and binaurally aided conditions.

For speech in quiet, scores among the different devices were similar at the high- and the mid-intensity levels. However, they were significantly different when speech was presented at the lowest input level. In Figure 2.13, the left half displays the average speech recognition scores for soft speech in quiet for the multiband compression device and for subjects' own aids. With the ReSound devices in a compression mode, over 85% of the words were perceived correctly, whereas with traditional sound processing, the average recognition score was less than 40%. These results demonstrate that MBFDRC allows speech to be understood over a wide intensity range without volume control adjustment. The ability to understand speech in the presence of background noise was improved significantly with the use of the fast-acting two-band compression system when compared to the unaided condition and to subjects' own hearing aids. It should be noted that most linear hearing aids do not improve the intelligibility of speech in moderate and high noise levels (Duquesnoy and Plomp, 1980; Festen and Plomp, 1986; McAlister, 1990). Nor have other noise reduction hearing devices performed well under noisy conditions (Van Tassell et al., 1988; Fabry et al., 1990). The advantage of compression over linear processing varied across subjects; patients with small dynamic ranges at high frequencies (<27 dB) tended to benefit more than subjects with wider dynamic ranges. The appearance of a significant binaural advantage, both when speech and noise were spatially separated and when they were coincident, demonstrated that independent compression at the two ears did not adversely affect the use of binaural cues.

The right half of Figure 2.13 shows the results of speech recognition testing in the presence of multitalker babble. For a 3 dB signal-to-noise ratio, the average score with ReSound compression was greater than 60%, whereas with the previous devices, it was less than 30%. Going from a monaural linear condition (worst case) to binaural compression (best case) corresponded to a greater than 75% increase in speech recognition under very difficult listening conditions. Questionnaires on the subjects' experiences with the aids in everyday life indicated that they generally preferred compression over linear aiding in a variety of environments.

A second study, by Benson, Clark and Johnson (1992), was carried out in a busy hearing aid dispensary. Eighteen patients with sensorineural hearing impairment compared the MBFDRC hearing devices with their previous conventional hearing aids. They represented a broad age range and a variety of hearing loss configurations ranging from mild to severe. A battery of audiologic tests measured clinical performance, and questionnaires investigated patients' hearing ability in a variety of different listening situations. Hearing devices were matched in real-ear response up to 3200 Hz.

The mean dynamic range of hearing was broader with the MBFDRC devices than with previous hearing aids. Additionally, speech recognition scores were significantly better with ReSound than with patients' previous hearing aids at both 50 and 65 dB SPL presentation levels. The results highlight the dissimilarities in how the different sound processing technologies handle low- and high-intensity inputs. With MBFDRC, the weakest components of speech were boosted more than the more intense sounds. The low compression knee allowed for more gain to be given to sounds near threshold and, at the same time, less gain to more intense sounds — in contrast to previous hearing aids that, for the most part,

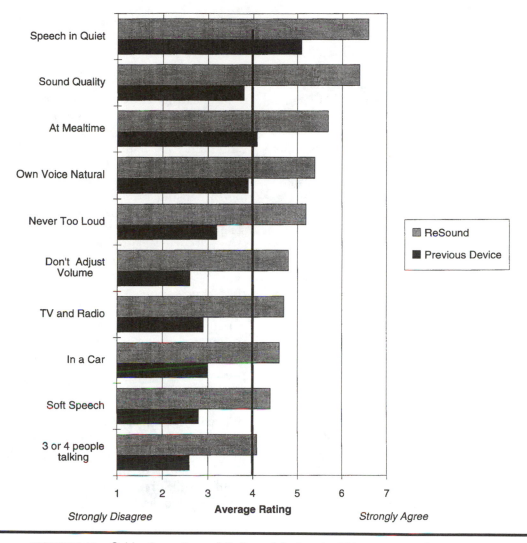

FIGURE 2.14.   Subjective ratings of ReSound devices by 300 customers. See text for explanation.

provided linear amplification throughout all or most of the dynamic range of speech (45–85 dB SPL).

Overall, patients rated the ReSound devices more favorably than they did their previous hearing aids. In particular, the patients reported that they heard soft speech better, that speech was never too loud, that they rarely needed to make volume changes,

that sound quality was very good, and that their own voices sounded natural. Clinical tests and subjective patient responses were in good agreement.

Similar results were obtained from questionnaires completed by over 300 patients. A series of positive performance statements was proposed and each patient recorded agreement or disagreement on a scale of 7 to 1.

A short summary of each statement is indicated on the left side of Figure 2.14. For example, "Speech in Quiet" is short for "I could easily understand in quiet." The average scores show a neutral to positive average in each category for the multiband full dynamic range compression devices, and a negative average in most categories for the previously owned devices. It is to be noted that the latter devices were well fitted and of recent design.

A third study addressed the flexibility and reliability of Resound's programmability feature by utilizing real-ear measures (Moore et al., 1991). The results affirmed that it is possible to configure this programmable instrument to suit patients having a wide variety of patterns of hearing impairment. Furthermore, the correspondence between gains programmed in the device and the gains actually achieved in situ was very close. By providing level- and frequency-dependent gain characteristics, the system increased the usable dynamic range of hearing beyond that of more conventional hearing devices.

CONCLUSION

A new generation of hearing instruments has been developed and is being dispensed today whose design and implementation are based upon a psychoacoustic rationale. In the case of the multiband full dynamic range compression system, controlled measures of patient performance, as well as information from field use of the device by thousands of users, indicate that the design goals have been achieved. Hearing-impaired patients are being provided with a significantly broader range of listening comfort than was possible with conventional hearing devices. By ensuring adequate amplification at frequencies where it is needed most, MBFDRC allows them to hear and understand softer levels of speech while at the same time avoiding overamplification where little gain is needed. Evidence demonstrates that appropriate hearing devices can clearly improve the ability to understand speech in a variety of typical noisy environments.

Certainly there are some areas that merit further attention. The success of these new devices is highly dependent on the skills of the dispensing professional. Training techniques are being improved so as to facilitate a steeper learning curve and to avoid some pitfalls and early frustrations. New fitting algorithms, based on auditory research, will provide better starting points, while improved procedures undoubtedly will evolve to assist in fine-tuning devices to more closely suit individual hearing requirements. Automated psychoacoustic measures that could lend accuracy and efficiency to clinical procedures have been developed by several research groups and must find their way into the clinical setting.

Finally, hearing devices suffer from numerous drawbacks not solved by electronic sound processing, for example, acoustic feedback, the discomfort of tightly fitting shells and earmolds, the ubiquitous occlusion effect, and reliability problems created by cerumen and perspiration. These problems must be addressed with the same technological commitment devoted to the electronics. Only then will the patient's expectations truly be met.

Acknowledgments: The author wishes to thank Dr. Jeannette Seloover Johnson for proofreading the manuscript and suggesting numerous improvements.

REFERENCES

Allen, J.B., and Jeng, P.S. (1990). Loudness growth in 1/2-octave bands (LGOB): A procedure for the assessment of loudness. *Journal of the Acoustical Society of America* 88:745–753.

Benson, D., Clark, T.M., and Johnson, J.S. (1992). Patient experiences with multiband full dynamic range compression. *Ear and Hearing.*

Duquesnoy, A.J., and Plomp, R. (1980). Effect of reverberation and noise on the intelligibility of sentences in cases of presbycusis. *Journal of the Acoustical Society of America* 68:537–544.

Duquesnoy, A.J., and Plomp, R. (1983). The effect of a hearing aid on the speech-reception threshold of hearing-impaired listeners in quiet and in noise. *Journal of the Acoustical Society of America* 73:2166–2173.

Fabry, D.A., and Walden, B.F. (1990). Noise reduction hearing aids. *ASHA* 32:48–51.

Fabry, D.A., Leek, M.R., and Walden, B.E. (1990). Do "adaptive frequency response" (AFR) hearing aids reduce upward spread of masking? *Journal of the Acoustical Society of America* 87 (Suppl. 1):S87.

Festen, J.M., and Plomp, R. (1986). Speech reception threshold in noise with one and two hearing aids. *Journal of the Acoustical Society of America* 79:465–471.

Killion, M.C. (1979). Design and evaluation of high-fidelity hearing aid. Ph.D. dissertation, Northwestern University.

Laurence, R.F., Moore, B.C.J., and Glasberg, B.R. (1983). A comparison of behind-the-ear high-fidelity linear hearing aids and two-channel compression aids, in the laboratory and in everyday life. *British Journal of Audiology* 17:31–48.

McAlister, P.V. (1990). The effect of hearing aids on speech discrimination in noise by normal-hearing listeners. *Journal of Rehabilitation Research and Development* 27:33–42.

Moore, B.C.J., Clark, T.M., Buckles, K.M., and Johnson, J.S. (1991). Processing frequency/intensity information: Programmable versus conventional hearing instruments. Presented at the ASHA Annual Convention, Atlanta.

Moore, B.C.J., Johnson, J.S., Clark, T.M., and Pluvinage, V. (1992). Evaluation of a dual-channel full dynamic range compression system for people with sensorineural hearing loss. *Ear and Hearing.*

Moore, B.C.J., and Glasberg, B.R. (1986). A comparison of two-channel and single-channel compression hearing aids. *Audiology* 25:210–226.

Moore, B.C.J. (1987). Design and evaluation of a two-channel compression hearing aid. *Journal of Rehabilitation Research and Development* 24(4):181–192.

Pearsons, K.S., Bennett, R.L., and Fidell, S. (1976). Speech Levels in Various Environments. Report No. 3281. Cambridge, MA: Bolt, Beranek and Newman.

Pluvinage, V. (1989). Clinical measurement of loudness growth. *Hearing Instruments* 39.

Pluvinage, V., and Benson, D. (1988). New dimensions in diagnostics and fitting. *Hearing Instruments* 39:28, 30, 39.

Skinner, M.W. (1976). Speech Intelligibility in Noise-Induced Hearing Loss: Effects of High-Frequency Compensation. Ph.D. dissertation, Washington University, St. Louis, MO.

Van Tasell, D.J., Larsen, S.Y., and Fabry, D.A. (1988). Effects of an adaptive filter hearing aid on speech recognition in noise by hearing-impaired subjects. *Ear and Hearing* 9:15–21.

Villchur, E. (1973). Signal processing to improve speech intelligibility in perceptive deafness. *Journal of the Acoustical Society of America* 53:1646–1657.

Zurek, P., and Rankovic, T. (1990). Potential benefits of varying the frequency-gain characteristic for speech reception in noise. Presented at the 119th Meeting of the Acoustical Society of America, May 1990, State College, PA.

CHAPTER 3

PRINCIPLES AND APPLICATION OF THE WIDEX MULTIPROGRAMMABLE HEARING AID SYSTEM

Søren Westermann

The application of digital technology to hearing aid devices has sparked considerable interest among electroacoustic engineers, audiologists, and hearing instrument dispensers. While the application of true digital technology (wherein the input signal is digitized, processed, and reconverted into an acoustic event) has not been commercially successful, other forms of digital application are promising.

This chapter deals with the development of a hearing aid system (Widex Quattro) (Figure 3.1) that employs a form of digital technology in which various parameters affecting the acoustic performance of the hearing aid can be mediated by digital control. The reader should remember that in present digital hearing aid devices the signal path remains analog at all times.

While the basic technology underlying the development of the Quattro has been available for some time, it is the method by which this technology is employed that gives a uniqueness to performance. Essentially, the system provides for four separate acoustic responses, each at the immediate command of the user. By providing more than one acoustic response to the user, it is highly probable that a best-fit response can be found to meet the acoustic needs for a specific listening environment.

The entire premise upon which the Quattro was developed rests on the observation that conventional hearing aids provide a single acoustic response, which represents, in part, a compromise for all listening environments. Thus, a multiprogrammable system providing a different hearing aid response as the listening environment changes seems infinitely more utilitarian.

The chapter presents a technical description of a multiprogrammable system that has proven to be of value to most individuals with hearing impairment. Further, it offers some suggested fitting protocols to the reader, which may facilitate their clinical experiences with the Quattro. Although it is realized that there is no definitive, or agreed-upon, number of programs needed by the user to perform at optimal levels in specific listening environments, four programs seem to be adequate for most persons. One realizes, also, that there is no one single fitting philosophy for multiprogrammable hearing aid devices.

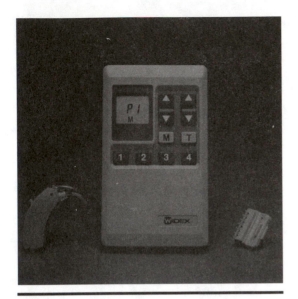

FIGURE 3.1. The Widex Quattro hearing aid system.

cessful implementations of digital technology in hearing aids. Inasmuch as it is a digitally controlled analog hearing aid, the digital technology has been applied to achieve functions unattainable if using only analog technology. As it is essentially a linear device, true digital technology (digital processing of the acoustic signals) was considered unnecessary. In that true digital technology, due to the state of technology at the time of the development of the Quattro, would cause serious problems with respect to power supply, power consumption, costs, and so on, the digitally controlled analog approach was chosen from the start. The system is now available as a complete series of behind-the-ear (BTE) instruments and as small in-the-ear (ITE) instruments. The system is an example of applying new (digital) technology in order to realize a completely new idea.

Those fitting recommendations offered in this chapter are based on our research with hearing-impaired subjects responding to various acoustic signals in different environmental backgrounds. From these data, we have drawn several conclusions and present a "cookbook" fitting strategy. Obviously, as one gains more clinical experience with the system, variations in methodology may be formulated. Finally, this chapter reviews pertinent research conducted in Europe and in the United States that supports the use and application of multiprogrammable hearing aids in general and the Quattro system in particular.

In the absence of general consensus of what technological interface the pathologic ear needs to best process an incoming acoustic signal in different listening environments, the introduction of a digitally controlled multiprogrammable hearing aid device may serve as an initial step in arriving at a rational answer. The Quattro multiprogrammable system is one of the first commercially suc-

HISTORICAL BACKGROUND

The idea of a digitally controlled, multiprogrammable hearing aid developed from a research project internally designated the "831" project. The 831 arose from the conclusion of a technical-acoustic meeting in Scandinavia in August 1982. One of the conclusions was that "the final setting of the hearing aid should be decided by the patient by utilizing a subjective judgment of the sound reproduction" (14th Nordic Hearing Aid Technical Meeting, 1982). This statement was of course in opposition to calculating the response by using a fitting rule and emanated from the confusion experienced by many hearing aid specialists when they had to decide which of the many fitting rules would be the correct one in each particular case.

For two decades numerous prescriptive formulas have been suggested, most of these being based on experiences from undertaking a large number of actual fittings of hearing aids. Formulas such as half-gain rule (Lybarger, 1963), NAL (Byrne and Tonisson, 1976), Berger (Berger, Hagberg, and Rane, 1977), and POGO (McCandless and Lyregaard, 1983) were all applied to the fitting procedure in order to improve the final result. Since 1982 several other formulas have been added, such as $\frac{1}{3}$–$\frac{2}{3}$ rule (Libby, 1985 and 1986) and New NAL (Byrne and Dillon, 1986), among others. While many of these rules normally would yield a useful result, confusion would prevail merely from the very number of rules. They simply could not all be right. On the other hand, no single rule stood out as being "the best rule." The feeling in 1982 was, therefore, that the prescriptive rules could form a useful basis for the selection of the hearing aid and an initial adjustment thereof. But in

order to obtain an optimal fitting, the user should have influence on which fine-adjustments should be made. The 831 offered this opportunity by having all adjustments as four trimmers in the back of a BTE instrument, and the hearing aid specialist would have a remote control with a Bowden control cable that would snap into the trimmer panel of the hearing aid, thus allowing easy remote operation of the trimmers (see Figure 3.2).

A laboratory set-up was established in order to undertake a clinical evaluation of the system. Three loudspeakers were used in a dampened room (see Figure 3.3). Two of the loudspeakers were used for presenting different noises in stereo, and the third (middle) loudspeaker was used for presenting speech material. The prototype 831 had low-cut, output compression and preset gain controls (see Figure 3.4).

The first experiment, in which the patients were allowed freely to adjust all four controls while different sound material was pre-

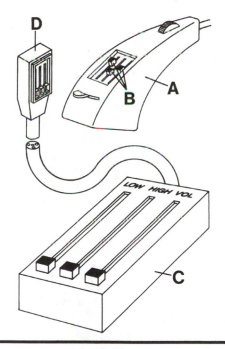

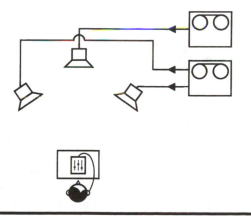

FIGURE 3.2. The 831. This philosophy used a BTE instrument (A) with a number of trimmers (B) that could be manipulated from a mechanical remote control (C) with a bowden cable and a snap-in connection (D) to facilitate easy, final adjustment of the instrument by the user.

FIGURE 3.3. Laboratory setup for testing the 831 philosophy clinically. The two side loudspeakers presented different types of background noises, and the middle speaker mainly presented speech in order to simulate different listening situations. The user sat with the remote control in front of him and adjusted for optimal setting.

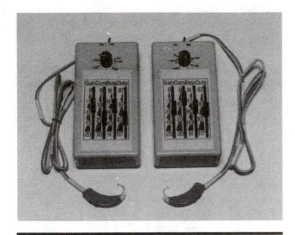

FIGURE 3.4.   The prototype 831s. These instruments were built electronically (analog) and offered preset gain, compression, low-cut and output control trimmers. The volume control was also built into the remote control.

sented, demonstrated that it was completely impossible for patients to select one optimal setting. Often when a new sound environment was presented, patients would prefer a setting very different from the previous setting, just as they would choose almost the same setting the next time that same sound environment was presented.

A second experiment was conducted in which patients concentrated on one adjustment control at a time and were taken through a step-by-step procedure with one or more listening environments for each control (see Figure 3.5). This procedure gave a very consistent, complete setting if repeated. However, if the patients were presented some of the listening environments from the first experiment, the setting would in many cases be unacceptable and a better one (one for each environment) could be found.

All in all, the 831 concept did not offer significant advantages to previous hearing aid fitting strategies. On the other hand, it was clear that in each environment the patients were quite easily able to choose a favorite and more optimal setting.

NEW FITTING PHILOSOPHY

The conclusion was that all patients should be given control of specific program selection from a number of different distinct responses. This idea should prove to have far more extensive consequences than originally assumed.

Previously, the hearing impaired were offered only one single response. This response had been either calculated according to one of the many fitting rules or adjusted by the hearing aid specialist according to his or her clinical experience and some type of trial-and-error method. These methods would always result in a compromise between maximum intelligibility and a comfortable sound quality.

Maximum intelligibility is achieved by emphasizing the high frequencies (above 1000 Hz) and attenuating the low, and often noise-contaminated, frequencies, which tend to make the sound quality hard and tinny. A comfortable sound quality will, on the other hand, normally require emphasis in the low-frequency range (100–500 Hz) and a roll-off towards higher frequencies. Seen from the point of view of the hearing impaired, several other factors (transients, overall loudness, the purpose of listening, etc.) influence the optimal response.

In fact, the above compromise incorporated into a traditional hearing aid could very well turn out to be less than optimal in any specific environment and only offer poor performance in most environments. However, by providing the hearing impaired with a series of different preprogrammed responses each optimized to a particular hearing loss in specific environments, significant improvements may be experienced. Additionally, by offering a simple and easy selection mechanism to facilitate rapid interchange between preprogrammed responses, an improved

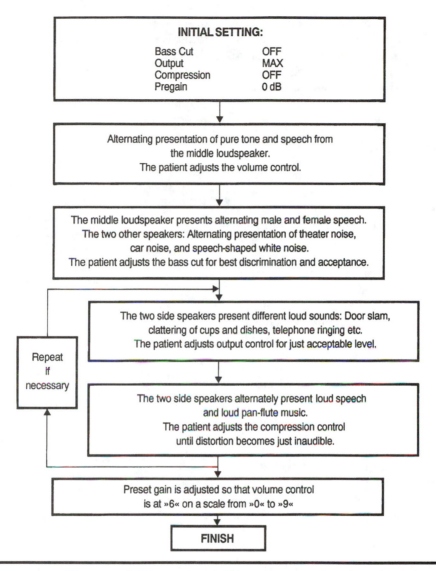

FIGURE 3.5.   The second 831 experiment. The patient was taken through a strict fitting procedure in order to systematize the patient's adjustments. While the procedure was highly reproducible, it never resulted in a setting acceptable in all listening situations.

hearing rehabilitation system would evolve, facilitating *optimal* response in any listening situation. The fitting procedure would, of course, require the adjustment of many more parameters corresponding to a complete hearing aid adjustment for each environment.

The 831 research demonstrated that it was easy for the hearing impaired to choose an optimal setting in a given specific listening situation. Therefore, by using prerecorded sound examples, speech material, background noise, word lists, and so on, fitting of a multiple-response hearing aid could be a simple procedure.

DESIGN PHILOSOPHY

At an early stage of development much consideration was given to how many different responses should be available to the user. Too many responses would cause more confusion than help, and too few would result in poor performance in a number of listening situations. As the name Quattro implies, four individual responses were chosen.

The next question that arose was how to adjust or program all the parameters in each of the four programs. The 831 would have had four slide trimmers. Multiplied by four programs this would result in 16 trimmers and a four-position program selection switch. It goes without saying that such an instrument would be difficult to develop, particularly with reference to a reasonable size. Small ITEs would obviously be out of the question. Furthermore, it was expected that operating the four-position switch would cause difficulties relative to patient manipulation of the controls. In light of this, it was concluded that all response parameters had to be stored digitally and recalled easily by a simple maneuver of the hearing impaired. This in turn implied that some kind of programming device would have to be made available to facilitate adjustment and storage of the many parameters.

Soon it was realized that by incorporating a remote control in the design concept, a number of advantages could be obtained:

• By having one push button on the remote control for each of the four programs, the user could easily and randomly select any pro-gram appropriate in specific listening situations. Without the remote control it would be difficult for the user to know which program is active and which is chosen.

• By equipping the remote control with a display and a powerful microprocessor, the remote control could become the programming tool as well. In mass production this could be realized at a reasonable price, and no expensive external programming equipment would be necessary to achieve the advantages of multiprogrammability.

• As the hearing aid would need no trimmers, volume controls, and so on, the instrument could be made smaller, provided that the electronics could be made small as well. This would be particularly beneficial if a small in-the-ear instrument could be made.

Thus it was decided that the system should consist of a hearing aid and a remote control. The hearing aid would not need any external controls. The hearing aid should be able to wirelessly receive a set of parameters, which in turn would control the different functions (volume control, filters, output control, etc.). The hearing aid should be capable of receiving such parameter sets at any time and without making errors (such as false adjustments, erroneous program changes, etc.).

For the wireless transmission, three basic principles were possible for implementation:

1. *Infrared transmission.* This technique is well known from remote controls for television sets but has the disadvantage that the receiver (hearing aid) must be in visible contact (line of sight) with the transmitter (remote control).

2. *Ultrasound transmission.* This technique is known from a few hearing aids with remote-controlled volume control. It has a transmitter that transmits ultrawave frequencies (higher than 20,000 Hz), and the system uses a microphone in the hearing aid that is able to pick up these high frequencies. Unfortunately, ultra-

sound has a very directional dispersion, which in practice means that the remote control often must be held at ear level. So both infrared light and ultrasound require in most instances that the remote control be held at ear level. This in turn implies that in the case of binaural fitting, either two separate remote control units are needed or one remote control must be shifted from side to side to adjust one side at a time.

3. *Radiowave transmission.* This technique is known from radio-controlled toy cars and other devices. It has the advantage that radio signals spread much more uniformly in most directions and can easily penetrate material such as fabrics and flesh. This means that a remote control using radiowave transmission can be held in almost any position and can be operated even from the inside of a pocket or handbag. The disadvantage of this technique is that it requires an antenna in both the remote control and the hearing aid. It also requires more sophisticated electronics in the transmitter and receiver.

It was decided that a radiowave system should be attempted.

The remote control should transmit a new set of parameters to the hearing aid at the user's command. If the user is wearing two instruments, the remote control should be capable of transmitting two individual parameter sets simultaneously so that the user can switch programming at each ear simultaneously.

Four dedicated push buttons for program (environment) selection, two separate up/down volume controls for left and right ear, a separate microphone, and telecoil on/off switches should be available (see Figure 3.6). Furthermore, the previously mentioned display should show the daily use status of the system and assist the hearing specialist in programming the parameters. The remote control should be made small and yet easy to operate. Despite the small number of push buttons and the limited size of the display,

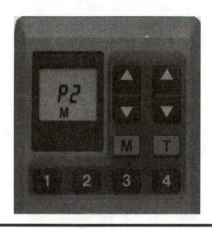

FIGURE 3.6. The remote control. Four program selection switches (1, 2, 3, and 4), two up/down digital volume controls, an M switch, a T switch, and a display are required.

user operation should be simple and the programming procedure should be as logical and easy as possible.

Obviously, the above design goal could never be achieved by using only conventional analog technology. The hearing aid would most conveniently be a digitally controlled analog amplifier with analog filter functions. The remote control should be an all-digital instrument with a microprocessor, a microprocessor program and display, push buttons, and batteries.

DESCRIPTION OF THE QUATTRO HEARING AID AND REMOTE CONTROL

Quattro Wireless Communication

The Quattro system uses a one-way wireless communication technique. The remote control can send "packages" of control information to one hearing aid or two hearing aids simultaneously. The radio frequency transmission is a frequency shift modulated signal and works as described in the following paragraphs.

Two different frequencies, 137 kHz and 148 kHz, can be transmitted/received. The signal is divided into short time slots, and each time slot contains either 137 kHz or 148 kHz, never both. Binary digits (0 or 1) are transmitted as two different time slot patterns, and any binary pattern could be transmitted by repeating these time slot patterns as appropriate.

All transmissions in the system respect a fixed rule. A transmission from the remote control forms a well-defined package that consists of five sub-blocks of data (Figure 3.7). The first block is a start bit block that holds a fixed bit pattern. The start bit block, which is used for synchronizing the receiver, informs the receiver that the present signal is a package and not just noise. The next four blocks are the actual data blocks. The transmitter data consist of parameters (i.e., volume control setting, filter setting, maximum output and compression setting, etc.) and an identification code (ID-code).

The ID-code is necessary for two reasons. First, in order to operate two individual hearing aids (for a binaural fitting), each hearing aid must be able to distinguish which data package is meant for it and which package is meant for the other aid and, therefore, should be ignored. Second, in order to avoid the situation that two Quattro users that meet influence each other's hearing aids, each hearing aid should have one single ID-code out of a great many numbers. Presently the system allows 250 different ID-codes, but this number could easily be expanded.

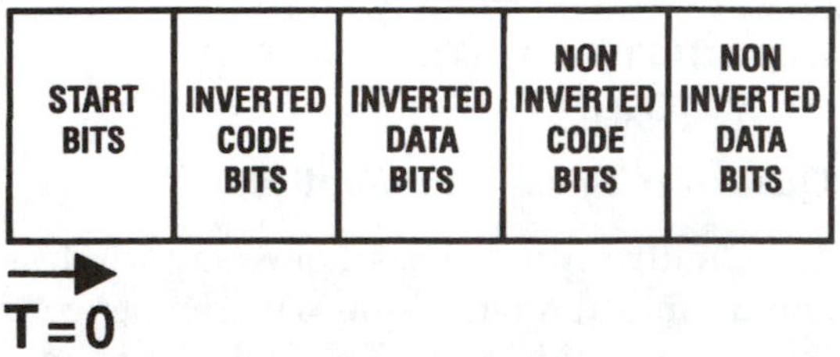

A parameter block has 18 bits split up as follows:

Number of Bits	Function	Number of Settings
1	AGC on/off	2
2	Maximum output	4
2	High-cut filter	4
2	Low-cut filter	4
2	IPA filter	4
2	Telecoil function	3
1	Microphone on/off	2
6	Volume control setting	40

Each parameter function is described in the section on Quattro Chip Description.

Both the ID-block and the parameter block are transmitted twice within a complete package (Figure 3.7). First the start bit block is transmitted. Next the ID-code is transmitted in inverted form—that is, zeroes (0) have become ones (1) and ones have become zeroes. Then the complete parameter block is transmitted, also in inverted form. Finally, both the ID-code and the parameter block are transmitted again, but this time in a noninverted form. So, for each transmission package all data bits are transmitted twice (both inverted and noninverted). This format ensures a tremendous security since all data bits must be received correctly both as inverted and noninverted bits. Otherwise, the entire package will be rejected by the hearing instrument.

START BITS	INVERTED CODE BITS	INVERTED DATA BITS	NON INVERTED CODE BITS	NON INVERTED DATA BITS

T = 0

FIGURE 3.7. Data sub-blocks. Each time a change to the hearing aid setting is desirable, the remote control sends a digital package consisting of five blocks. The entire package is transmitted in less than 1/10 second.

QUATTRO CHIP DESCRIPTION

At this stage it was obvious that the Quattro hearing aid electronics would have to consist of a radio frequency receiver part, an analog amplifier and filter part including a large digital control section. As the hearing aids should work with a single 1.5-volt battery cell, the design possibilities within integrated circuits are very limited.

From the beginning it was believed that at least two custom-made integrated circuits would be needed since the analog part would need one technology and the digital part another technology. Fortunately, after some time a bipolar technology was identified, allowing a single chip to implement both digital and analog functions down to approximately 1.1 volts and at the same time using very little power.

Figure 3.8 shows a block diagram of the chip, and Figure 3.9 is a detailed picture of the actual chip. The chip is approximately 4 mm by 5 mm (0.15 inch by 0.2 inch) and contains 450 transistors, 1,500 digital gates, and 250 passive components (resistors and capacitors). Functionally, this corresponds to more than 100 times the number of transistors in a standard BTE or ITE instrument. The chip typically consumes 1.5 mA.

As can be seen from Figure 3.8, the microphone and telecoil signals are connected to input amplifiers that can be switched on and off independently. The outputs of these amplifiers are combined and pass through three programmable filters: IPA (inverse presbycusis adaptation, an electronic simulation of stepped-response microphones designed primarily to correct typical presbycusis types of hearing losses), low-cut filters, and high-cut filters. Figure 3.8 also shows that each filter is controlled by two digital control lines. This in turn results in the four different settings of each filter. The function of each filter and their combinations are shown in Figure 3.10.

From the filters, the signal enters the digitally controlled volume control. The volume control is controlled by six lines, and theoretically this would enable $2^6 = 64$ different settings. In practice, there are a number of redundant settings (i.e., several settings resulting in the same gain), meaning that 40 distinct gain settings are available. As there are 1.5 dB between each step of the volume control, the full range of the volume control is

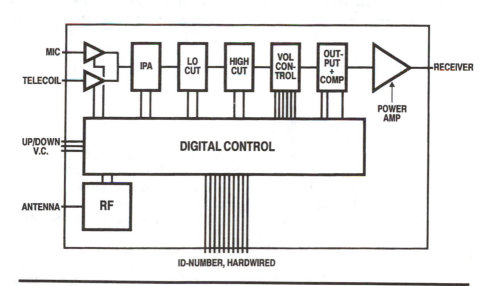

FIGURE 3.8. Block diagram of the Quattro chip.

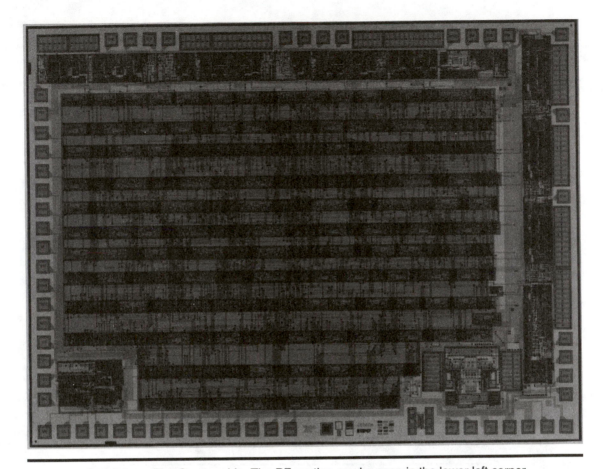

FIGURE 3.9. The Quattro chip. The RF section can be seen in the lower left corner, the analog amplifier and filter circuitry is located along the upper and rightmost edges, and the huge central part is the digital control section.

almost 60 dB (58.5 dB). In daily use, only 30 of these steps will normally be available to the user. This is mediated by the remote control.

From the volume control, the signal passes through a programmable output limiter and compression stage. Two digital control lines allow the maximum output to be reduced by 0, 3, 6, or 10 dB. A third line can switch an output compression function on and off. Figure 3.11 shows the influence of the compression on the input/output characteristic. The last circuit block in the signal path is a class

A/B power amplifier that drives the acoustic receiver.

The RF (radio frequency) receiver circuitry is connected to a very small loop-type antenna resting inside the hearing aid. It extracts clock and data information from the RF signal and presents these to the digital control section.

First the controller (Figure 3.12) demodulates the pulse width modulated signal and checks for correct pulse widths. Then it synchronizes to the start bits and checks that the

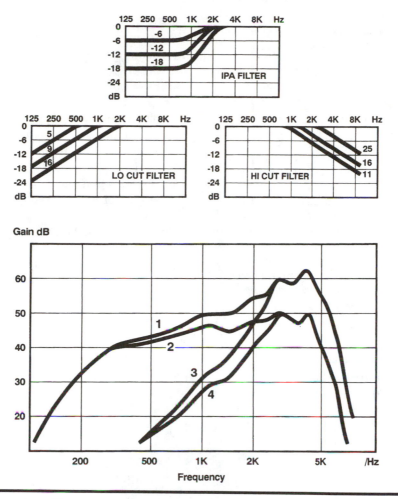

FIGURE 3.10. The relative effect of the three programmable filters (upper half) and frequency responses obtainable with the Q8 (lower half). Curve 1: all filters inactive; curve 2: hi-cut filter at maximum (1100 Hz); curve 3: IPA filter at maximum (−18 dB) and low-cut at maximum (1600 Hz); and curve 4: all three filters at their maximum cutoff. Practically any response between response 1 and response 4 can be programmed (all responses measured on IEC 711 coupler).

start bit sequence is correct. If this is the case, the inverted ID-code and data are collected in a register. Next the noninverted code and data are taken into a similar register. When the entire package has been received, the data part can be transferred to the final control register that controls the analog signal path.

This does not happen, however, unless some very strict conditions are met.

The controller checks that the inverted and noninverted ID-codes correspond exactly to one another, that the inverted and non-inverted data correspond exactly to one another, and that the noninverted ID-code

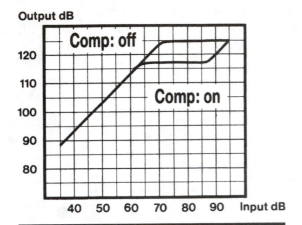

FIGURE 3.11. Input/output characteristics showing the effect of the compression circuitry. In practice (where input levels rarely exceed 85 dB SPL), the compression also acts as an output reduction of approximately 15 dB.

exactly matches a bit pattern that is hard-wired to the chip (this is how the ID-code is coded into the hearing aid during production). Only if all three criteria are met will the controller latch the data part into the control register and thus change the characteristics of the hearing aid. In all other cases, the entire information package is completely ignored and the digital controller will await a new start bit sequence.

In case the hearing aid user wants to change the volume and does not have the remote control at hand, the digital controller has inputs for an optional up/down volume-control switch. In addition, the controller section contains some initialization and "household" functions that ensure proper operation after power-on and so on.

In all models of the Quattro system, the chip is mounted on a dual-sided thick-film substrate, together with the approximately twenty necessary external components (Figure 3.13). Due to the ultra-high power capacity of the Q32, a separate output stage is added to the circuitry and mounted onto a second dual-sided thick-film substrate, and both substrates are "sandwiched" into one unit. Having removed all trimmers and switches from the hearing aids, a very smooth and elegant design results (Figure 3.14).

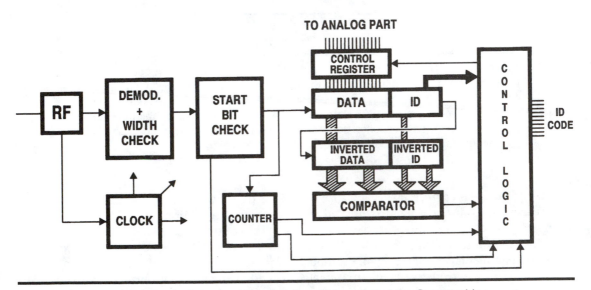

FIGURE 3.12. Block diagram of the digital control section of the Quattro chip.

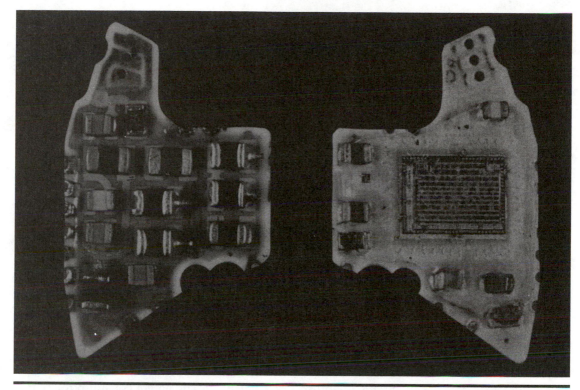

FIGURE 3.13.   View of both sides of the thick-film substrate holding the entire Q8 circuitry. The Quattro chip is easily identified on the substrate to the right.

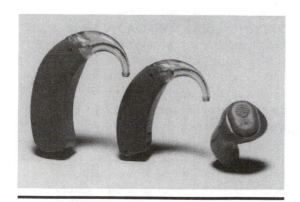

FIGURE 3.14.   Quattro hearing instruments. No trimmers are present on the instruments, and the volume control is only optional as it can be operated from the remote control. Shown are (from left to right) the Q32 and Q8 BTE models and the QX small ITE model.

REMOTE CONTROL DESCRIPTION

The remote control serves both as the user's means of adjustment and as the hearing aid specialist's programming device. This means that no external programming device or computer is necessary as the remote control is also a complete self-contained programmer. It is, however, *possible* to program the Quattro system from a computer. This will be discussed in the section on Interfacing with Computers.

The remote control is built around a powerful 8-bit CMOS microprocessor (80C51) (see Figure 3.15). The microprocessor has 4 KB program memory, 128 bytes RAM (random-access memory), a programmable full duplex serial interface, and 32 input/output lines.

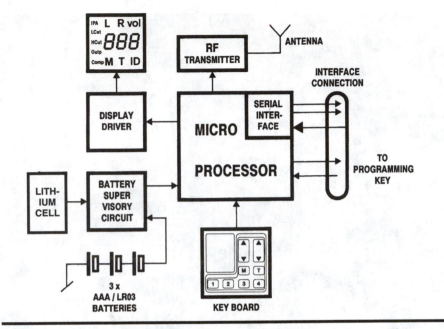

FIGURE 3.15.   Block diagram of the entire remote control.

The architecture of 80C51 is shown in Figure 3.16 but will not be discussed in detail here (interested readers can consult data books from Intel, OKI or other 8051/80C51 manufacturers).

The microprocessor program is written exclusively for the Quattro. It takes up the entire 4 KB program memory and is burned into the microprocessor chip at chip-processing time (the microprocessor is mask programmed). The microprocessor communicates with several peripherals: the keyboard, the LCD (liquid crystal display), the RF transmitter circuitry, a battery supervisory circuitry, and a complete duplex serial interface. The keyboard can be scanned whenever convenient, and the microprocessor performs a number of checks to ensure that erroneous interpretation of the keypresses is avoided.

The LCD is controlled by sending bit streams to an extremely low power consuming display driver, which in turn controls the display itself. The power consumption of this display driver is very important because the driver is always active (the display is always showing something), whereas the microprocessor "goes to sleep" (power-down mode) five seconds after each normal keypress and in this mode consumes virtually no power.

As Figure 3.17 shows, the display has a common group of segments (used by both the user and the hearing aid specialist) and a group of programming segments that is relevant only when the hearing aid specialist programs the Quattro. Each time the microprocessor recognizes a keyboard action that calls for a new setting of the hearing aid(s), it activates the RF circuitry and transmits a new parameter setting in accordance with the previously mentioned rules. The RF circuitry has been specifically designed to use as little power as possible.

In the event that the three mini-penlight batteries run out of power, it is important that

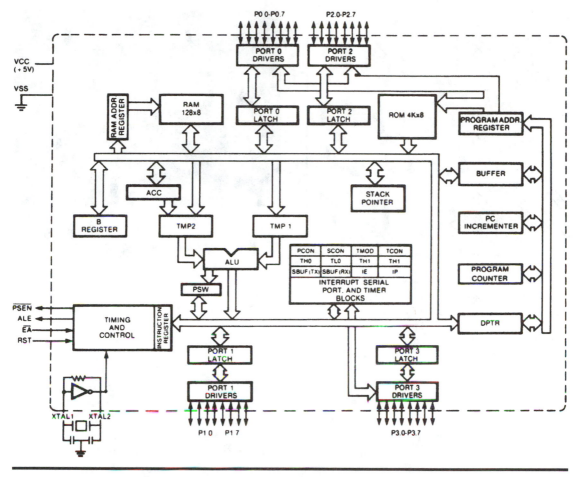

FIGURE 3.16. Block diagram of the 80C51 microprocessor, the heart of the remote control. Reprinted with permission from Philips Semiconductors, The Netherlands.

the microprocessor does not loose all the preprogrammed parameters that are stored in the microprocessor's RAM. A battery supervisory circuitry is thus present to ensure that if the normal batteries go low, a backup lithium battery takes over and thereby keeps the programmed parameters intact. As the lithium cell has a limited capacity once the microprocessor is switched to the lithium cell, the microprocessor refuses to perform most normal operations until new batteries have been inserted into the remote control. Still, without normal AAA batteries the lithium cell is capable of preserving any stored parameters for at least one to two years. The remote control gives the user a number of visual warnings once the normal batteries are about to run out of power.

The microprocessor has a built-in full duplex serial interface that enables the remote control to communicate with other computers. In particular, by attaching a rather inexpensive adapter, the remote control can directly communicate with a personal computer (IBM compatible). (See the section on Interfacing with Computers.)

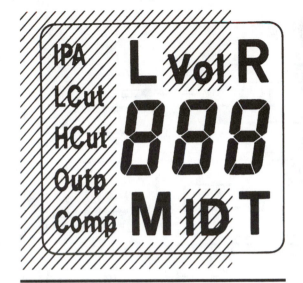

FIGURE 3.17. The remote control display. The display is separated into two groups, a common group for both the user and the hearing aid specialist (unhatched area) and a programming group for the specialist only (hatched area).

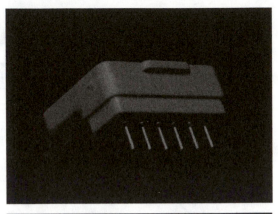

FIGURE 3.18. Close-up of the programming key. The key is approximately one inch wide.

The final peripheral element that the microprocessor recognizes is the programming key. This key (shown in Figure 3.18) is inserted in the back of the remote control (Figure 3.19) into a small six-pin connector (this connector also serves as the serial interface).

One of the first things the microprocessor does upon any keypress is to check if a programming key has been inserted, and if this is the case the microprocessor goes into programming mode (the programming mode is extensively described in the Quattro manual and briefly discussed in the section on Using the Quattro). The programming key is only meant to be used by the hearing aid specialist as its use requires the understanding of the various parameters of the system.

In order to obtain a logical and easy operation of the remote control (for both the user and the programmer/hearing specialist), the entire behavior of the remote control was simulated on a CAD/CAM workstation. All of the procedures, programming features, and input/output functions were simulated and tried out on a number of skilled and nonskilled people. Figure 3.20 shows a snapshot of the (at that time not yet existing) remote control on the workstation screen.

The entire electronics of the remote control is assembled on one double-sided, dual side-mounted printed circuit board. All the different parts of the remote control are shown in Figure 3.21. The RF radiation level is very low (less than 15 microvolts/meter at a distance of 100 feet), and the mini-penlight batteries are expected to last for more than one year of daily use.

USING THE QUATTRO

The practical use of the Quattro system is split up into two parts: (1) the user operation and (2) the programming.

The User Operation Mode

This mode is very straightforward and is accomplished whenever neither the programming key nor the serial interface is attached to

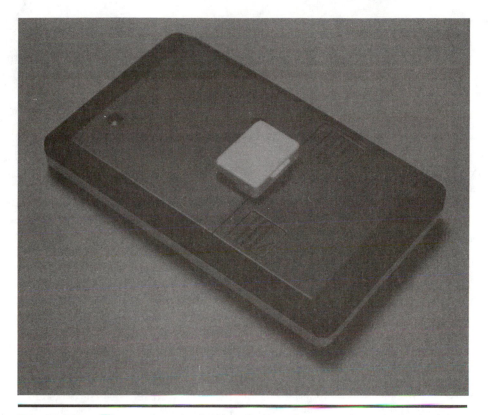

FIGURE 3.19.   The programming key inserted into the connector at the back of the remote control.

the remote control. The user can simply operate two volume controls (left and right), a microphone ON/OFF switch (M), a telecoil ON/OFF switch (T), and the four program selection keys (1, 2, 3, and 4).

The volume controls are digital and of the UP/DOWN type. If the fitting is binaural, each volume control will influence only its respective hearing aid side. If the fitting is monaural, the remote control can be programmed to have both volume controls react (in parallel) on the one hearing aid.

The M and T switches allow the user to turn the microphone and telecoil (if present) on and off freely. The four program switches (1, 2, 3, and 4) perform the function that to the

user makes the big difference between a traditional hearing aid and the Quattro system: At the touch of any of these four keys, the hearing aid can dramatically change its transfer characteristic in order to obtain a better adaptation of the hearing impaired to the present listening situation. It takes the Quattro system approximately 0.2 seconds to change to any new setting.

If the four programs have been properly set to the particular needs of the hard of hearing (his or her four most relevant listening environment types), moving from one situation to a very different situation will require only one single press on the appropriate program selection key, and a completely new and

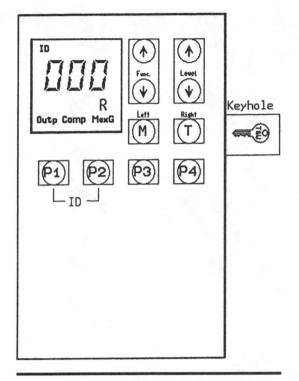

FIGURE 3.20. The workstation screen displaying the simulated remote control. The operation was simulated by using a computer mouse to click on the different switches, and the computer would then display the actions taken.

more suitable transfer function is operational in the hearing aid.

The Programming Mode

This mode is accomplished by inserting the programming key in the back of the remote control and pressing any key on the remote control. The complete programming procedure is described in detail in a programming manual (*Widex Quattro Manual*, 1989), but certain design features will be discussed in the following section.

As *all* parameters are adjusted by activating the volume controls (the left volume control adjusts the left-side parameters and the

right volume control operates the right-side parameters simultaneously), there are both an up and a down change in all parameters. Therefore, internally to the microprocessor all parameters have been arranged in a cyclic manner so that while operating the volume control in one direction and reaching the upper or lower limit of the actual function, this function will automatically roll over to the opposite lower or upper limit and start all over again.

This cyclic behavior is even more pronounced when it comes to the selection mechanism that points out which parameter is to be changed next. As can be seen in Figure 3.22, all seven parameters for each of the four programs are arranged in separate seven-step cycles, and getting from one parameter to another in the same program circle is accomplished simply by pressing the corresponding program key a sufficient number of times. Once the relevant parameter of the appropriate program has been reached, both its right- and left-side settings can be easily changed simply by activating the volume controls. If the parameters in one of the other programs are to be programmed, all that is necessary is to activate the corresponding program key a number of times.

The display will always tell which parameter, which program, and which side (left or right) is being changed. Once the desired parameter combination has been selected and programmed, the removal of the programming key will freeze this selection, and the programming will not change unless the key is reinserted.

An important issue is that each time any parameter is changed in the remote control, the entire relevant program is transmitted to the hearing aid(s) so that the hearing impaired can immediately listen in on all the changes made by the hearing aid specialist. The entire programming procedure was also programmed and simulated on the CAD/

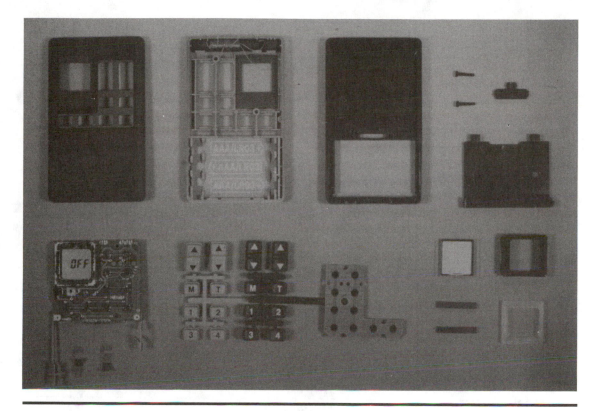

FIGURE 3.21.   All the components necessary for building a remote control. The electronics are mounted on the dual-sided printed circuit seen at the lower left corner.

CAM workstation in order to reach the simplest possible procedure of the remote control in the programming situation.

INTERFACING WITH COMPUTERS

The Quattro remote control includes a full duplex serial interface and thereby facilitates communication between the remote control and any programmable computer that conforms to the following specifications:

- The serial interface is RS232C compatible.
- The baud rates are 1200/1200 bits per second.
- Each byte is transmitted as 8 bits with *no* parity and 1 stop bit.

- The electrical connections follow the Quattro Serial Protocol (*Quattro Serial Protocol*, 1989).
- The communication runs in packages, the syntax of which conforms to the Quattro Serial Protocol.

In principle, the remote control could communicate with any computer from the smallest home computer to the largest mainframe as long as the serial interface of the computer can be programmed to the above specifications. In practice, IBM Personal Computers and compatibles are normally used.

In order to overcome some simple level and power requirements, a specially developed inexpensive interface is required to con-

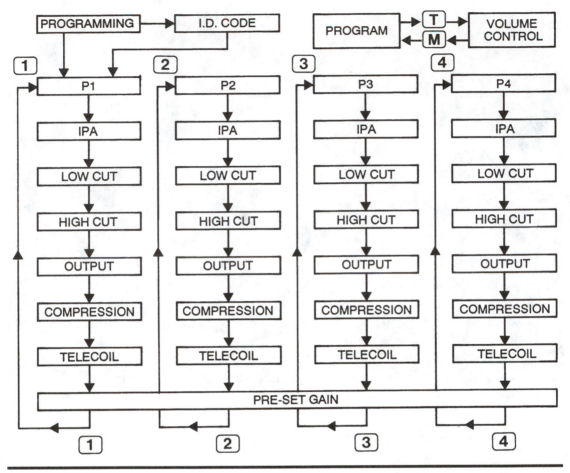

FIGURE 3.22.   Flow diagram illustrating the cyclic behavior of the programming procedure. The illustration is taken from the Quattro Manual, where the procedure is described in detail.

nect the remote control to the computer (see Figure 3.23). The interface has a standard RS232C connector with a cable that plugs into a computer, and at its top is a six-pin connector that plugs right into the connector at the back of the remote control when the remote control is placed on top of the interface. At the touch of any of the remote control keys, the remote control will now enter into a communication mode, in which the host computer has complete control of the behavior of the system.

The parameters already stored in the remote control can be transmitted (uploaded) to the host computer for inspection, storage, or change. New parameters can be downloaded from the host to the remote control, and if a new parameter set is downloaded to the program that is presently the active program in the remote control, this parameter set is immediately transmitted to the hearing aid(s) so that the user can hear the changes at once. A few other communication functions are available to the programmer. The specifi-

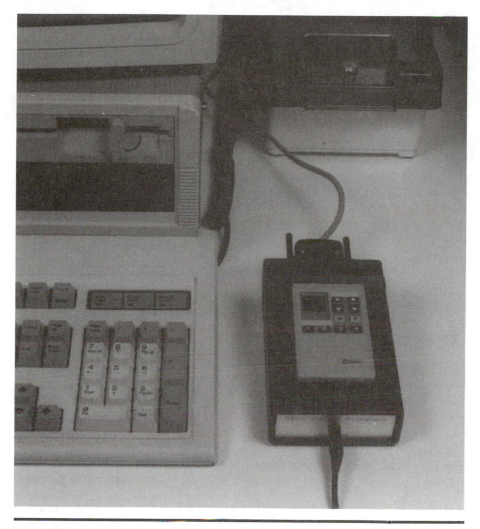

FIGURE 3.23.   PC interface. A simple, inexpensive interface box will connect the remote control to any personal computer. The remote control is simply plugged into the interface box.

cations of these are also described in the Quattro Serial Protocol.

For the hearing aid specialist, a specially developed ready computer program, WQ, is available for the IBM Personal Computers and compatibles (*Widex Quattro Programming Manual*, 1991). This program enables remote operation of the remote control and easy calculation and download of the parameters for the four programs based on a well-proven fitting rule that is specially developed for the Quattro system. Furthermore, all data (personal, audiometric, parameters, etc.) can be stored to disk for later retrieval and/or printed out for archive/documentation purposes. The serial communication is very easy to program and can be useful, for example, for research experiments using the Quattro system.

FITTING STRATEGIES

In contrast to conventional hearing instruments, where a single response must be optimized as a compromise for all listening situations, the Quattro system now allows a number of very different fitting strategies. The common feature of these strategies is that compromises are no longer necessary. For each of the user's four most important listening environment types, a dedicated program can be optimized for performance and acceptance.

The ultimate procedure would have the hearing aid specialist follow the patient into his or her actual daily environments and optimize each of the four programs in situ. This being an unrealistic task, one or more procedures that simulate the in situ procedure are necessary The most obvious solution would be to use tape or compact disc recordings of numerous environmental sounds, select and play the most suitable examples in the offices of the hearing aid specialist, and adjust the four programs to the satisfaction of the patient.

Another procedure is based on experience from the types of settings that, on average, would yield the best result given a specific audiogram and a certain set of environment groups. Normally, program 1 is first fitted for quiet situations (this being convenient as this is the environment the patient is in during the fitting procedure). Next, the remaining three programs are constructed based on program 1 and a table of corrections. For each of the seven different environmental groups, a set of predefined corrections can be added to the setting of program 1, thus obtaining a new setting that in turn can be stored in one of the remaining programs. This procedure and variations thereof are described in detail in the Quattro Manual. Table 3.1 lists the environmental corrections.

Finally, a procedure calculating the settings directly from the audiometric data and the correction table is based on a new general fitting rule (in press). This rule is implemented in the previously mentioned WQ computer program.

QUATTRO-RELATED RESEARCH

Goldstein and colleagues (1991) conducted a study to determine if one recommended prescriptive fitting strategy was superior to another when hearing-impaired subjects listened to male and female talkers in changing acoustic backgrounds. The authors reasoned

Table 3.1. Corrections necessary to calculate the three remaining programs, based on program 1 having been programmed for the quiet situation. Further details can be found in the Quattro Manual.

Environment	Parameter				
	IPA	LCut	HCut	Max. Outp	Comp
1. Quiet	same	same	same	same	same
2. Music	Δ1 step	same	Δ1 step	same	same
3. Party	same	∇2 steps	Δ1 step	∇1 step	same
4. Traffic	∇1 step	16	16	∇2 steps	On
5. Industry	same	9	11	∇3 steps	On
6. Office	same	5	Δ1 step	same	On
7. High freq.	same	same	11	∇2 steps	On

that if one fitting protocol was indeed superior to another in determining the best electroacoustic response, then all subjects would select it as preferable to all others. That is, they would select that specific fitting strategy regardless of the environment in which listening takes place. Four currently used prescriptive formulas were evaluated in this study. They were (1) Libby ⅓–⅔ method, (2) National Acoustic Laboratory-Revised (NAL-R) method, (3) Memphis State University method, and (4) Berger method.

Ten hearing-impaired subjects were used in the study. The Quattro Q8 was selected because of its ability to provide four separate programs, immediately accessible to the user. For each subject, the target gains for each of the selected formulas were placed in one of the four programs. In this manner, each of the fitting methods could be compared by having the subject simply press the appropriate response key and have immediate access to any of the four prescriptive responses stored in the Quattro system. Each subject listened to a male and female talker under different conditions of background noise and selected that response (fitting formula) which was best. The conditions for listening were quiet, multitalker babble, cafeteria noise, and environmental backgrounds.

An analysis of the subjects' ratings indicated quite clearly that no one prescriptive fitting yielded the electroacoustic response appropriate for all listening environments. That is, different prescriptive fittings were judged to be best under specific listening conditions. Subject ratings were influenced, also, by a male or female talker. The Goldstein study provided clear evidence that no one fitting formula response was the unanimous choice of any subject for all listening conditions. This study demonstrated clearly that multiprogrammable hearing aid systems may be of significant value to those hearing-impaired persons who must listen under

changing environmental background conditions on a fairly frequent basis.

Kuk (1990) reports on the hearing aid amplification needs of two hearing-impaired groups. Nine subjects in group A had threshold sensitivity at 250 Hz and 500 Hz at 40 dB HL or less. In group B, eight subjects had a threshold at 250 Hz and 500 Hz greater than 40 dB HL. The primary intent of this study was to determine the preferred insertion gain of hearing aids in listening and reading-aloud situations. All subjects were fitted binaurally with Quattro Q8 multiprogrammable hearing aids. They listened to a continuous discourse spoken by a male talker, as well as listening to their own voices as they read aloud the same passage. Insertion gain was determined for each of the listening and reading-aloud conditions. Word recognition and subjective impressions were elicited for all subjects. As would be expected, the required insertion gain for the listening task was greater than that for the read-aloud condition for both groups. Different insertion gains led to different objective and subjective performances.

Kuk concluded: "Assuming the primary purpose of a hearing aid is for amplifying the speech of others, these findings suggest that one should not adjust the gain of a hearing aid using one's own voice as the reference. In addition, one should be careful in soliciting subjective comments from hearing-impaired patients during hearing-aid fittings to avoid underamplifying those individuals in the low frequencies. Multimemory hearing aids may be necessary for some hearing-impaired patients to use their hearing aids satisfactorily in listening and speaking conditions."

One of the critical issues in any innovation relative to hearing aid technology is that of determining whether or not hearing-impaired persons benefit. That is, in a field-trial format, how does the new technology compare with existing technology? Endo et al.

(1991) conducted a study in which 17 bilaterally hearing-impaired subjects were involved in a field-trial evaluation. The four programs of the Q8 were set for four different listening environments determined by the subject assessment. All subjects were experienced binaural hearing aid users, and all were fitted binaurally with multiprogrammable hearing aid devices.

Following an audiological evaluation, subjects were fitted with the programmable hearing aids and given appropriate instructions relative to the manner in which their own hearing aids and the Quattro system were to be compared during normal, daily activities at home and at work. On day one of the study, all subjects utilized their own hearing aids, and on the next day they used the programmable aid. This alternating schedule was followed over a two-week evaluation period. At the conclusion of the evaluation period, each subject rated subjective differences between the two systems. Ratings included (1) listening in quiet environments, (2) listening while others were talking, (3) listening in noise, (4) sound quality, and (5) ease of manipulation.

Most subjects rated the Quattro as yielding superior performance over their own hearing aid devices for ease of manipulation, sound quality, understanding in noise, and overall performance. When listening in quiet environments, there was no statistical difference between the subject's own aids and the programmable system. In general, when speech discrimination function was measured in the presence of background noise, the Quattro yielded superior scores, compared to the individual's own hearing aids assessed under the same conditions.

Sandlin and Meltsner (1989) reported on four selected case studies of hearing-impaired individuals for whom the Quattro Q8 provided response characteristics not available in more conventional hearing aid systems. One of the cases described the value of multi-

programmability for a judge who had difficulty discriminating female voices in the courtroom, as well as other voices at a distance from the bench. One of the Quattro programs was dedicated to improved audibility of the female voice, the other to provide greater audibility for distant voices. The remaining two programs were set to yield different response characteristics to meet specific needs.

In another case study, the value of multi-programmable aids for a physically impaired, arthritic patient was discussed. The patient found the remote control easier to manipulate than her conventional behind-the-ear hearing aid device. Further, in that the patient lived a very sedentary life, only two of the four available programs were utilized to meet her acoustic needs.

In yet another case, the Quattro proved to be of value for a patient who desired improved performance in environments of quiet listening, theater, music, and normal competing noise background. In that his previous experiences with binaurally applied postauricular hearing instruments had proven less than satisfactory in all environments, significant gains were realized through multiprogrammable hearing aids.

Finally, multiprogrammable hearing aids were of benefit to a 58-year-old attorney needing a number of different electroacoustic responses to function best in courtroom and social environments. In that luncheon meetings were rather frequent occurrences, one program of the Quattro was designated for that specific environment. Other programs were set according to need.

In an unpublished paper, Born (1990) reports on the results of an analysis of 63 questionnaires completed by experienced Quattro users. All respondents to the questionnaire received their hearing aids between April 1989 and April 1990. Hearing loss ranged from mild to severe. No effort was made to control for age, sex, or socioeconomic levels. Of those completing the questionnaire, 73% were fitted binaurally, and 61% had used hearing aids prior to being fitted with the Quattro (33% had used behind-the-ear devices and 22% had used in-the-ear hearing aids). The instruments were individually programmed for speech in quiet backgrounds, speech in noise backgrounds, and selected work-related and traffic noise environments, and one program was used for listening to music.

The conclusions of this study suggested the following: The majority of patients used their hearing aids during waking hours. Patients changed from one program to another from three to five times a day. Eighty-five percent reported that the remote control unit, which is part of the Quattro hearing system, was easy or very easy to operate. All patients reported that they changed programs more often than they adjusted the volume of the hearing aid. Eighty-nine percent of those reporting stated that having four listening programs meant better listening comfort and, in many environments, better speech discrimination function. Finally, 92% of all respondents reported that they would not consider returning to the use of hearing instruments that provided only a single program.

Sweetow and Mueller (1991a, b) investigated the utility of programmable hearing aid devices in meeting target gain of the NAL-R fitting formula. Using four hearing-impaired subjects, three clinical questions were addressed. They were: (1) Is the range of responses for specific electroacoustic parameters altered in the real ear as a function of various earmold coupling systems? (2) Do programmable systems facilitate achieving target gains for a variety of audiometric configurations? and (3) How can the dispenser incorporate the increased flexibility of user control, inherent in certain programmable hearing aids, to the fitting strategy?

Clear evidence was presented that closed-mold and various vent configurations greatly affect the magnitude of response changes provided by the programmable system. With a closed mold, greater response changes can be generated than with open or vented molds. Equally compelling evidence was presented suggesting that a programmable system (Quattro Q8) could reliably achieve recommended target gain better than, or at least equal to, single-response, conventional hearing instruments. Question 3 was answered in the affirmative by suggesting that controlling the various acoustic parameters can be most advantageous to the desired acoustic performance as a function of the listening environment. The authors cautioned, however, that confirmation of the acoustic modifications be confirmed by real-ear assessment.

Sweetow and Mueller maintain: "Programmable hearing aids therefore have provided the dispenser and the user with the ability to rapidly adjust the hearing aid to compensate in an individually determined manner for different acoustic environments." Assuming that target gains can pertain to more than a single hearing aid response, a multiprogrammable instrument can provide several target gain criteria as a function of the listening environment.

The reader should keep in mind that the utility of digitally controlled, multiprogrammable hearing aids are just emerging as instruments of choice in meeting the electroacoustic needs of hearing-impaired persons. Extant evidence supports the application of these systems in reducing difficulties experienced when listening conditions change. There is no general consensus suggesting what parameters of acoustic performance should be programmable, nor is there consensus of how the acoustic input into the hearing aid device should be processed prior to its output at the receiver stage. However, there are clear and positive indications of the value of multiprogrammable instruments. The Widex Quattro system is representative of that perceived value.

QUATTRO, DIGITAL TECHNOLOGY, AND THE FUTURE

The present line of Quattro multiprogrammable hearing aids should not be considered as just another line of hearing instruments. The Quattro instruments form a completely new concept based on the philosophy that the hearing-impaired person needs several hearing responses in order to obtain an optimal adaptation to different listening situations.

The present system involves both analog and digital technology. Without digital technology, it could simply not have been realized. Without the analog technology, the system would have been extremely costly and much too power consuming. When digital technology drops farther in power consumption and cost, we will see new hearing systems based on the Quattro idea and using true digital technology throughout. The future may bring variations to the Quattro principle—fewer or more responses programmed into the remote control, different filter designs and functions, and so on—but the principle is fully exploited by the present system.

REFERENCES

Berger, K., Hagberg, E.N., and Rane, R.L. (1977). *Prescription of Hearing Aids*. Kent, OH: Herald Publishing Co.

Born, S. (1990). Are four listening programs better. Presented at the International AKUSTIKA Congress, Montreux, Switzerland.

Byrne, D., and Dillon, H. (1986). New procedure for selection gain and frequency response of a hearing aid. The National Acoustic Laboratories (NAL). *Ear and Hearing* 7(4):257–265.

Byrne, D., and Tonisson, W. (1976). Selecting the gain of hearing aids for persons with sensorineural hearing impairments. *Scandinavian Audiology* 5:51–59.

Endo, J., Lake, T.M., McFarland, W.H., and Sandlin, R.E. (1991). Self-assessment of a programmable BTE hearing instrument system. *Hearing Instruments* 42(4):9–10, 44.

Goldstein, D.P., Shields, A.R., and Sandlin, R.E. (1991). A multiple memory, digitally-controlled hearing instrument. *Hearing Instruments* 42(1):18–21.

Intel 8051 Manual. Intel Corporation.

Intel Microcontroller Handbook (1986). Intel Corporation.

Internal Memorandum (1982). 14th Nordic Hearing Aid Technical Meeting.

Kuk, F.K. (1990). Preferred insertion gain of hearing aids in listening and reading-aloud situations. *Journal of Speech and Hearing Research* 33(3):520–529.

Libby, E.R. (1985). State-of-the-art of hearing aid selection procedures. *Hearing Instruments* 36(1): 30–38, 62.

Libby, E.R. (1986). The shift toward real ear measurements. *Hearing Instruments* 37(1):6–7, 50.

Lybarger, S.F. (1963). Simplified fitting system for hearing aids. In: *Radioear Specifications and Fitting Information Manual* (pp. 1–8).

McCandless, G.A., and Lyregaard, P.E. (1983). Prescription of gain/output (POGO) for hearing aids. *Hearing Instruments* 34(1):16–21.

MSM80C31/MSM80C51 User Manual (1985) OKI Elektric Industri Co., Ltd.

OKI 80C51 Manual. OKI Elektric Industri Co., Ltd.

Philips User Manual (1986): Single-Chip 8-Bit-Microcontrollers. Philips Electronic Components and Materials Division.

Sandlin, R.E., and Meltsner, R. (1989). Clinical trials with a remote control, programmable hearing instrument. *Hearing Instruments* 40(10): 34–39.

Sweetow, R.W., and Mueller, H.G. (1991a). The interfacing of programmable hearing aids and probe microphone measures, part I. *Audecibel*, Spring: 11–12.

Sweetow, R.W., and Mueller, H.G. (1991b). Interfacing of programmable hearing aids and probe microphone measures, part II. *Audecibel*, Summer: 19–22.

Quattro Serial Protocol (1989). Widex ApS.

Widex Quattro Manual (1989). Widex ApS.

Widex Quattro Programming Manual (1991). Widex ApS.

CHAPTER 4

PMC™ AND TRITON™: AN EXPANDING, COMPREHENSIVE PROGRAMMABLE PRODUCT LINE

Pamela L. Burton

Although digitally programmable technology has progressed remarkably in recent years, hearing instrument professionals are searching for more efficient and cost-effective systems. At this time, there are numerous digitally programmable hearing instruments available to the hearing-impaired public, and this number is constantly increasing. It is expected that many more hybrid digital, or digitally controlled analog, instruments will be introduced.

It is interesting to note that all of the current instruments on the market fall into the digitally controlled analog (DCA) or digitally programmable category (with the exception of the Nicolet Phoenix.) This refers to the fact that they are not true digital hearing aids—that is, they have no analog–digital conversion (and vice versa), nor do they have any true digital signal processing. In our current definition, the hearing instrument signal follows an analog path. However, they are digitally programmable by some external means, and the instruments contain digital memory. Some are programmable via a hard-wire connection to a stationary or portable programmer, while other instruments are programmed via remote control by a small transmitter that is hand held. In some cases, the remote control is given to the consumers so that they may make modifications based on environmental changes. In these cases, initially the remote control is utilized by the dispenser to designate the initial acoustic parameters of the instrument.

Due to the difficulties in miniaturizing the components, the lack of satisfactory power supply, and some other factors, approximately 30% of the instruments are represented in custom product applications at this time. As the technology progresses, it is expected that this percentage will increase significantly. As a matter of fact, at least two products are now available in canal configurations.

The practical applications of each aid are unique. Each manufacturer has focused on one or two segments of the hearing health care market, concentrating either on the degree or type of hearing loss or on the utilization of the programming system(s). There are instruments that are alleged to be more appropriate for patients with primarily high-frequency hearing loss, and others with specific applications for narrow dynamic ranges and/or tolerance difficulties, as well as a host of other applications.

Unless otherwise noted, figures and photographs in this chapter are reprinted with permission of Siemens Hearing Instruments, Inc., 10 Constitution Avenue, Piscataway, NJ.
™Trademarks of Siemens Hearing Instruments, Inc.

THE PMC PROGRAMMING SYSTEM

The Concept of Standardized Programming

Since there is a patent lack of standardization, it appears that a substantial portion of programmer development has progressed with considerable limitations. The most conspicuous of these limitations is the absence of flexibility most programming systems can offer (Branderbit, 1991).

A typical dispensing professional is bombarded with information about many of the available programming systems and their corresponding hearing instruments. This tends to create some justifiable confusion on the part of the dispenser in regard to which system, or combination of systems, will prove to be the most practical for his or her particular setting.

In a perfect world, it might be optimal to have three, four, or even more programming systems to assure that there will be an appropriate programmable hearing instrument available for every hearing-impaired patient who is referred to the facility. Even if this were feasible, however, most dispensing offices have neither the financing nor the space for multiple programming systems and accessories. At this time, the costs for obtaining a programmer and the accompanying paraphernalia range from slightly less than $500 to upwards of $14,500. The costs typically reflect the extraneous functions that are performed by the system, in addition to standard programming of the hearing instrument parameters. These might include the ability to perform probe tube microphone measurements and personal computer software to store individual patient parameters and maintain a data base, among other features. If the dispensing office is already furnished with any of this equipment, the programming system may create a redundancy. If the office is not currently utilizing such equip-

ment, there is the risk that the system that is obtained will not allow the generalization of certain functions to other programmable, and even nonprogrammable, hearing instruments, thus rendering it limited in its usefulness.

For example, several programming systems involve the use of probe tube microphone measurements. However, the probe tube system may not be suitable to validate results with hearing instruments from other manufacturers. For many professionals who have chosen to be multiline dispensers, this may necessitate the purchase of another probe tube system that can be used with all other hearing instruments. On the other hand, if real-ear measurement is not part of a dispenser's repertoire of procedures, a programming system like the one described above may not be convenient or appropriate.

Financial considerations often play a dominant role in the selection. Due to the sometimes exorbitant costs of this instrumentation, it can be difficult, especially for large clinics and hospitals operating under strict administrative control, to obtain the approval for the necessary equipment. In addition, if approval is obtained for the purchase of a particular system, this limits the dispenser to one manufacturer's programmable product line. As flexible as some of these hearing instruments may be, they cannot be expected to meet the needs of the majority of cases seen in a facility. On any given day, the hearing health care professional will evaluate patients who present very different audiologic profiles and listening requirements. Based on their current communication skills and resulting amplification necessities, flexibility is essential in determining which of the many instruments available will provide significant benefit to the consumer. A solution that permits the greatest number of options will presumably allow the most flexibility for the dispenser.

It has been noted that programmers, and programming systems, do not constitute a business for either the manufacturer or the hearing health care professional (Branderbit, 1991). The ultimate benefit in programmability of any kind lies in the hearing instrument and its capabilities. The consumer of hearing health care products should not have to be interested or concerned with the number and kind of programmers housed in his or her dispenser's office. Although many consumers of hearing health care products are impressed with new technology and "bells and whistles," it would be ludicrous to suggest that a dispenser with the three most expensive programming systems has a greater ability to satisfy his patients than the dispenser who deals with one or two of the less-expensive manufacturers.

Therefore, the bulk of research and development should be directed at better, more sophisticated processing circuitry in the hearing instrument, rather than elaborate (and expensive) hardware systems. Certainly, the consumer can be expected to agree with this philosophy. Of course, there are always those patients who would be initially impressed with equipment that appeared to be very complex and elaborate. However, the shortcomings of the hearing instrument, when discovered, would surely overcome these positive feelings.

Perceived versus expected benefits play a major role in the acceptance or rejection of a hearing instrument, programmable or otherwise. Patients have very definite images of what, and how much, they feel a particular hearing instrument may provide and which aids might be more beneficial for their hearing problem. This idea is supported by a study carried out at Letterman Army Medical Center by Mueller (1991). The study allowed patients to rate the potential benefits for their hearing loss for programmable and nonprogrammable hearing instruments. The study indicates that the consumer, when presented with a visual collection of programmable and nonprogrammable in-the-ear and behind-the-ear hearing aids, will rate the programmable in-the-ear aid as the most technologically advanced instrument. Consumers also feel that the programmable in-the-ear aid will provide the most benefit for their hearing loss, regardless of the type or degree of hearing loss they exhibit. The nonprogrammable behind-the-ear instrument was consistently rated as the least progressive, least beneficial, and least appropriate aid.

Does programmability truly provide the dispenser the ability to supply superior quality fittings for the hearing-impaired individual? The answer to that question is likely to be found in the hearing instrument's capabilities and flexibility, rather than the programmer or programming system.

The PMC Philosophy

The Programmable Multichannel (PMC™) system was conceived as a standardized approach to programmable technology. It allows for the adjustment of digitally programmable hearing instruments from as many as 32 different manufacturers with a single programming unit. The unit is shown in Figure 4.1.

Originally developed by Siemens Audiological Engineering in Erlangen, West Germany, the PMC has been accepted by many manufacturers, among them, Siemens, Rexton, Philips, Phonak, Qualitone, Danavox, Argosy, 3M, and Hansaton. Each manufacturer has already introduced or can develop programmable instruments to be used with the PMC system. Discussions are continuing with other manufacturers to optimize the PMC concept by including as many companies as possible. This, of course, allows the dispenser to have the most flexibility with one piece of equipment at greater cost savings. In other words, the cost of the PMC is

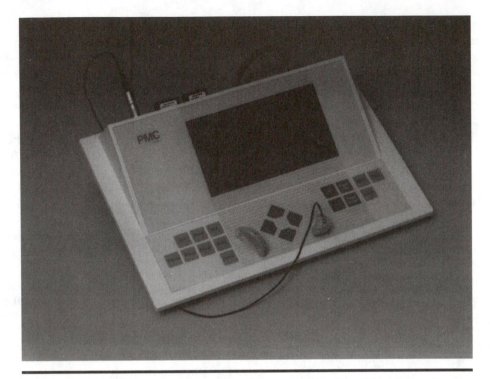

FIGURE 4.1. The PMC programmer with standardized keyboard functions, allowing programming of many different manufacturer's hearing instruments.

amortized very quickly over the purchase of hearing instruments. In addition, many of the manufacturers have developed arrangements that permit the dispenser to acquire the PMC equipment through the purchase of programmable hearing instruments without any initial outlay of cash.

Since the PMC allows programming of many different instruments, the system answers the dispenser's need for a single, standardized fitting approach with minimal investment. The microprocessor-supported programmer makes it possible to program all system-compatible single- and multichannel instruments. In addition, a PC software version with interface is being developed by Siemens to perform the same functions as the PMC programmer.

Software Requirements

The programming unit uses interchangeable software modules to program the hearing instruments. Each module contains programming instructions for a single manufacturer, regardless of the number of programmable instruments offered by that manufacturer. For any future developments, only updated software modules are required, rather than entirely new hardware systems. Up to five separate manufacturer-specific modules can be simultaneously inserted into the PMC and catalogued by the system's master module. The PMC system is capable of updating software to accommodate as many as 32 different hearing instrument manufacturers' software. The ability to expand the functions of the

PMC and the individual instruments is easy and inexpensive via these module replacements, as opposed to potential hardware changes and updates that may be necessary with other systems. The system module and company-specific modules are identical and very simple to insert and remove from the PMC.

Display Characteristics

All fitting parameters are displayed on a 16-line LCD display window. The fitting process is made simpler by the graphic illustration and textual explanation of performance specifications shown on the same screen. The contrast may be adjusted by a control, which is located on the back of the PMC unit.

Depending upon the manufacturer, the parameters that can be programmed may be exhibited in various ways. For example, it is possible to display a parameter or set of parameter values using a graphic representation, such as an ANSI or KEMAR frequency response curve. It would be possible to see the same information represented numerically on the same screen, next to the graph. The manufacturers may also program their software so that this same information is separated onto two or more pages. Another example of diversity in display types occurs with AGC-I threshold settings. The dispenser may display a bar graph depicting the threshold settings, as well as the actual threshold in numeric form.

In the setup phase of the PMC, the dispenser may choose from several configurations for the graphic display. Selecting the KEMAR display will provide graphics that would be most similar to the probe tube microphone measurements obtained for the patient. In preliminary evaluation of the PMC, several dispensers found that the difference in gain between the probe tube results and the PMC graphic display was less than 2–3 dB. If the dispenser is not utilizing real-ear measurement as a validation procedure, the ANSI 2cc coupler display may be chosen. Other choices that exist include language selection (English, German, French, or Spanish) and configuration for the RS232C interfaces (9 pin and 15 pin).

Audiogram Data Entry

In researching methods of validation for hearing instrument fittings, it becomes apparent that professionals dispensing hearing instruments are not a homogeneous group and are prone to use a variety of methods to determine the success, or failure, of a fitting. The use of probe tube microphone measurements has become more and more popular over the last five to ten years, as have numerous prescriptive fitting methods (Preves, 1987; Libby, 1987; Mahon, 1986). In order to cater to the various types of validation procedures available, it was necessary to design into the system a variety of choices for programming the hearing instrument of the dispenser's choice. The use of a standardized programming system such as the PMC does not necessitate the use of ancillary equipment, nor does it preclude the use of potentially useful instrumentation.

The dispenser has a choice of several different prescriptive fitting formulas to assist in programming the hearing instruments compatible with the PMC. Prescriptive fittings, in addition to enjoying long-standing popularity, have proven to be valuable tools for clinicians involved in dispensing hearing instruments (Braida et al., 1979; McCandless and Lyregaard, 1983). The PMC software update allows the dispenser to enter the parameters of the patient's audiogram (air, bone, UCL) at discrete frequencies between 125 Hz and 8000 Hz (Figure 4.2) and choose one of

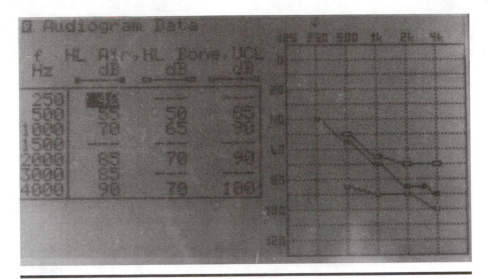

FIGURE 4.2.   Audiogram data entry screen for the PMC.

the following fitting rules: Berger, Pogo II, ½ gain, ⅓ gain, NAL, or Special Method (Figure 4.3). After entering key data and selecting one of the fitting rules listed above, the PMC software, in conjunction with the company-specific software, will program the hearing instrument to the specifications of the chosen formula.

It is possible, by touching a multifunction (MF) button, to view the written formula of any formula programmed into the PMC; however, the Special Method formula can be re-

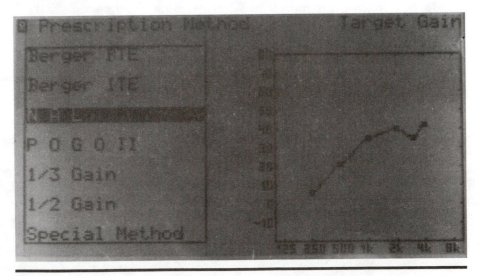

FIGURE 4.3.   A choice of 7 fitting rationales allowed by PMC.

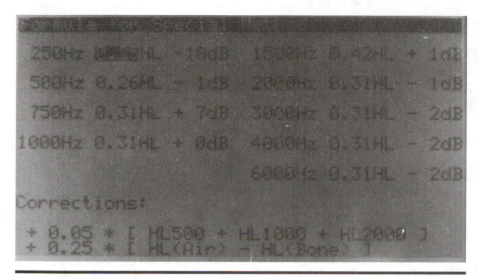

FIGURE 4.4. Special Method. Hearing instrument professionals may program their own prescriptive formulas onto this screen.

programmed by the dispenser to reflect his or her own fitting biases and philosophies. Therefore, Special Method becomes the individual dispenser's own fitting rationale, or prescriptive formula (Figure 4.4).

PMC Memories

Although it has been demonstrated to be successful in many applications, a large number of dispensers do not subscribe to the concept of prescriptive fittings. For this purpose, there are three different memory banks associated with the PMC system. These memory banks are present consistently, regardless of the individual manufacturer's company-specific module. The first bank allows the control settings to be preselected, using nine basic preset options. These nine preset parameter sets are referred to as the *A memory*, and are labeled "A1" through "A9." The A memory is permanent and cannot be reprogrammed by the dispenser.

The hearing instrument dispenser can also preset up to nine of his own control settings,

according to individual fitting preferences. These nine parameter sets are referred to as the *B memory*, and are labeled "B1" through "B9." The B memory is semipermanent. In other words, the parameter selections will remain intact until the dispenser chooses to reprogram different parameter sets for any or all of the nine locations.

The PMC system offers immediate comparison of different parameter values by allowing up to 15 temporary settings, or memories, to be used during the fitting. These memory locations are referred to as the *C memory* and are labeled "C1" through "C15." The C memory is a volatile memory. As soon as the power source is eliminated (e.g., the power is turned off), the information stored in these memory locations is erased. When power is restored to the PMC, the memory locations can be programmed for a new client. There are 15 locations for each side—right and left. In this way, the dispenser can offer each individual patient a number of different control settings and then store the optimum setting in the hearing instrument permanently or until additional change is necessary for any reason. In utilizing the C memory locations during the fitting, it is also possible for the dispenser or patient to assign a rating to each of the programmed settings. The rating is assigned using the + and – keys on the PMC. The ratings that may be given are as follows: ++, +, no rating, –, and – –. These ratings may be assigned on the basis of objective (speech discrimination scores in noise, probe tube microphone measurements, etc.) or subjective results and can be used for comparison later in the fitting.

PMC Standardized Functions

The rear of the PMC programmer is pictured in Figure 4.5. Two connector cable interfaces are shown for connection of the PMC. (It may

be necessary to obtain different connector cables for custom products and BTE instruments from the same manufacturer due to size restraints.) During the entire fitting process, one or both instruments are worn by the user so that he or she can be aware of all changes in the response characteristics. The programmer will have the ability, through two RS232C interfaces (one 9 pin and one 15 pin), to connect to a personal computer and/or printer.

The programmer's key functions are uniform, regardless of the hearing instrument that is being programmed. The configuration of the function keys and their designations allow easy-to-understand and systematic operation of the programming unit. Logically related functions are automatically called up and executed at the touch of a key. For example, touching the READ function key will

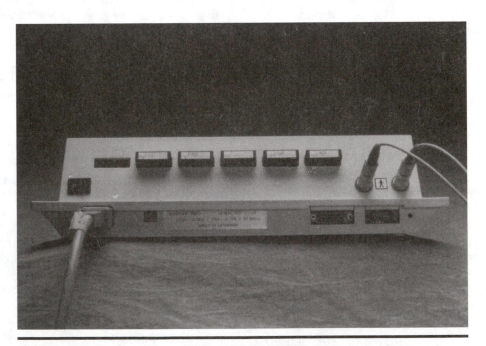

FIGURE 4.5. Rear view of the PMC: PMC systems master module, programming cables, power-on button, and RS232C interfaces.

automatically display all parameter values from any hearing instrument that is connected to the programmer. Other function keys are used to modify parameters such as gain and AGC-I, as well as any other parameters that have been rendered programmable by the manufacturer, to store complete sets of control settings and to recall the settings for quick comparison. Due to this organization of key functions, learning only one method of programming is required for a large number of hearing instruments.

STATE OF THE ART IN COMPRESSION TECHNOLOGY

Purposes of Compression

Compression technology has long been utilized in other applications for the objective of reducing the dynamic range of a signal to fit into a less-than-perfect signal channel. For the telephone, compression is utilized to keep the volume of the speech signal, which is weaker, above the unavoidable circuit noise that is encountered. In analog audio recordings, the technique of Dolby Noise Reduction, a form of compression, is employed to keep the band of weak signals above the magnetic tape noise. With Dolby, during the playback of recordings, the signal is expanded to reestablish the original dynamic range. Radio stations also use compression limiting to automatically prevent overload of their transmitters, which allows for an increase in the average output signal level.

Compression applications for hearing instruments are generally associated with two areas: protection and noise filtering. For the protection of overamplification of intense sounds for patients with tolerance problems, it is imperative that compression limiting be incorporated into the hearing instrument. Several studies have indicated the impor-

tance that hearing aid users place on this particular parameter. Franks and Beckmann (1985) studied groups of geriatric hearing aid users. Of the group that eventually rejected their hearing aids, 88% indicated that the aid "makes sounds too loud." Even in considering the group that kept their hearing aids, 32% also indicated that "sounds are too loud." The problem of tolerance and restricted dynamic range will be explored later in this chapter.

For the purpose of noise filtering, compression technology has also been employed in many different forms. Signal processing, or automatic noise reduction, can appear in the form of compression-limiting circuitry. It is widely accepted that a foremost goal in the majority of hearing aid fittings is to improve speech intelligibility when background noise is present. In fact, many hearing-impaired persons seek help only because of difficulty in troublesome listening situations.

Conventional ASP circuitry reduces background noise by automatically attenuating most low-frequency amplification whenever background noise is present somewhere in the frequency range. Conventional AGC-I circuitry does not reduce gain dependent upon frequency; rather, it reduces gain across the entire frequency range of the hearing instrument.

In a study by Schum (1990), different types of noise reduction were evaluated. The results indicated that noise reduction technology improved performance for most elderly hearing aid candidates when compared with simple, broadband, linear amplification. More importantly, however, this study demonstrated that different hearing losses required different types of processing techniques. Some of the subjects performed more favorably with traditional ASP circuitry, and some with more high-frequency reduction. This research also suggested that the incorporation of more than one noise-reduction technique might lead to even more improvement of speech discrimination.

Compression: Frequency-Dependent Limiting

Since the dynamic range for the hearing impaired listener usually varies by frequency, it may be assumed that the presence of intense, low-frequency sounds should not be allowed to control compression action for middle and/or high frequencies and vice versa. Perhaps what is necessary is multichannel compression, which would allow the different segments of the frequency range to be addressed individually. Of course, the tendency is to assume that increased compression in the low-frequency range is desirable for reduction of background sounds. Stein and Dempsey-Hart (1984) obtained speech recognition scores from hearing-impaired subjects for word lists presented in various noise environments. The hearing aids contained an adaptive filter that could be switched out of the hearing aid circuit when desired. In both studies, the largest improvement in speech recognition scores from filter-off to filter-on conditions occurred in a narrowband (600-800 Hz) low-frequency noise, while the least improvement occurred with either white noise or in babble (Wolinsky, 1986). In the narrowband noise, adaptive filtering would produce attenuation in a restricted area of low frequencies, presumably leaving high-frequency speech information intact. With the broadband babble and white noise, the filters apparently attenuated both speech and noise across a wide range of frequencies. The authors concluded that optimal results with noise reduction are obtained when the noise is restricted in frequency content and when it does not interfere with regions where important speech information is located (specifically, high frequencies).

The effects of spectral shaping on speech recognition were also researched for hearing-impaired listeners with either flat or steeply sloping audiometric configurations (Kamm and Dirks, 1982). One of the responses selected was shaped relative to each subject's loudness discomfort curve. This response incorporated a high-pass filter but also provided an amplification increase for frequencies above 1000 Hz. By doing so, the speech spectrum paralleled the curve for the subject's loudness discomfort levels for ⅓ octave bands of noise. This response allowed maximum amplification levels in the regions where hearing loss was greatest and was similar to the "optimal response" described by other researchers (Pascoe, 1975; Skinner, 1976; Barfod, 1972; Lippman, Braida, and Durlach, 1981).

Research on a digitally controlled adaptive filter (Van Tasell, Larsen, and Fabry, 1988) measured aided speech recognition thresholds in noise, with and without a filter. The performance of the subjects also demonstrated that effects of the filters were related both to the frequency spectrum of the noise and to the distribution of speech information by frequency.

Even when not found to improve significantly the speech recognition or discrimination ability in a conclusive manner, noise reduction is justified simply by user preference. Kuk et al. (1989) demonstrated that, in low to moderate noise levels, noise reduction circuitry was subjectively chosen by the subjects involved in the study. It is important to realize that hearing-impaired individuals are affected by negligible amounts of background noise and that even slight increases in intelligibility or perceived ease of listening are noted and appreciated. From the existence of past and current research, it is apparent that compression limiting has been sought as a means to increase comfort and provide superior speech intelligibility to hearing instrument users.

TRITON

The Need for Multichannel Compression Technology

Researchers have, in the past, experimented with different prototypes of multichannel compression technology (Braida et al., 1981; Yanick, 1976; Yanick and Drucker, 1976).

In order to explore the potential benefits of multichannel compression, Siemens Hearing Instruments, Inc., commenced development of a three-channel compression integrated circuit. After years of product development, the Triton 3000 was introduced to the industry. This is the first three-channel AGC-I instrument in which it is possible to separate and modify the low-, mid-, and high-frequency ranges. Each compression channel can now be accurately and precisely programmed to respond to individual hearing impairment. The Triton 3000 hearing instrument Figure 4.6 was introduced in the fall of 1990 as a PMC-compatible hearing instrument.

The development of a single hearing instrument with three separate channels is a significant breakthrough, made possible by an exclusive, digitally programmable amplifier chip. This IC contains a three-channel AGC amplifier and requires only 1.1 volts of operating power (Hohn, 1990).

The technology features three independent amplifier channels using switched capacitor (SC filter) technology. It contains adjustable crossover frequencies and an independent AGC-I for each channel, with varying attack and recovery times. A cross-section of the hybrid is shown in Figure 4.7. Utilizing the crossover frequencies and independent gain in each channel, the dispenser has an almost unlimited amount of flexibility with regard to frequency response. It is already accepted that programmability alone offers great benefit in the area of frequency response changes that are significant and easy to accomplish. With the Triton, there are liter-

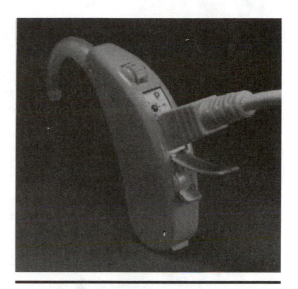

FIGURE 4.6.   Triton 3000, the world's first three-channel compression instrument, introduced by Siemens Hearing Instruments, Inc., in October, 1990.

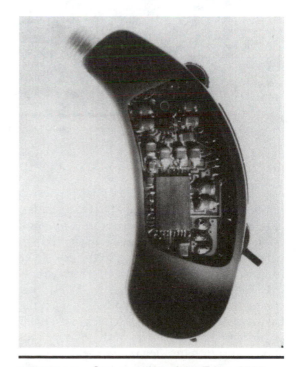

FIGURE 4.7.   Cross-section of the Triton 3000 amplifier, which utilizes SC filter technology.

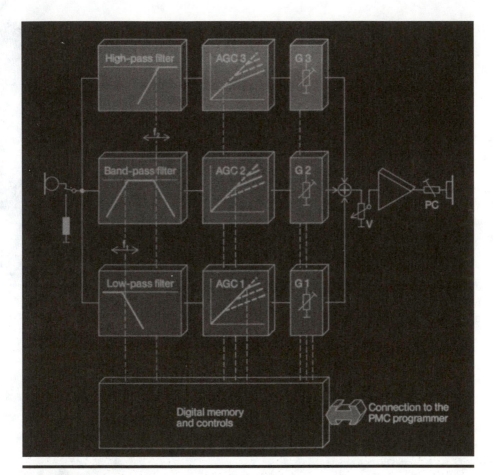

FIGURE 4.8.   Block diagram of the Triton with digital memory.

ally hundreds of thousands of possibilities, as not only can the dispenser adjust the relative gain in three frequency areas, but also the boundaries of those three areas can change constantly with adjustments to the crossover frequencies. For example, each time a crossover frequency is moved, even by 50 Hz, this creates new possibilities for adjustment of the frequency response and gain in each channel.

More precise definition of the required response through multichannel signal processing is an improved solution to the problems of degraded speech discrimination. This defi-

nition also utilizes the dynamic range available in the critical speech frequency ranges to a greater degree. The three independent AGCs optimally reduce background noise to allow selective amplification of specific sound signals and maximize speech discrimination ability.

Processing of the Signal via Three-Channel Compression

Figure 4.8 shows a block diagram of the Triton circuit and its digital memory. The microphone or telephone signal is first divided into low-, mid-, and high-frequency channels within the critical speech range. Using the PMC programmer and the audiological parameters of the hearing loss, two crossover frequencies are selected (F1 and F2) by which the three separate frequency ranges are defined.

The signal then passes through individual gain controls (G1, G2, and G3) and AGC-I controls (AGC-I-1, AGC-I-2, and AGC-I-3), which are also digitally programmed, to be recombined and transmitted by means of the volume control (which is operated by the patient as usual) to the output amplifier. The maximum achievable sound pressure level on the hearing instrument can be limited using the external PC control, although the necessity for this has been infrequent, with appropriate setting of the programmable parameters.

The crossover frequencies, separate AGC thresholds, and the individual gain control settings for each channel can then be transferred to and stored in the hearing instrument's digital memory. The complete spectrum of programmed and stored electroacoustic characteristics can be recalled and altered by the PMC programmer at any time. The parameter memory and the control electronics operate in 1V digital technology. The Triton is especially suitable for moderate to severe, flat to sloping high-frequency hearing loss and is appropriate for a wide range of hearing loss configurations. See Figure 4.9 for examples of response characteristics that may be attained using the Triton.

Since its introduction, the Triton series has been updated with two new models. The Triton 3004 BTE and Triton 3004i ITE contain all of the programmable parameters that had been available with the Triton 3000 BTE, with the addition of a situation button. This button is very important for the hearing-impaired user, as it allows the wearer to maneuver between four different responses programmed into the instrument by the dispenser, based on different listening requirements. Responses may be programmed for such personal requirements as the telephone or listening to music, as well as for a classroom situation, party noise, or work-related noise, as well as numerous other situations (Burton, 1992). Figure 4.10 pictures the Triton 3004i ITE and Triton 3004 BTE, with the situation button located near the top of the ITE instrument and the covered programming connector located at the bottom of the faceplate.

Factors Influencing Determination of Compression Thresholds

The setting of the parameter values is accomplished by first evaluating the audiological information, including the slope of the hearing impairment. Calculation of the Articulation Index (AI), previously regarded as strictly a research tool, can be used to optimize setting of the filters and determine the boundaries of each channel. In recent years, studies have demonstrated the ability of the AI to predict the proportion of the average speech signal that is audible to a particular patient.

The concept of the AI can serve to explain much of the difficulty encountered by hearing-impaired persons in understanding speech. Pavlovic (1991) referred to five different procedures of calculating the AI in his research. Recently, a simple method for calculating the AI has been published (Mueller and Killion, 1990). In addition to outlining the "Count-the-Dot" method of calculating the AI, the authors state that the AI has at least three important potential uses, including the prediction from unaided audiograms of the amount of patient communication handicap for normal-level conversational speech, the prediction of benefit that will be realized from a given hearing instrument, and a comparison of potential benefit between any two hearing aids.

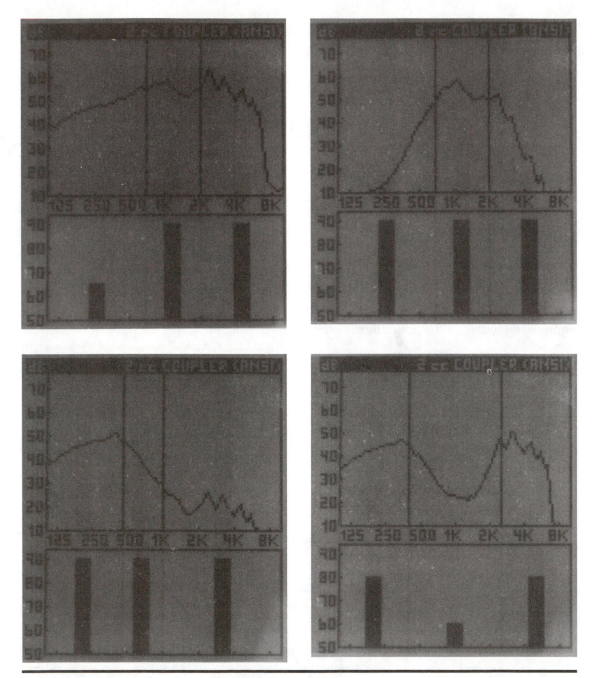

FIGURE 4.9.   Four examples of the thousands of responses that can be attained with the Triton, using the PMC programmer to modify parameters.

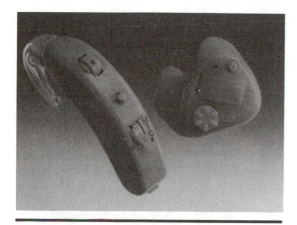

FIGURE 4.10. Triton 3004b BTE and Triton 3004i three-channel ITE, with size 13 battery.

According to Popelka and Mason (1987), it is possible to quantify speech audibility for both unaided and aided conditions with the AI. In the AI, considerably more importance is placed on the 2 kHz range. Unfortunately, it is in this area of the frequency range where most hearing-impaired persons experience poor hearing. With the Triton, it is possible to make individual, precise adjustments in the area where the patient is experiencing the most difficulty. It is very important to allow optimum utilization of any residual dynamic range of the hearing-impaired person. This involves attenuating in some areas and enhancing others.

Conventional hearing instruments are not able to provide the degree of differentiated fitting that is easily achieved with multichannel compression. For example, if an AGC effect is optimized for the high-frequency range, it may no longer be appropriate for the mid- or low-frequency ranges, where most disruptive background noise occurs. The three independent AGC-I circuits make it unnecessary for the patient to operate a switch or other control in the event of sudden onset of background noise. AGC-I-1 (low frequency) and AGC-I-2 (middle frequency) will react automatically in

this situation. If incoming signals in the AGC-I-3 (high frequency) region do not occur with sufficiently high intensity to make the patient uncomfortable, the compression action is confined to the low- and mid-frequency range, where critical information necessary for discrimination is not concentrated.

Differentiation, or the automatic discrimination between useful sounds or signals and disruptive background noise, is obviously very important for the hearing-impaired individual. Those with normal hearing do this naturally and almost subconsciously. Manufacturers are constantly searching for better solutions to provide the optimal signal-to-noise ratio. Current ASP instruments equipped with special filters continue to be somewhat effective in improving speech discrimination, if only subjectively in some cases (Kuk et al., 1989).

With three-channel compression, speech discrimination requirements for each individual hearing loss can be met more precisely. Recent studies have shown improvement in speech discrimination using two-channel compression (Moore, Laurence, and Wright, 1985; Villchur, 1973). Field-test results suggest that the improvement that is possible with three-channel compression is even more significant.

How the Triton Functions

Conventional noise-suppression hearing instruments typically reduce background noise by automatically reducing all low-frequency amplification whenever background noise is present in the frequency range. Conventional AGC-I instruments do not reduce gain dependent upon different frequency ranges; typically the gain is reduced across the entire response. One of the most significant advantages of the Triton is the independent AGC-I functionality of the three channels. In addition, there is a considerable reduction in the effects of background noise—all without affecting the amplification in the higher frequency ranges that are most important for speech discrimination.

The independent high-frequency range AGC ensures that consonants spoken with relatively weak energy remain audible, even as other sounds are filtered out. At higher input levels, the AGC prevents amplification from exceeding the patient's UCL. For compensation of a precipitous high-frequency loss, the unusually steep filter edges (up to 26 dB, in some cases) of the three frequency ranges offer a much better opportunity for a successful fitting.

The Impact of Tolerance Problems

Although most hearing instrument professionals do not assign sufficient importance to the aspect of loudness discomfort levels (LDL) or uncomfortable loudness levels (UCL), we have seen that this parameter is probably the one most closely associated with the acceptance or rejection of amplification (Franks and Beckmann, 1985; Walker et al., 1984). According to Mueller and Hawkins (1990), there are significant negative consequences of exceeding LDLs, the most severe being the outright rejection of amplification. Hawkins (1984) reported several other results that were observed, including reduction of the volume control wheel by the patient (automatically) to a less-than-optimum level for good signal-to-noise ratio, constant manipulation of the volume control wheel, and restricted use of the hearing aid to quiet environments only. It is obvious that in view of the potential consequences, in order to optimally utilize the multichannel compression technology available with the Triton, it is imperative that frequency-specific UCL measures be obtained.

Morgan et al. (1974) performed two investigations to determine a reliable procedure for obtaining UCL measurements and to ob-

serve the effects of frequency on the UCL. Of the methods studied, the most reliable judgments were obtained for a programmed method of constant stimuli. The UCL was measured utilizing this method for pure tones from 125 Hz to 4000 Hz and for narrow and wide bands of noise. The UCL results across frequency compared closely with results from loudness-contour studies. Other programmable instrument manufacturers have also utilized loudness-contour curves in developing programming systems (ReSound, 1989). This finding also suggests that frequency-specific UCL measurement is essential to accurately program the three AGC-I thresholds for the Triton.

When the UCL is the same as or lower than that for normal-hearing individuals, sounds across the frequency spectrum that are amplified without AGC are often perceived as uncomfortably loud. Because high-frequency tones in the majority of hearing losses typically require greater amplification than mid- and low-frequency tones, the high-frequency AGC response must have a shorter attack time. In the three-channel Triton, the AGC response for the mid- and low-frequency channels can be set for a minimum AGC threshold. The available dynamic range can then be utilized to maximum effectiveness. The three AGC channels function independently of each other in all listening situations. The attack and recovery times vary, providing additional improvement. Mueller and Hawkins (1990) state that two of the characteristics of compression that are important are the attack and release times. Since the response of any compression system does not occur instantaneously with the onset of the offending noise, a longer attack time in the low-frequency area is desirable so that the listener does not perceive the compression action when it occurs. The Triton incorporates this philosophy into its specification with an attack time of approximately 60 milliseconds in the AGC-I-1 (low frequency) channel, but the attack times in the AGC-I-2 and AGC-I-3 (middle and high frequency) channels are less than 10 milliseconds. Also according to the above authors, release time should be longer than attack time to eliminate a "flutter," which may be heard by the hearing aid user. This requirement is reflected in the Triton, with a release time of 700 milliseconds in the low-frequency channel and 100 milliseconds in the mid- and high-frequency channels.

To ensure the programming of optimal responses and AGC-I thresholds, it is recommended that the dispenser utilize probe tube microphone measurements to validate parameter settings in the patient's ear. The complexity of multichannel compression indicates the necessity for assurance that the programmed response, which is seen in either 2 cc coupler or KEMAR form on the screen, is providing usable gain and restricting potential tolerance problems across the frequency range. Probe tube microphone measurements provide an ideal means of obtaining objective data on the efficacy of these types of instruments. Most recent research has indicated the effectiveness of real-ear measurement in verifying results with different hearing instrument settings, as well as establishing desired gain values during the initial fitting (Hawkins, 1988; Mueller, 1990).

Initial Field-Test Results

In a preliminary field test, subjects who were currently wearing other compression instruments were chosen and tested with the Triton. Approximately 68% of the users were previously fitted with BTE instruments, and 32% were previously fitted with custom products. It was requested that all participants be asked to purchase the product(s) on a trial basis to eliminate positive bias due to the lack of monetary involvement. One hundred ears were fitted with the Triton at six

locations around the country. The dispensers were requested to provide probe tube microphone measurements for each patient, indicating that desired target gain values were attained. This was accomplished in 92% of the cases. In the 8% that did not meet the original target gain, the patient insisted on changes that were based on the responses in their prior fittings.

Subjective evaluation of the instrument's performance by the patient was weighted heavily in this field test, as there have been instruments that have shown objective improvement in threshold evaluation, yet have been rejected by the patient. Each patient was asked to evaluate his or her current hearing instrument (prior to fitting with the Triton) and, later, the Triton, in eight listening situations. In addition, the patient was requested to provide a rating for overall speech discrimination and overall tonal quality. In evaluating other instruments, tonal quality has been named as a primary issue that requires attention.

The eight listening situations were as follows: quiet room, TV/radio, supermarket/store, car, music, restaurant/party, workplace/conference room, and telephone. The rating scale had the following designations: 1 = poor, 2 = fair, 3 = average, 4 = good, 5 = very good, and 6 = excellent. The results are shown in Figure 4.11. Subjective evaluations by the patients indicated superior performance by the Triton in all eight situations, in addition to overall ratings of speech discrimination ability and tonal quality of the instrument (Figure 4.11).

SUMMARY

Programmable technology has placed demand upon the dispensing community to accept additional responsibility in the fitting process (Staab, 1990). In many cases, in the ini-

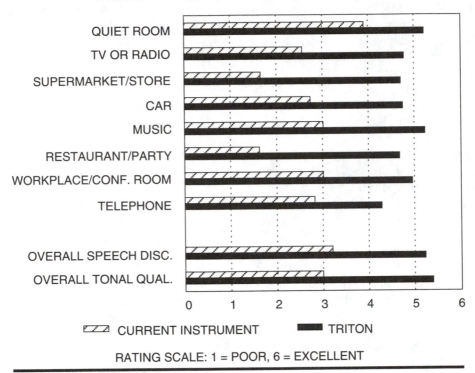

FIGURE 4.11.   Average subjective patient ratings for different listening situations in field-trial evaluation.

tial stages of accepting programmable technology, increased time is required to accomplish these fittings. However, the positive benefits of programmability far outweigh the potential negative aspects.

It is essential for all clinicians to become familiar with the technology in order to improve the service that is currently being provided to the hearing-impaired population. The flexibility offered by programmable hearing instruments allows instant diagnosis and correction of problems during the fitting process and beyond. By having the ability to solve problems in the office, as opposed to sending the instru-

ment to the manufacturer, the dispenser is established as the expert, and the confidence level of the patient increases accordingly.

Difficult or complex losses, which are evaluated every day in various facilities by hearing health care professionals, and the difficulty of significantly improving speech discrimination in real-life situations with amplification are certainly challenges of the future. The Triton circuitry, coupled with the flexible fitting procedures of the PMC programmer, offers dispensers a custom fitting system today that is designed to accommodate them in the future.

REFERENCES

Barfod, J. (1972). Investigations on the optimum corrective frequency response for high-tone hearing loss. Report No. 4. The Acoustic Laboratory, Technical University of Denmark.

Braida, L.D., Durlach, H.I., Lippmann, R.P., Hicks, B.L., Rabinowitz, W.M., and Reed, C.M. (1979). Hearing aids–A review of past research on linear amplification, amplitude compression and frequency lowering. *ASHA Monographs No. 19.* Rockville, MD: American Speech-Language-Hearing Association.

Branderbit, P.L. (1991). A standardized programming system and three-channel compression hearing instrument technology. *Hearing Instruments* 42(1).

Burton, P.L. (1992). Expanding the use of digitally programmable technology. *Hearing Instruments* 43(1).

Franks, J.R., and Beckman, N.J. (1985). Rejection of hearing aids: Attitudes of a geriatric sample. *Ear and Hearing* 6:161–166.

Hawkins, D.B. (1984). Selection of a critical electroacoustic characteristic: SSPL90. *Hearing Instruments* 35:28–32.

Hawkins, D.B. (1988). Some opinions concerning real ear probe tube measurements. *Hearing Instruments* 39:7.

Hohn, W. (1990). Fitting with the three-channel technique–Easy as ABC. Siemens Audiologische Technik GmbH. Promotional literature (SC 04918.0/70258).

Kamm, C.A., and Dirks, D.D. (1982). Some effects of spectral shaping on recognition of speech by hearing-impaired listeners. *Journal of the Acoustical Society of America* 71:1211–1224.

Kuk, F., Tyler, R.S., Stubbing, P., and Bertschy, M. (1989). Noise reduction circuitry in ITE instruments. *Hearing Instruments* 40(7).

Libby, E.R. (1987). Real ear considerations in hearing aid selection. *Hearing Instruments* 38(1):14–16.

Lippmann, R.P., Braida, L.D., and Durlach, N.I. (1981). A study of multichannel amplitude compression and linear amplification for persons with sensorineural hearing loss. *Journal of the Acoustical Society of America* 69:524–534.

Mahon, W.J. (1986). Real ear probe measurements. *Hearing Journal* 39(5):7–11.

McCandless, G., and Lyregaard, P. (1983). Prescription of gain output (POGO) for hearing aids. *Hearing Instruments* 34:16–21.

Moore, B.C.J., Laurence, R.F., and Wright, D. (1985). Improvements in speech intelligibility in quiet and in noise produced by two-channel compression hearing aids. *British Journal of Audiology* 19:175.

Morgan, D.E., Wilson, R.H., and Dirks, D.D. (1974). Loudness discomfort level: Selected methods and stimuli. *Journal of the Acoustical Society of America* 56:577–581.

Mueller, H.G. (1990). Probe tube microphone measures: Some opinions on terminology and procedures. *Hearing Journal* 43:1.

Mueller, H.G. (1991). Seven reasons for fitting programmable hearing aids. Presented at the American Academy of Audiology Programmable Workshop, Denver, CO, April.

Mueller, H.G., and Hawkins, D.B. (1990). Three important considerations in hearing aid selection. In: R. Sandlin (ed.), *Clinical Considerations in Hearing Aid Fitting, Volume II.* San Diego: College Hill Press.

Mueller, H.G., and Killion, M.C. (1990). An easy method for calculating the articulation index. *Hearing Instruments* 43:9.

Pascoe, D.P. (1975). Frequency responses of hearing aids and their effects on the speech perception of hearing-impaired subjects. *Annals of Otology, Rhinology, and Laryngology* 84:523.

Pavlovic, C.V. (1991). Speech recognition and five articulation indexes. *Hearing Instruments* 42(9): 20–23.

Popelka, G., and Mason, D. (1987). Factors which affect measures of speech audibility with hearing aids. *Ear and Hearing* 8(Suppl.):109(S)–118(S).

Preves, D.A. (1987). Some issues in utilizing probe tube microphone systems. *Ear and Hearing* 8(Suppl.):82(S)–94(S).

ReSound (1989). The ReSound digital hearing system.

Schum, D.J. (1990). Noise reduction strategies for elderly, hearing-impaired listeners. *Journal of the American Academy of Audiology* 1:31–36.

Skinner, M.W. (1976). Speech intelligibility in noise-induced hearing loss: Effects of high-frequency compensation. Ph.D. dissertation, Washington University, St. Louis, MO.

Staab, W.J. (1990). Digital/programmable hearing aids—an eye towards the future. *British Journal of Audiology* 24:243–256.

Stein, L., and Dempsey-Hart, D. (1984). Listener-assessed intelligibility of a hearing aid self-adaptive noise filter. *Ear and Hearing* 5:199–204.

Van Tasell, D., Larsen, S., and Fabry, D. (1988). Effects of an adaptive filter hearing aid in speech recognition in noise by hearing impaired subjects. *Ear and Hearing* 9:15–21.

Villchur, E. (1973). Signal processing to improve speech intelligibility in perceptive deafness. *Journal of the Acoustical Society of America* 53:1646–1657.

Walker, G., Dillon, H., Byrne, D., and Christen, R. (1984). The use of loudness discomfort levels for selecting the maximum output of hearing aids. *Australian Journal of Audiology* 6:23–32.

Wolinsky, S. (1986). Clinical assessment of a self-adaptive noise filtering system. *Hearing Journal* 39:29–32.

Yanick, P. (1976). Effect of signal processing on intelligibility of speech in noise for persons with sensorineural hearing loss. *Journal of the American Audiological Society* 1:229–238.

Yanick, P., and Drucker, H. (1976). Signal processing to improve intelligibility in the presence of noise for persons with ski-slope hearing impairment. *IEEE Transactions on Acoustical Speech and Signal Processing* ASSP-24:507–512.

CHAPTER 5

PRIZM™ PROGRAMMABLE HEARING SYSTEM

Thomas A. Powers

Programmable hearing instruments have been introduced into the hearing industry over the last few years. Programmable hearing instruments can be defined as those systems in which the electroacoustic response of the hearing instrument can be changed using an external programming device. The programmable market can be divided into four distinct groups, depending on the type of programmer that is used with the hearing instrument (Powers and Fry, 1990). These approaches include:

1. Those that require a dedicated system to program their instrument
2. Those that use a dedicated system to program the instrument *and* use a remote control
3. Those that use a remote control with adjustable features in the remote
4. Those that use the remote control both as the programmer and as the remote control for the patient

A complete review of the commercially available programmable systems has been accomplished by several investigators (Sammeth, 1990; Bentler, 1991).

The signal processing of the programmable systems can be characterized as having an analog signal path and a digital control circuit that perform the frequency shaping and compression functions. These systems are commonly referred to as digitally programmable hearing systems. None of the current systems on the market are using a full digital implementation. In a fully digital system, the input signal would be subjected to an analog-to-digital conversion, digital signal processing, and a digital-to-analog conversion. The application of digital signal processing to hearing instruments is well described by Levitt (1987).

The programmable systems can also be classified on the basis of the number of unique frequency responses available to the patient. The systems provide either a single response or multiple responses for the patient. The single-response philosophy creates the optimal electroacoustic response for the patient to use in all listening environments. The multiple-response systems provide different response characteristics for different listening environments. These multiple responses can be accessed by the patient either through a push button on the instrument or via a remote control device.

The programmable PRIZM Hearing System from AudioScience, Inc., is a remote-con-

™Trademark of AudioScience, Inc., Minnetonka, MN.

trolled, programmable, multi-environment hearing system. It was designed to give the dispenser the most flexibility in fitting and adjusting the hearing instruments, together with the most advanced technology possible. The development goals for the PRIZM system were:

1. No hardware or programming equipment for the dispenser to purchase
2. Improved compression circuitry
3. The need for multiple environments for the user
4. The need for the patient to have access to these environments via a remote control

In order to optimize the hardware requirements, the remote control would serve as the programmer for dispensers to relieve them of the financial burden of purchasing a dedicated programming system and as the patient remote control. The product development began in September, 1989. The system required a proprietary, custom-designed integrated circuit (IC) for the hearing instrument and also proprietary software and hardware for the remote control.

The PRIZM system is based on the rationale that the hearing-impaired individual is placed in many acoustically different listening environments every day. In order to optimize patients' residual hearing, their amplification system must be able to accommodate these listening environments. This is the core of the multiple-environment fitting rationale. The patient that has the need for these different acoustic responses must also have a simple way to access these response characteristics. This is most easily accomplished using a remote control, since the patient using the remote will have easy access to volume adjustments, as well as a choice of listening environments.

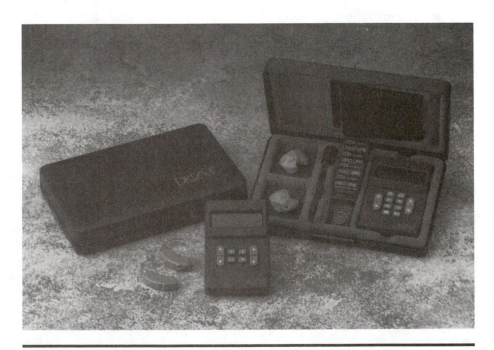

FIGURE 5.1. The PRIZM™ Hearing System. Reprinted with permission from AudioScience, Inc., Minnetonka, MN.

SYSTEM OVERVIEW

The PRIZM system is available in both behind-the-ear (BTE) and in-the-ear (ITE) models. The PRIZM system is shown in Figure 5.1. The ITE instrument has a smooth contoured convex faceplate with no external controls. It features a standard select-a-vent system and a choice of three custom colors (pink, tan, and brown). The full-on gain of 50 dB and 118 dB of output (SSPL90) is appropriate for up to moderately severe hearing losses. The mini-BTE instrument has a full-on gain of 60 dB and output of 125 dB (SSPL90). It is available in three colors (beige, brown, and gray), has a standard telecoil, and can be modified to accept direct audio input (DAI). The DAI connection is especially important for access to other assistive devices that may be available to the hearing impaired under the American Disabilities Act.

The ITE and BTE instruments can be combined with either a full-function PRIZM remote control (PRC-1) or a reduced-function model (PRC-2). The result is four systems that the dispenser can select to provide the optimal system based on the lifestyle needs of the patient.

PRIZM CUSTOM INTEGRATED CIRCUIT

The IC for the PRIZM system contains two separate amplifiers, one for the low-frequency spectrum and one for the high-frequency spectrum. Each channel can be independently controlled by the dispenser. The system is a digitally controlled analog CMOS circuit. The two-channel design allows for independent adjustment of response parameters for the low and high channels. Multichannel compression with independent AGC circuits was described by Villchur (1973) and Waldhauer and Villchur (1988). Multichannel compression systems should be most appropriate for individuals with severely restricted dynamic ranges. Multichannel compression separates the compression characteristics so that low-frequency noise should only affect the low-channel compressor and cause a gain reduction in the low channel. In this way, high-frequency energy would be relatively unaffected and could provide increased speech intelligibility (Kates, 1986) Multichannel systems have been shown to have increased speech intelligibility over single-channel compression systems (Moore, 1987; Laurence, Moore and Glasberg, 1983). Results with multichannel compression using more than two channels have not demonstrated significant improvements in speech intelligibility (Bustamante and Braida, 1987; Levitt and Neuman, 1991).

The programmable features of the PRIZM system in each channel are shown in Table 5.1. In addition, there are system parameters available to the dispenser. These include SSPL90 of the system and default gain level (SETVOL). In all there are 14 programmable parameters that define the electroacoustic response characteristics. These programmable parameters are combined into a number of preprogrammed matrix curves that are stored in the remote control. Any of these curves can be loaded into the specific listening environments of the remote.

COMPRESSION OVERVIEW

The most important element of the PRIZM system is the compression system. The primary use of compression, or automatic gain control (AGC), is to automatically reduce the gain of the circuit. The advantage compression circuits have over peak-clipping systems is that the compression systems introduce considerably less harmonic distortion. The amount of distortion has been shown to be related to loudness discomfort levels (Fortune and Preves, 1992). A hearing instrument with lower distortion levels should be more

TABLE 5.1. Programmable features of the
PRIZM™ system.

Low Channel	High Channel
Gain	Gain
Low break frequency	Low break frequency
High break frequency	High break frequency
Low slope	Low slope
High slope	High slope
Compression ratio	Compression ratio

comfortable to use and may lead to increased intelligibility.

Historically, compression systems have been required to perform two functions: protect the user from high-intensity, short-duration signals and provide recruitment compensation (Kates, 1993). These two functions require different performance characteristics. The element of protection requires that the circuit have a rapid attack time in order to respond as quickly as possible to a short-duration sound (door slam). The circuit should also have a high compression ratio so as to limit the maximum output level. The second function of compression, recruitment compensation, attempts to map the dynamics of speech to the reduced dynamic range of the impaired ear. This function of compression requires the circuit to respond more slowly to accurately reproduce the speech signal envelope (Plomp, 1988; Boothroyd et al., 1988). By separating these functions, each block of the circuit can be optimized for the function required. This approach is at the core of the PRIZM compression system.

The Integrated Compression System (ICS)™ of the PRIZM is composed of three major sections: the input limiter, the dynamic range compression (DRC) circuit, and the output compression system. The input limiter has two main functions: to prevent circuit saturation and to provide protection for short-duration signals. The limiter is the first circuit block

after the microphone. The output of the limiter is maintained at 85 dB. The limiter provides the input to the filters and compression circuits. By maintaining an 85 dB input to the filters and compression circuits, distortion is reduced. By reducing distortion, sound quality and user comfort are improved.

The second major section, the DRC circuit, is designed to operate over a wide range of intensity and frequency-based signals that are encountered by patients every day. The compression threshold is fixed at 50 dB input for both the low and high channels. The dispenser can select from four compression ratios for each channel independently. These ratios are 1.5:1, 2.0:1, 2.5:1, and 3.0:1 dB. The choice of compression ratios is the subject of much debate. Kates (1992) presents a model for determining compression thresholds based on auditory physiology. In a healthy cochlea, the outer hair cells provide approximately 50–60 dB of gain (Kiang and Moxon, 1974). As the signal level increases, the gain of the outer hair cells is reduced to 0–10 dB. Kates proposed that in a healthy cochlea an input of 0 dB would get 60 dB of gain, while an input of 100 dB would receive 0 dB of gain. This corresponds to a compression ratio of 2.5:1. This would suggest that the maximum compression required is 2.5:1, since the cochlea with complete outer hair cell damage is providing 0 dB of gain and therefore is acting linear. Lower compression ratios would be required for lesser amounts of hearing loss and hair cell damage.

The compression ratio strategy evolved from this analysis would suggest that the maximum compression ratio required is 2.5:1. Hearing losses above 60 dB should require the same compression ratio; however, additional gain would be required to compensate for inner hair cell damage (Liberman and Dodds, 1984). The compression strategy of the PRIZM system allows the dispenser access to four compression ratios in each channel between 1.5:1 and 3.0:1 to optimize the characteristics for the individual patient.

The third section of the ICS is the output compression circuit. The output limitation is programmable to 5, 10, or 15 dB below the SSPL90 of the hearing instrument. The output compression system acts as the final check on the output signal to insure that the patient tolerance level is not exceeded. Output compression was chosen to reduce the harmonic distortion in this stage of the ICS.

PRIZM REMOTE CONTROL

The PRIZM Remote Control (PRC) is the vehicle for all dispenser programming and patient use. The PRC is a small, hand-held device (3.6" L × 2.3" W × 0.7" H) that contains a liquid crystal display (LCD) screen and the keypad. The LCD screen provides two 12-character lines of alphanumeric characters and a small graphics area that displays the environmental icons. The intelligence of the remote is its EEPROM (electrically erasable programmable read-only memory) circuit. All changes in hearing instrument performance are initiated by a key press on the PRC.

The two styles of the PRC are based on the needs of the individual. The full-function PRC-1 has five "environments" to choose from, including WIDE RANGE, TYPICAL, NOISE 1, NOISE 2, and TELEPHONE. In addition, the PRC-1 has an ON/OFF key, an INFORMATION key, and an OPTIONS key. Each of these keys serves specific purposes for the user. The environment keys are designed to reflect the general listening needs of a hearing-impaired individual. Communication in face-to-face situations is usually the role of the TYPICAL key. It is programmed for the response and compression requirements of listening in quiet environments. The needs of the user for communication in noise environments are controlled by the NOISE 1 and NOISE 2 keys. The response characteris-

tics recalled by these keys have been programmed to respond to low to moderate levels of noise and contain appropriate low-frequency suppression and overall compression characteristics.

The appreciation of music may require a different set of parameters that can be recalled by use of the WIDE RANGE key. The TELEPHONE key activates the telecoil of the BTE instrument, and in the ITE instrument activates an acoustic response change to couple the instrument to the telephone.

The PRC-2 was designed for the individual that has a somewhat more limited need for listening environments. The PRC-2 has the ON/OFF and the INFORMATION keys, as well as the TYPICAL and NOISE 1 keys. It also has two volume keys that adjust the gain for each ear (either volume key can be pressed in a monaural setting).

In each listening environment (TYPICAL, NOISE 1, etc.), there are two memory locations for the dispenser to store preprogrammed response curves. These are designated Rx A and Rx B, or prescriptions A and B. These contain the matrix selection (frequency response) and the specific compression characteristics for that listening situation. The PRC-1 can contain up to ten distinct response programs, while the PRC-2 contains up to four distinct response programs.

PROGRAMMING OVERVIEW

The PRC also serves as the programming device for the dispenser. This does not require the dispenser to invest in dedicated programming systems. The PRC is placed in the programming mode by inserting a programming key into the left side of the device. In programming mode the volume control keys are function keys controlling the programming action of the PRC. The LCD displays the user-friendly screens that prompt the dispenser through the programming.

Programming is divided into three major areas: setup, information, and environments. Setup programming is the first area to be addressed. This section contains screens for system-wide functions, such as the presence of a confirmation tone for each press of an environment key. The confirmation tone is a 165 msec tone that alerts the user that the remote has successfully sent a new listening environment to the hearing instrument. It does not send a confirmation tone for volume changes. The second setup screen relates to the display time of the LCD screen and can be set to either 5, 10, 15 or 20 seconds, depending on the need of the user.

The next setup screens relate to binaural or monaural fitting screens. If this screen is set to NO, the system asks if the fitting is for the right or left ear. If the binaural is set to YES, then it will prompt the dispenser in all successive screens for information on the right and left ears. The system also asks for information on the symmetric nature of the hearing loss to determine if identical settings should be placed in both ears. In addition, the binaural setup screen allows for the linking of the volume controls to a preset offset. The dispenser can, for example, set the one volume to be always a fixed number of dB higher than the other, and this relationship will be maintained through all volume control adjustments by the patient. The volume controls can also be set to be totally independent.

The final part of the setup is related to the default gain setting for changes between environments. The nature of a multi-environment system indicates that there will be considerable difference in response and gain characteristics between environments. Changing between the NOISE 2 (considerable low-frequency reduction) and the TYPICAL or WIDE RANGE environment (increased low-frequency gain) could result in excessive gain increases for the patient. The SETVOL feature allows the dispenser to program a specific volume control step as the default for changes between environments. The user then can adjust the gain up or down from the default (SETVOL) level to achieve a comfortable listening level. The SETVOL can also be turned off to allow the gain to adjust based on the response characteristics of the selected environment.

Information programming allows the dispenser to enter up to 20 lines of text that can be recalled by the user. Information that could be stored includes the patient's name, address or phone number of the dispensing location, battery size, instrument and remote serial numbers, next appointment, and so on. The text can be entered in two-line increments with 12 characters available on each line.

Environment programming is activated by inserting the programming key and then pressing any environment key. The screen will display the current matrix curve selection, as well as the compression characteristics for each of the A and B responses. The matrix curves are contained in the *PRIZM Programming Matrix Guide* and also are resident in the remote control. Any of the predetermined matrix curves can be loaded into any memory location simply by entering the matrix number. In addition, the compression ratio for the low- and high-channel response can be selected. The current ratios are 1:1 dB (off), 1.5:1 dB, 2.0:1 dB, 2.5:1 dB, and 3.0:1 dB. The resulting electroacoustic response can then be recalled by the user by pressing any environment key. The response characteristics can be loaded into the remote at the factory or at the dispensing office. In either protocol, the response can be easily modified by inserting the PRIZM programming key and making the necessary changes. When the programming key is removed, all changes are saved and the PRC is returned to the user mode.

PATIENT USE OF THE REMOTE

The PRC was designed to provide the patient with easy access to the preprogrammed responses contained in its memory. Any key press turns the hearing instrument on to the listening environment selected. The patient can then select changes to the listening environment or access the information screens. Volume changes are easily accomplished by pressing the appropriate volume control. By pressing any environment key once, the patient enters the A response of that environment. Successive key presses toggle the response between the B and the A responses. This may also be a useful tool for the dispenser to allow for paired comparisons between two similar responses. The patient may also refresh the LCD display by pressing the OPTIONS key. This does not change the setting but merely brings the current settings to the screen. Any key press activates the LCD screen for the amount of time established in the setup programming.

SELECTION OF RESPONSE CHARACTERISTICS

The PRC can recall the appropriate frequency responses and compression characteristics for up to ten listening environments. The two environments that are the most intuitive are the TELEPHONE and WIDE RANGE. The TELEPHONE key in the BTE instrument is linked to a telecoil circuit that allows electromagnetic coupling of the telephone or other inductive systems. In the ITE system the coupling is acoustic. Terry et al. (1992) have recently investigated telephone coupling with hearing instruments and indicated that for mild hearing losses, frequency shaping of the input signal can lead to increased intelligibility. Their results indicated that a simple 6 dB/octave emphasis in the frequency shaping

was most effective. Unfortunately, Terry et al. also found that while most of their subjects were currently wearing hearing instruments, they took them off when they used the telephone. Clearly much work needs to be done in this area.

The WIDE RANGE key is intended to be used while listening to music or at any time when a broad frequency response is desired. The compression characteristics for this environment may be very different from that of the other environments. An iterative process with patients and their perceptions will be required to define this environment fully.

The TYPICAL, NOISE 1, and NOISE 2 environments are intended to be used by the dispenser to define the scope of frequency shaping and compression characteristics that will optimize the intelligibility of each patient. Any of the standard fitting rules, NAL-R, POGO, Berger, and so on, could be used to define the TYPICAL key. The dispenser must then decide on the patient need and has two options for setting the remaining environment keys. Each environment has an A and B memory location. The dispenser could keep the frequency response constant and vary the compression ratio characteristics. The second option is to vary the compression characteristics and to maintain the frequency shaping. A third option is to vary both the compression and the frequency shaping characteristics. The *PRIZM Matrix Guide* provides suggestions on the selection of the response and compression characteristics for hearing impairments within the fitting range of the system. These guidelines will assist the dispenser in selecting the family of curves that is appropriate for the patient. The flexibility of the programmable systems on the market provides the dispenser with many more options than ever before. The challenge for the manufacturer and the dispenser is to work together to optimize the amplification system for the patient requirements.

CANDIDATES FOR THE PRIZM SYSTEM

The PRIZM was designed for those individuals with an active lifestyle or who encounter varied listening environments. There is no single set of auditory performance problems experienced by hearing-impaired individuals; they are as variable as hearing impairment. The PRIZM system offers a unique set of signal processing strategies to optimize the amplification devices to the patient. In addition, the patient must be able to use the remote effectively and be willing to make it an integral part of his or her hearing system. The gain and output characteristics of the PRIZM make it appropriate for losses up to moderately severe. The single most important factor is the motivation of the patient to address his or her hearing loss through amplification. Second,

the hearing system must easily accommodate to patients' hearing difficulties.

CONCLUSION

The PRIZM Hearing System utilizes each patient perception of his or her listening experience as an integral part of the fitting formula by providing the ability to utilize a real-time paired-comparison technique. Toggling between environment prescriptions makes comparisons quick and reliable. The hearing professional can choose to contrast different frequency responses or identical frequency responses with changes in compression ratios to fine-tune each environment to fit the individual's perception and hearing needs. These subjective measurements, along with objective clinical analysis, such as sound field and probe tube measurements, allow the hearing professional to continually optimize the PRIZM performance for each individual based on his or her lifestyle, perception, and hearing needs.

REFERENCES

Bentler, R.A. (1991). Programmable hearing aid review. *American Journal of Audiology: A Journal of Clinical Practice* 1:25–28.

Boothroyd, A., Springer, N., Smith, L., and Schulman, J. (1988). Amplitude compression for the hearing impaired. *Journal of Speech and Hearing Research* 31:362–376.

Bustamante, D., and Braida, L. (1987). Principle component—Amplitude compression for the hearing impaired. *Journal of the Acoustical Society of America* 82:1227–1242.

Fortune, T.W., and Preves, D.A. (1992). Hearing aid saturation and aided loudness discomfort. *Journal of Speech and Hearing Research* 35:175–185.

Kates, J. (1986). Signal Processing for hearing aids. *Hearing Instruments* 36:19–22.

Kates, J. (1993). Hearing aid design criteria. *JSLPA Monograph* (Suppl. 1): 15–23.

Kiang, N., and Moxon, E. (1974). Tails of tuning curves of auditory-nerve fibers. *Journal of the Acoustical Society of America* 55:620–630.

Laurence, R., Moore, B.C.J., and Glasberg, B. (1983). A comparison of behind-the-ear high-fidelity linear hearing aids and two-channel compression aids, in the laboratory and in everyday life. *British Journal of Audiology* 17:31–48.

Levitt , H. (1987). Digital hearing aids: A tutorial review. *Journal of Rehabilitation Research and Development* 24(4): 7–19.

Levitt, H., and Neuman, A. (1991). Evaluation of orthogonal polynomial compression. *Journal of the Acoustical Society of America* 90:241–252.

Liberman, M., and Dodds, L. (1984). Single neuron labeling and chronic cochlear pathology III: Stereocilia damage and alterations of threshold tuning curves. *Hearing Research* 16:55–74.

Moore, B.C.J. (1987). Design and evaluation of a two-channel compression hearing aid. *Journal of Rehabilitation Research and Development* 24(4): 181–192.

Plomp, R. (1988). The negative effect of amplitude compression in multichannel hearing aids in light of the modulation-transfer function. *Journal of the Acoustical Society of America* 83:2322–2327.

Powers, T.A., and Fry, D. (1990). An environmentally sound hearing system. *Hearing Instruments* 42:34–39.

Sammeth, C. (1990). Current availability of digital and digital-hybrid hearing aids. *Seminars in Hearing* 11(1):91–100.

Terry, M., Bright, K., Durian, M., Kepler, L., Sweetman, R., and Grim, M. (1992). Processing the telephone speech signals for the hearing impaired. *Ear and Hearing* 13:70–79.

Villchur, E. (1973). Signal processing to improve speech intelligibility in perceptive deafness. *Journal of the Acoustical Society of America* 53:1646–1657.

Waldhauer, F., and Villchur, E. (1988). Full dynamic range multi-band compression: From concept to reality. *Hearing Journal* 29:29–31.

CHAPTER 6

3M PROGRAMMABLE HEARING INSTRUMENTS

Paul H. Stypulkowski

The use of digital circuitry in hearing instruments represents an evolutionary, rather than revolutionary, advance in technology. As in many other areas, including medical and consumer electronics, digital circuits were first utilized to perform specific functions as components of larger systems, and this same development pathway holds true for hearing instruments. A good comparison can be found in the consumer audio marketplace, where today's compact disc (CD) technology represents the current concept of digital sound. CD technology evolved from earlier analog systems that began with the phonograph and evolved through several generations of magnetic recording tape technology. Original analog systems used mechanical counters to display tape position, analog VU meters to display recording levels, and analog potentiometers to adjust various parameters. Second-generation systems incorporated digital circuits for many of these applications and by definition were therefore hybrid systems, employing digital circuitry for control, accuracy, and convenience, and analog circuitry for signal processing. Farther along the audio analog-digital continuum

emerged the CD player, which added digital circuitry to the actual signal processing pathway as well.

This same evolutionary path can be seen in the development of today's hearing instruments. Conventional hearing aid designers utilize different analog circuits to create various hearing instrument responses by altering discrete components to change frequency shaping, gain, and output. In some cases the dispenser has limited control over these parameters through adjustable potentiometers within the circuit. The hearing aid user typically has access to an analog volume control and in some cases to a tone control that alters frequency shaping.

Digital-analog hybrid hearing instruments, commonly called programmable instruments, represent the next generation in amplification technology. In their simplest form, programmable hearing instruments utilize digital circuitry to provide limited control of an analog signal pathway, in some sense functioning as a digital screwdriver. These designs allow the dispenser to adjust various hearing aid parameters, providing access to a variety of conventional circuits within one

Unless otherwise noted, figures and photographs in this chapter are reprinted with permission of the 3M Company, St. Paul, MN.

package. In this type of programmable system, the standard analog volume control (if present) remains as the only available adjustment option for the end-user.

A more advanced application of digital circuitry in programmable instruments is the inclusion of multiple memories (i.e., the ability to create and store more than one hearing aid response within the same hearing instrument), thereby allowing the user to select the most appropriate response, which may differ in frequency shaping or signal processing, for a specific listening situation, rather than simply being able to change volume. Another level of programmable technology is represented by instruments that interface with personal computer–based fitting systems, allowing the clinician to take advantage of the speed and power of the PC in the hearing aid fitting process.

The next era in hearing instrument evolution is the fully digital signal processing (DSP) instrument. Although a number of DSP instruments have been designed and developed, and a few marketed, they have yet to receive widespread acceptance. In the case of DSP instruments, the cost/benefit ratio becomes particularly relevant. In this case, cost refers more to practical considerations than to financial ones. Although the expectation of dramatically improved sound quality exists for DSP instruments, that promise is typically unfulfilled. Those expectations are created in part by the sound quality associated with consumer audio CD technology. It must be remembered, however, that prior to the introduction of the CD player, extremely high quality sound recordings could be achieved with older, analog, magnetic tape technology. In reality, a high-end tape system produces a sound quality that is comparable to a digital CD system, and in fact, most CDs are mastered from analog tape systems. This same comparison holds true for today's hearing instruments: High-quality analog signal processing circuits produce sound quality as good as or better than DSP systems.

The true promise of DSP, the ability to utilize advanced signal processing, remains for the most part unrealized. Signal processing algorithms that can cancel feedback or reduce background noise have been under development for a number of years (Engebretsen, Morley, and Popelka 1987; Kates, 1991), and it seems likely that feedback cancellation will be the first practical application of DSP in hearing instruments. It is also likely that this implementation of DSP will be in the form of a circuit added to an existing analog signal processing instrument (i.e., an analog-digital hybrid). True noise reduction remains difficult to implement even on large computers, particularly with single-microphone systems (Levitt, 1991), and even when marginally successful (on the basis of speech intelligibility) may be rejected by the hearing aid user due to diminished or artificial sound quality. From a practical point of view, digital systems are typically larger and require higher power than most of today's hearing instruments, meaning that cosmetic appearance and battery life suffer. Thus the true promise of digital sound for hearing instruments remains an area that awaits further development in both design and practical implementation.

On the other hand, analog-digital hybrid instruments are well into their development cycle, and their impact is now only beginning to be felt in the hearing health care field. Programmable instruments at the present time represent a small percentage of the hearing aids dispensed annually; however, various estimates (ranging from 20%–80%) exist regarding the growth curve for programmable instruments into the next decade. By any estimate, the growth trend for this technology is very positive, and programmable instruments represent the leading edge of amplification technology for the immediate future.

3M PROGRAMMABLE HEARING INSTRUMENTS

Design Considerations

The 3M programmable hearing instruments represent the most flexible analog-digital hybrid instruments available today. When the concept for these instruments was originally conceived, a number of clinical, as well as practical, considerations guided their design and development. One primary design goal was to allow maximum flexibility in tailoring hearing aid characteristics with respect to gain, output, frequency shaping, and compression parameters to meet the needs of different hearing losses, as well as the needs of different individuals. In addition to the amplification requirements dictated by differing degrees of hearing loss, clinicians have long recognized that individuals with similar audiograms may have different listening preferences and require different hearing aid fittings to achieve optimal user performance and satisfaction (Martin, 1973; Leijon, Eriksson-Mangold, and Bech-Karlsen, 1984; Cox and Alexander, 1991).

Moreover, the designers of the 3M system recognized that for a given individual, a hearing aid with a single signal processing mode simply could not meet the needs of many different listening situations. Clinicians are well aware that, in many cases, a hearing aid response that produces maximum speech intelligibility may not be the same response that results in optimal sound quality (Mangold and Leijon, 1979; Mangold, 1982). With a single response instrument, the dispenser is left with the dilemma of compromising one or the other consideration or of selecting a set of parameters that apply to some average listening condition. These clinical considerations led to a series of research investigations whose results revealed that, if available, users would select different patterns of hearing aid characteristics based on the particular listening environment or the source material (e.g., speech, speech in noise, or music) (Mangold and Leijon, 1979; Mangold, 1982; Johnson et al., 1988; Ringdahl et al., 1990). Thus, in addition to fitting flexibility, the envisioned hearing instrument design also included the capability to create and access multiple hearing aid responses (i.e., multiple memories) within the same instrument.

With these design considerations in mind, a number of state-of-the-art technologies were evaluated for the necessary characteristics that would lead to the proposed hearing instrument. Different technologies such as DSP and digitally controlled analog systems were considered, along with different forms of filter technology, including finite-impulse-response (FIR) filters, switched capacitor filters, and resistor-capacitor filters. Engineering performance considerations, such as low power consumption and low processing noise, were also factored into the design equation. The optimum combination of available technology yielded two integrated circuits: a very flexible analog signal processing circuit that could be digitally controlled and a memory-logic chip for storing the programming variables of the multiple hearing aid responses. To achieve the goal of very low levels of circuit noise, a major design decision was to utilize resistor-capacitor filters for the signal processing IC, rather than the typical switched capacitor filters used in most hearing aid applications. Switched capacitor filters, as their name implies, function as a collection of rapidly operating switches and in doing so generate circuit noise. By contrast, resistor-capacitor filter circuitry operates with a continuous nature on the audio signal and generates very low levels of noise. This design consideration is reflected in the equivalent input noise levels of the 3M programmable instruments, which are among the lowest available in a programmable instrument. This measure and other technical specifications are listed in Table 6.1.

TABLE 6.1. ANSI S3.22-1987 specifications for the 3M programmable ITE and BTE hearing instruments.

	ITE	BTE
Output (HFA SSPL 90)	118 dB	122 dB
Gain (HFA full-on gain)	48 dB	55 dB
Frequency range	200–8000 Hz	250–5200 Hz
Equivalent Input Noise	<24 dB	<24 dB

Features of the 3M Instruments

The 3M programmable hearing instruments that represent the culmination of this design and development effort are two-channel, multiple-memory, multiband compression designs (Johnson et al., 1988; Mangold et al., 1990; Stypulkowski, Raskind, and Hodgson, 1992). On both the in-the-ear (ITE) and behind-the-ear (BTE) models shown in Figure 6.1, the user has access to the multiple memories of the instruments via a selector switch located on the instrument. Because the programming variables are stored directly in the memory of the hearing aid, there are no additional remote controls or other hardware needed by the user. This design concept represents an important practical consideration for most users who object to having to carry an additional piece of hardware to adjust

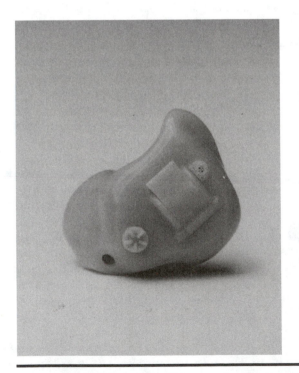
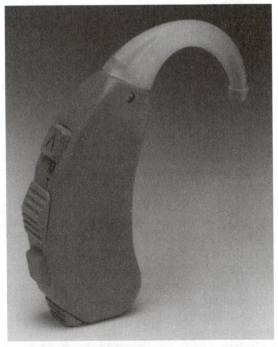

FIGURE 6.1. The 3M programmable hearing instruments: ITE and BTE models.

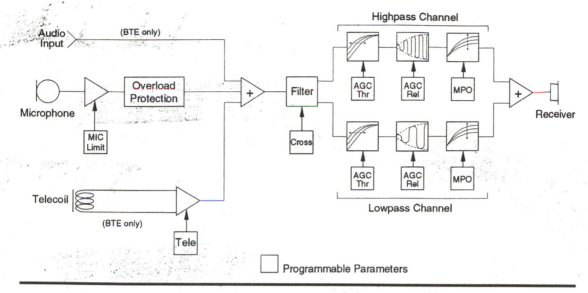

FIGURE 6.2.   Block diagram of the signal processing pathway.

their hearing instruments. This view was recently documented in a study of another multiple-memory hearing aid by Kuk (1992), where more than one-half of the subjects listed the requirement of using a remote control as the major disadvantage of the system.

The analog signal processing pathway of the instruments, with the dispenser-controlled programmable parameters highlighted, is shown in Figure 6.2. As indicated in the block diagram, the behind-the-ear (BTE) instrument accepts microphone, telecoil, or direct audio input, and the (ITE) uses microphone input only. The input stage contains a programmable microphone limiting adjustment that functions as a transient remover, preventing impulsive sounds from exceeding the user's tolerance level and also providing overload protection for the filter circuitry. Following this variable-gain input stage, the incoming signal is divided into two channels by 24 dB/octave filters. The programmable crossover frequency, variable between 400–4000 Hz, defines the dividing point between the low-pass and high-pass

channels. Each channel contains an independent compression circuit with variable AGC threshold and AGC release time. The gain and maximum power output (MPO) in each channel are also programmable. These various programmable parameters can be independently adjusted in each of the eight programs of the 3M instruments. This programming flexibility affords the opportunity to provide a variety of hearing aid responses, differing in frequency shaping and compression characteristics, within the same instrument for use in various listening environments. The individual programmable parameters, the functions served by these parameters, and the adjustment ranges available are listed in Table 6.2.

A unique feature of the 3M programmable instruments is a memory circuit within the hearing aid that records information about the use pattern of the instrument. This function, known as datalogging, was designed into the instrument as a means to better understand and refine the fitting process by providing the clinician with feedback as to exactly how the hearing aid is being used. Datalogging records

TABLE 6.2. Programmable parameters.

Parameter	Function	Range
Mic limiting	Input overload protection	85–112 dB
Crossover frequency	Separation between LP and HP channels	400–4000 Hz
Gain	Independent LP and HP channel gain	48 dB (ITE) 55 dB (BTE)
MPO	Independent LP and HP channel MPO	87–118 dB (ITE) 87–122 dB (BTE)
AGC threshold	Independent LP and HP AGC thresholds	54–104 dB
AGC release	Independent LP and HP AGC release times	LP: 0–500 ms HP: 0–150 ms

the number of times that each memory is accessed, the total duration of use for each program, and additional hearing instrument data, as shown in Figure 6.3. This information provides insight into which responses are most useful for the patient, which responses require modification, and potential directions for such modifications. In combination with user reports, the datalogging results assist the dispenser in fine-tuning the instruments and in optimizing the programs for each individual user. In addition, datalogging serves as a unique research tool for academic investigators, as well as fitting system designers, by collecting information about the performance and user preference of various fitting algorithms. Because the 3M fitting system is software based, research findings on successful fitting strategies can be rapidly and easily incorporated into new fitting algorithms.

Of the many design features incorporated into the 3M programmable instruments, three components—the two-channel compression system, the multiple memory capability, and the PC-based fitting system—differentiate them from others and provide the instruments with their range of fitting and signal processing flexibility. Separately, each of these components adds important capabilities and advantages to the system; however, it is the

combination of these features that ultimately allows the clinician, and the user, to fully access the performance and flexibility that was designed into these hearing instruments. The design rationale and a detailed description of each of these system components are presented in the following sections.

Multiple Memories

A good analogy regarding the practical utility of multiple memories in a hearing instrument is the wearing of eyeglasses. In fact, several analogies can be drawn between the use of eyeglasses to correct for visual deficits and the use of amplification to correct for an auditory impairment. Even though the underlying cause of the impairment is very different in these two situations and from a physiological basis, much more complex in the case of hearing loss, it nonetheless serves as a useful comparison to highlight the practical considerations addressed by a multiple-memory hearing instrument.

Most vision corrections are necessitated by the eye's inability to focus at different distances—that is, nearsightedness or farsightedness. In many cases, particularly as individuals age, the ability to focus on both far and near objects deteriorates, and correc-

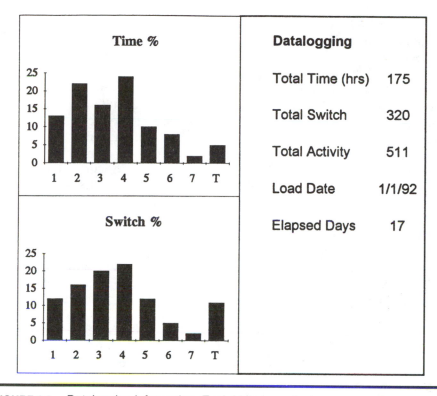

FIGURE 6.3.   Datalogging information. Each histogram displays a percentage distribution of activity: total time that each program was used (top), number of times that each program was accessed (bottom).

tions may be required for both situations. Years ago this meant having two pairs of glasses, one pair for distance and a second pair of reading glasses. Today those two pairs of glasses are often replaced by a single pair of bi- or trifocals. By choosing the viewing angle through the various parts of the composite lens, the user can select the correction most appropriate for the situation. For someone wearing hearing aids the ability to select a different correction for a different listening situation is just as important. For example, a user may select a particular frequency-gain and compression response for typical everyday situations at home or at the office. This selection may be based on sound quality, comfort, or other attributes. However, there may be occasions when speech intelligibility is critical (e.g., at a business meeting) and becomes the overriding consideration, rather than sound quality. With multiple-memory instruments the user can select a different hearing aid response tailored to improve speech intelligibility (e.g., additional high-frequency emphasis). Just as bifocals provide the ability to shift to a different lens when intelligibility (i.e., the ability to see words clearly) is the primary need, multiple-memory hearing aids afford the same opportunity to select the appropriate correction for a specific circumstance.

Upon entering a bright, sunny, outdoor

environment, the same individual might reach for a pair of sunglasses, another visual correction. The main purpose of the correction achieved by sunglasses is not really to improve intelligibility nor to improve focus, but more so to improve visual quality or comfort. For the hearing aid user a comparable circumstance might occur upon entering a noisy restaurant. The overall sound level in this situation may be much louder than the previous office environment, and the typical response would be to turn down the volume (gain). However, with the gain reduced the hearing aid may no longer amplify important speech components adequately, and speech understanding is degraded. In this situation the user has to compromise speech intelligibility for the sake of comfort. Rather than reducing the gain for all sounds, this situation requires an attenuation of low-frequency gain to reduce the amplification of background noise, but maintenance of adequate gain for lower-level, high-frequency speech components. In this circumstance, the user of multiple-memory instruments could select a response with decreased low-frequency gain and appropriate high-frequency gain, but reduced overall output, allowing both comfort and speech intelligibility considerations to be adequately addressed.

Attempts have been made to make these types of corrections automatic, both in the optical area as well as in a variety of hearing aids. Photogrey glasses represent the best example from the visual field. These lenses contain a light-sensitive pigment that varies in the amount of light transmission, depending on the level of incident light energy. They become darker in bright light and clearer in dim light (i.e., optical compression). Although this theoretically sounds like the ideal solution, for the most part these types of lenses are not in widespread use. Most eyeglass wearers prefer a discrete correction for each environment: sunglasses for the sun,

regular glasses indoors, each optimally designed to compensate for its main purpose, rather than attempting to fit all circumstances.

The same parallel holds true for hearing aids. AGC circuits have been designed that automatically reduce the gain in the presence of high levels of sound. Some of these circuits reduce overall gain, while others have frequency-specific actions, reducing either low-frequency or high-frequency gain. As might be predicted, such automatic systems work well in some types of sound environments, but not in others, and meet the user's needs in some, but not all, circumstances. For example, a compression circuit that reduces overall or high-frequency gain for high-level sounds might be excellent in reducing the annoying nature of paper rustling or dishes rattling, but may not be particularly advantageous in a noisy environment when the user's primary concern is speech intelligibility. The optimal solution is to have access to hearing aid responses designed specifically for these different types of circumstances, rather than a "one-size-fits-all" approach. Multiple memory capabilities, coupled with flexible signal processing, provide the opportunity to have several automatic responses, each of which adjusts gain appropriately and each of which is designed to optimize listening in specific types of situations.

Multiple Memories versus Volume Controls. Although hearing aids have been in use for decades and have undergone continual improvements in their sound quality and signal processing capabilities, conventional hearing aids still remain limited in their ability to adapt to the varying needs of the user. For the majority of hearing aid users, a volume control is the only available adjustment option to compensate for different listening situations, and in many cases, the volume control may create more problems than it solves. A classical dilemma for a hearing aid wearer is the situation with multiple speakers located at different distances. Typical examples of this situation might be a business meeting or dinner with the family. If everyone spoke at exactly the same level, the voice of the speaker located farthest from the listener would arrive at the hearing aid microphone at a lower level than other voices, based solely on the transmission of sound through the air. In the real world, however, that relatively small effect of distance is magnified by each talker's speaking characteristics—volume, enunciation, projection, and so on. If the individual at the far end of the table speaks softly and does not enunciate very well, the hearing aid user may have a difficult time understanding that person. The typical response in this situation would be to increase the volume (gain) of the hearing aid(s) to bring the talker's voice up to a level where speech is intelligible and comfortable.

However, when the person with the very loud voice who is seated next to the hearing aid wearer begins to speak, a new problem arises. Depending on the type of hearing aid, several possible scenarios, most of them bad, can occur. If these are linear circuits, or aids with input compression, where the output level changes with volume setting [Figure 6.4(a)], the output may reach intensities that become uncomfortable for the user. For aids with a limiting circuit or output compression, whose knee point varies with volume control setting [Figure 6.4(b)], the loud speech may become distorted, reducing both sound quality and intelligibility. In all of these cases, the user must choose among the trade-offs of comfort or speech understanding and/or continually adjust the volume in order to meet his or her listening requirements. The desired hearing aid response for this situation would be one that provided adequate gain, especially in the high frequencies, for quiet speech, but reduced the gain for higher-level sounds and whose output was independent of the gain (volume control). Having the ability to select a hearing aid response whose gain, frequency-shaping, and compression characteristics would optimize speech intelligibility and comfort in this situation provides the user with a superior alternative to a simple volume control.

The multiple-memory design of the 3M instruments is intended to address many of the common dilemmas faced by both the dispenser and the user of conventional hearing aids. Since the 3M instruments can be programmed with up to eight independent responses, if desired, some of the memories of the instrument can be programmed as simple gain changes of a preferred frequency response. This approach provides the individual with a digital volume control in situations where it is desired, yet insures that output can be independently controlled as needs dictate. Having up to eight memories available allows this type of user request to be easily met and avoids many of the complications created by analog volume controls. Ultimately, the number of memories used by each individual, as well as how they are programmed, varies depending on individual listening needs and lifestyle. The ability to provide a family of hearing aid responses custom tailored to an individual user's audiological requirements and specific listening environments provides solutions to many of the most common problems faced by the users of conventional amplification.

Compression System

The two-channel, syllabic compression system of the 3M programmable instruments provides tremendous flexibility in meeting the demands of different individuals, as well as different listening environments. Direct control of channel bandwidths, as well as gain, output, AGC threshold, and AGC re-

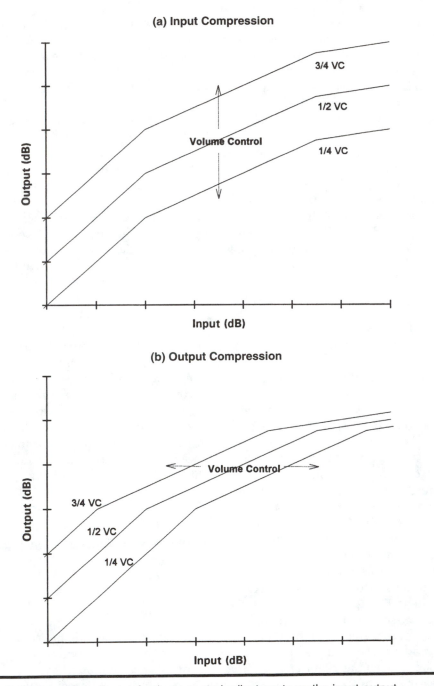

FIGURE 6.4.   The effects of volume control adjustments on the input-output relationship of different types of compression circuits. (a) Input-based compression. (b) Output-based compression. The arrows indicate the direction of shift in the input-output curves as the volume control (gain) is raised and lowered.

lease time in each channel, allows the clinician to accommodate a wide range of audiologic requirements. The independent two-channel design also ensures that the characteristics of each compressor, such as threshold and release time, can be tailored to maximize effectiveness in various types of listening environments. For example, in situations where typical low-frequency noise dominates, the low-pass channel can be programmed with a low compression threshold and long release time to reduce low-frequency gain without affecting the gain of the high-frequency channel, where important speech components are present. This type of two-channel compression design has been shown in a number of studies to provide enhanced speech intelligibility in noise (Mangold and Leijon, 1981; Moore, 1987; Moore and Glasberg, 1986; Johnson et al., 1988; Stypulkowski, Hodgson, and Raskind, 1992).

An example of the input-output characteristics of the 3M compression system is illustrated in Figure 6.5. Also shown are representative examples for a linear/peak-clipping circuit and a full dynamic range compressor, all three equated for comparable gain and output. Unlike typical compression circuits that operate according to a fixed compression ratio (log compression), the 3M system utilizes a variable compression ratio that continuously adapts across the input intensity range. Instead of all input levels being compressed at the same ratio (e.g., 2:1 or 3:1), the *intensity proportionate* design of the 3M compression system automatically adjusts the compression ratio, depending on the input level. Sounds that slightly exceed the compression threshold are compressed at a very low ratio (e.g., 1.3:1), while loud sounds are compressed at a much higher ratio (e.g., 4:1). The compression ratio varies in a curvilinear fashion (semilog compression) over the operating range of the compression circuit. This circuit design ensures a very smooth

transition into and out of compression, providing excellent sound quality, rather than an abrupt change from linear to nonlinear processing, which can create the typical pumping sensation common to compression circuits. The intensity proportionate design allows weaker sounds, especially low-level speech components, to be maximally amplified, while the loudest sounds receive the most compression, effectively mapping the intensity spectrum into the user's dynamic range. Rather than compressing all inputs at the same level, this approach to syllabic compression is intended to improve the intensity relationship between softer consonant sounds and the more intense vowels.

Numerous studies have shown that for most hearing-impaired individuals, improving the consonant-to-vowel ratio can improve speech understanding, since it is the consonant information that is not being accurately perceived (Montgomery and Edge, 1988; Freyman and Nerbonne, 1989; Gordon-Salant, 1987; Preves et al., 1991). Applying maximum gain to low-intensity speech components and reducing the gain proportionately for higher-intensity sounds provides a means to improve the intensity relationship between different speech sounds for the hearing-impaired listener. Finally, when equated for gain and output, this compressor design is also able to provide more usable gain for soft speech levels (50–60 dB SPL) compared to a ratio compressor, which is already into compression at these relatively low input levels (Figure 6.5). This advantage becomes more pronounced as the degree of hearing impairment worsens and gain requirements increase.

The ability to program gain and output independently in each of the two channels of the 3M instrument, combined with the multiple-memory capability, makes it possible to provide dramatically different types of signal processing in a single hearing in-

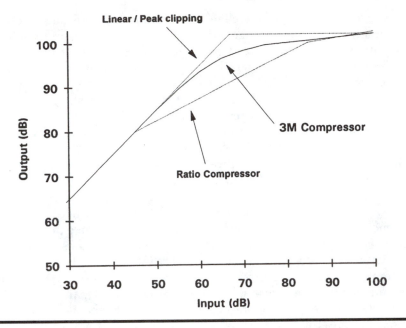

FIGURE 6.5. Representative input-output relationship for one channel of the 3M compression system. Also shown for comparison purposes are responses for a linear/peak-clipping circuit and a ratio (log) compression circuit equated for the same gain and output.

strument. Figure 6.6. shows a series of typical input-output curves for one channel of the hearing instrument that illustrate the relationship between gain, output, and AGC threshold. Curve B [Figure 6.6(a)] shows the I/O response of the high-frequency channel programmed to provide 25 dB of gain for low input levels and to have an output of approximately 100 dB SPL. Increasing the gain to 35 dB, without altering the output, results in the input-output relationship shown in curve A. And similarly, reducing the gain to 15 dB yields a different input-output response (curve C). These gain changes are accomplished without affecting the output of the channel by shifting the input level at which the AGC is activated (i.e., the AGC threshold). For the higher gain response (A) the

compression is activated at a lower intensity, maintaining the maximum output at the desired level. In the lower gain situation the AGC threshold has been increased, and the compressor is not activated until higher input intensities are reached, again maintaining the programmed output level.

The complementary situation, modifying the output independent of the gain, is illustrated in Figure 6.6(b). Curve B represents the identical input-output response of Figure 6.6(a), with a gain of 25 dB and an output of 100 dB. Adjustment of the programmable output parameter to 110 dB results in the I/O response shown in curve C. With these parameter settings, the output has increased by approximately 10 dB; however, the gain for lower-level inputs, as intended, remains at 25 dB. This has

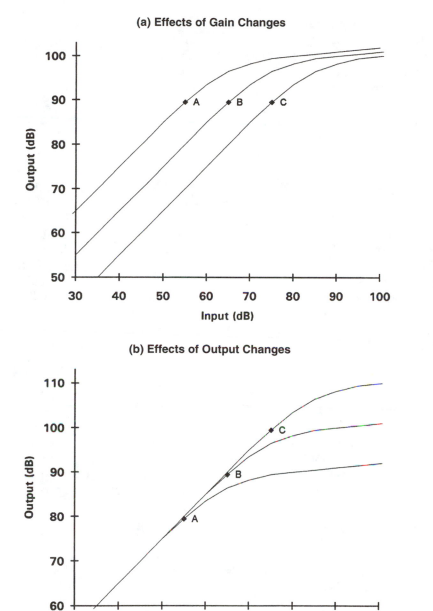

FIGURE 6.6.   Representative input-output curves for one channel of the 3M compression system illustrating the relationship between programmable gain, output, and AGC threshold parameters. AGC thresholds for the various curves are indicated by the diamonds.

been achieved by shifting the AGC threshold approximately 10 dB higher, delaying activation of the compression circuit until inputs reach approximately 75 dB. Conversely, if the MPO parameter is reduced to provide an output of 90 dB, the input-output response changes to curve A. In this case as well, gain has remained a constant 25 dB for low-level inputs, independent of changes to the output level. The AGC threshold has now been shifted downward to approximately 55 dB, resulting in activation of the compression circuit at lower input levels. Each of these programmed combinations of gain and output would provide equivalent gain for low-level sounds, but would respond quite differently as input levels increased.

The following section provides examples of how the ability to control gain and output in the two channels of the 3M instruments independently can be practically utilized to create different signal processing strategies that address different listening requirements in various situations. Four generic types of signal processing can be provided with a two-channel system: linear processing; low-frequency compression; high-frequency compression; and full-spectrum, two-channel compression. With the flexibility of the 3M compression system, each of these types of signal processing approaches is possible, and moreover, each can be custom tailored to varying degrees by adjustments to channel bandwidth, AGC threshold, AGC release time, and output in each of the two channels.

Examples of these four different types of signal processing schemes are illustrated in Figure 6.7. Each panel of Figure 6.7 contains a series of frequency-gain curves that represent the responses of four different memories of a 3M ITE instrument programmed to emulate a different type of signal processing. The programmed gain for each response at low input intensities (e.g., 55 dB) is identical and repre-sents NAL target gain (Byrne and Dillon, 1986) for a 65 dB flat hearing loss. In all cases the output has been programmed to remain below a speech-based UCL of 95 dB HL. Figure 6.7(a) shows the response of memory #1, programmed for a linear type of processing in both channels. In this case, as the input level increases from 55 dB to 80 dB SPL, there is little change in the response of the hearing aid (a small reduction in high-frequency gain occurs at 80 dB as the compression threshold in this channel is reached). At a 90 dB input level, the compression system has been activated in both channels and overall gain has been reduced, maintaining the output below the specified UCL. This type of linear processing generally provides excellent sound quality and would be useful for such situations as listening to music or in quiet environments where background noise is not a concern.

Figure 6.7(b) shows a different type of signal processing approach, characterized by low-frequency compression. This type of signal processing has been termed *bass increase at low levels* (BILL) (Killion, Staab, and Preves, 1990; Fabry, 1991) and is representative of circuits such as ANR (automatic noise reduction), AFR (automatic frequency response), or ASP (automatic signal processing). The similarity among these processing schemes is a reduction in low-frequency gain with increasing input levels (i.e., bass reduction at high levels) in an attempt to reduce the upward spread of masking, as well as hearing aid distortion (Van Tasell, Larsen, and Fabry, 1988). The responses shown in Figure 6.7(b), achieved by programming a low compression threshold in the low-frequency channel, illustrate this predominant low-frequency effect as input levels change. At higher input levels the high-frequency channel compressor is also activated to maintain appropriate output levels for this frequency band. This type of signal processing is advantageous in

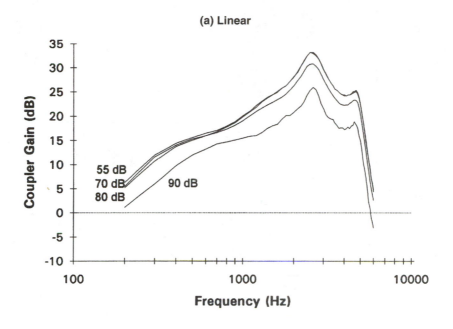

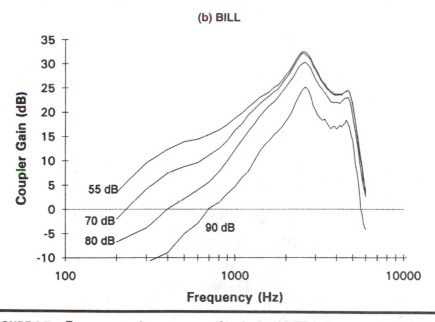

FIGURE 6.7.   Frequency-gain responses of a single 3M ITE instrument programmed for different signal processing schemes. (a) Memory #1: linear type of response. (b) Memory #2: BILL type of response. (c) Memory #3: TILL type of response. (d) Memory #4: full spectrum type of response. Output was measured in a 2 cc coupler with a speech-weighted composite noise input.

continues

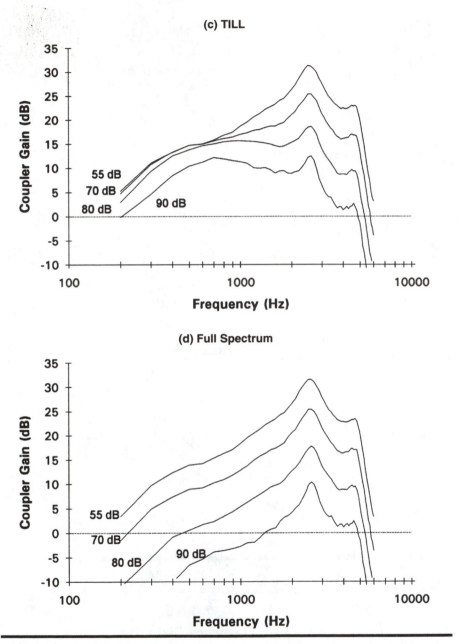

FIGURE 6.7.   Continued.

situations where typical low-frequency noise dominates, such as riding in an automobile or attending noisy social gatherings.

A third type of signal processing that can be implemented, in some regards the opposite of BILL, is known as *treble increase at low levels* (TILL) (Killion, 1990; Killion, Staab, and Preves, 1990). TILL processing, shown in Figure 6.7(c), is achieved with high-frequency compression and is characterized by providing maximum high-frequency emphasis for low input levels and reduced high-frequency gain for high input levels. The rationale underlying this signal processing approach is that some individuals, particularly those with less severe hearing losses, exhibit relatively normal loudness perception at high-level inputs and therefore require little or no gain in this range. With this type of compression processing, high-frequency gain is reduced as input levels increase, effectively flattening the frequency response. This signal processing approach is useful for mild to moderate hearing losses and is particularly well accepted by new users. Many of the typically annoying high-frequency sounds (e.g., paper rustling, dishes rattling) can be made tolerable with TILL processing. This signal processing may not be particularly advantageous in noisy situations where background noise will activate the compression and thereby reduce the gain needed for high-frequency speech sounds.

Finally, the BILL and TILL concepts can be combined into a full-spectrum, two-channel approach to compression. Figure 6.7(d) illustrates the response of memory #4 of the same instrument, in this case programmed to have low compression thresholds in both channels. In this example, as the input level increases, the overall gain is reduced, leaving only a small amount of gain being provided at 3 kHz with a 90 dB input. It should be noted that these test responses are generated using a broadband noise input signal that ac-

tivates both channels of compression simultaneously. This produces a response that might appear similar to that of a single-channel compression circuit. However, in the real world, the two channels of the compression system would act independently so that low-frequency gain would be reduced in response to loud sounds within that channel and the high-frequency compressor would respond specifically to inputs within its bandwidth.

These examples illustrate the variation in signal processing that can be provided for a given hearing loss with the combination of multiple-memory technology and a flexible, two-channel compression system. Although each of these four programmed responses provides the same amount of gain for low-intensity sounds, they each respond very differently as input levels increase. In use, these different programs would sound virtually identical for quiet speech or other low-level sounds, but would result in dramatically different sound quality, comfort, and intelligibility in various listening environments and in response to different types of inputs.

PC-Based Fitting System

The personal computer brings yet another level of digital technology and sophistication to the delivery of programmable hearing instruments. In particular, the computational power and speed of the PC is especially suited for use in fitting multiple-memory instruments. Manually creating multiple hearing aid responses varying in frequency-gain shaping and compression characteristics can be cumbersome and time consuming. 3M's PC-based Model 80 fitting system simplifies this process by automatically creating a family of hearing aid responses based on an individual's audiometric data, using predefined algorithms for different listening situations. The Model 80 system (Figure 6.8) consists of a small interface

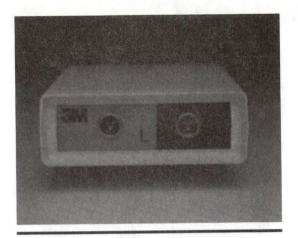

FIGURE 6.8.   The 3M Model 80 Fitting System.

unit and accompanying software that is compatible with most desktop and laptop personal computers.

The Model 80 system programs the multiple memories of the 3M instruments based on the dispenser's choice of prescriptive (e.g., NAL, 1/3 gain, POGO, etc.) and environmentally based fitting algorithms. These different target algorithms include responses designed for use in situations such as a restaurant, groups, listening to music, home/office, and others. The various environmental targets were developed based on several considerations: (1) typical acoustic characteristics of different environments; (2) the level and spectrum of typical background noise occurring in various environments; (3) the nature and source of the primary signal of interest (e.g., speech or music); and (4) practical field experience fitting the 3M hearing instruments.

Each of the environmental targets, like the prescriptive formulas, calculates a frequency-gain response based on the user's audiometric data. In addition, each target prescribes appropriate compression characteristics in each channel (AGC thresholds and release times; output levels; and microphone limiting) for the various environmental programs based on the considerations outlined above. The flexibility of the multiband compression system allows the fitting system (and the clinician) to program compression characteristics that are appropriate for different gain and tolerance requirements, as well as for different listening situations. By considering both the acoustic environment and the input signals to which the hearing aid must respond, in addition to audiological needs, user comfort, sound quality, and speech understanding can be optimized under a variety of listening conditions.

The Model 80 software is designed to reduce the complexity of the multiple-memory fitting process by allowing the clinician to modify the hearing aid quickly and easily. Adjustments can be made to the various programmable parameters of all programs at once or to individual programs, providing flexibility and ease in custom tailoring the instrument to the patient. During follow-up visits the dispenser can review the datalogging results and, in combination with user reports, modify any or all of the hearing instrument programs as necessary to better meet the needs of the user. In some cases this may mean changes to frequency-gain shaping or to compression parameters, or in others, simply reordering the programs for user convenience. Some individuals may have the need for a hearing aid response designed for a highly specialized situation, such as playing a musical instrument or working in a particularly noisy environment. Such requests can be easily addressed by modifying an existing program or creating a new program with appropriate frequency shaping, gain, and signal processing.

FITTING STRATEGIES

Prescriptive fitting is, in some sense, a compromise. Prescriptive targets are based on average hearing losses and the average speech spectrum. Precisely matching a prescriptive target, whether in a 2 cc coupler or the patient's real ear, does not guarantee either optimum speech intelligibility or optimum sound quality. As discussed earlier, most clinicians recognize that the frequency response that produces the best speech intelligibility may not be the same frequency response that yields the best sound quality as judged by the patient. For example, Harford and Fox (1978) reported that hearing aid wearers preferred reduced low-frequency gain and more high-frequency emphasis when listening to speech in noise. On the other hand, Franks (1982) reported that hearing-impaired listeners selected more low-frequency gain when listening to music than when listening to speech. With a single-response hearing aid, the dispenser is forced to select some compromise fitting between these different optimal responses.

Experimental studies evaluating the concept of multiple-response instruments have shown that listeners will select different frequency responses depending on the input signal and the listening environment (Sullivan et al., 1988; Ringdahl et al., 1990; Goldstein, Shields, and Sandlin, 1991). Recently, Fabry and Stypulkowski (1992) compared user-selected frequency responses to prescribed NAL target gain for three typical listening environments: speech in quiet, speech in noise, and music. In the laboratory, hearing-impaired subjects adjusted the gain in the low- and high-frequency channels of the 3M instrument to preference for each listening situation. Subsequently, the hearing aids were programmed with NAL target gain and one of the user-selected frequency responses. The subjects wore the instruments for two-week periods, but only for listening situations similar to the condition under evaluation. During this field trial the use patterns of the hearing aids were recorded with datalogging. The results revealed several interesting points: (1) In the laboratory,

the majority of subjects selected different frequency responses for the different listening conditions; (2) in the field evaluation, subjects utilized the user-adjusted frequency response more often than the NAL response; and (3) although definite patterns were evident in the changes to the NAL target for the different source materials, the magnitude of these changes varied considerably from individual to individual. These results suggest that users do indeed prefer, and use, different frequency responses for different listening situations and, moreover, that the use of interactive fitting procedures, coupled with the flexibility of programmable instruments, allows for accurate matching of different individual's sound quality preferences for various listening situations.

Frequency shaping represents only one dimension of the real-world performance of a hearing instrument. In addition to the more commonly recognized spectral domain, consideration must also be given to the dynamic performance of the instrument to maximize user comfort, sound quality, and speech intelligibility. Rather than fitting only in the static frequency domain, it is also important to consider the dynamics of sound—that is, the time-intensity domain.

Fitting strategies for the intensity domain encompass the same set of considerations that exist for the frequency domain, namely, the signal of interest, the background noise, and the listening environment. However, rather than focusing on spectral characteristics, it is the dynamic characteristics of these areas that must be analyzed and compensated for.

The practical application of these fitting concepts, in both the frequency and intensity domains, is where multiple-memory capabilities, flexible signal processing, and the power of the PC are optimally combined and utilized. The 3M fitting system software incorporates this multidimensional approach to hearing aid fitting and applies these concepts to each patient's specific hearing loss. The different environmental target algorithms generate a frequency response and compression parameters designed to compensate for the spectral and intensity characteristics of specific listening situations. For example, a response for listening to music would combine a broadband frequency response with a more linear signal processing approach to allow the full dynamics of the music to be realistically experienced while still maintaining appropriate output levels for the patient. Another program designed for use in a group situation would provide a frequency response with additional high-frequency emphasis and a full-spectrum, two-channel signal processing approach. In this case the user would have adequate high-frequency gain to hear a more distant, soft-spoken speaker, but would have appropriate compression so that transient high-frequency noise or a nearby loud talker would not create uncomfortable output levels. The environmental algorithms of the Model 80 software incorporate differences in frequency shaping and signal processing to create hearing aid responses that optimize sound quality, user comfort, and speech understanding in typical environments that are problematic for users of conventional amplification.

CLINICAL INVESTIGATIONS

The 3M programmable BTE and more recently the ITE instrument have been clinically evaluated in a number of studies (Johnson et al., 1988; Soli et al., 1990; Mangold et al., 1990; Ringdahl et al., 1990; Stypulkowski, Hodgson, and Raskind, 1992). The results of these various investigations have consistently indicated that users rate the sound quality and performance of the 3M instruments superior to conventional hearing aids, as well as other programmable instruments, in a number of different listening situations. A universal trend throughout these studies has been sub-

jective user reports that repeatedly highlight the noted performance difference of the 3M instruments in noisy environments.

For example, Figure 6.9 summarizes the subjective ratings of 34 individuals that compared their personal hearing aids to the 3M ITE instrument in various listening situations, using descriptive scales similar to those described by Gabrielsson, Schenkman, and Hagerman (1988) over a two-week trial (Stypulkowski et al., 1992a). For speech in quiet the mean ratings for the 3M instrument ranged between 3 and 4 in each category (grand mean = 3.80) and were higher than the personal aid ratings in all six categories (grand mean = 3.20). As might be expected, in the more difficult listening condition, speech in noise, the overall rating (grand mean) for each of the aids decreased considerably (3M ITE = 2.78 and personal aids = 1.88) . However, the ratings for the 3M instrument remained consistently higher than those of the personal aids, and these differences were statistically significant across all of the rating categories. By comparison to the speech-in-quiet condition, the overall rating decreased by 1.02 points (26.8%) for the 3M instrument and by 1.32 points (41.2%) for the personal aids in this more demanding listening situation. The fact that the overall rating difference between the two aids was nearly a full point higher for the 3M ITE in this condition suggests that more challenging listening environments actually served to highlight the performance differences between the hearing aids.

In this study, as well as many of the others cited, these subjective user reports were substantiated by laboratory speech-in-noise testing, which demonstrated significant improvement in subjects' test scores with the 3M instruments. Figure 6.10 illustrates the speech-in-noise testing results for the study described above. For this evaluation the subjects were first tested with their personal

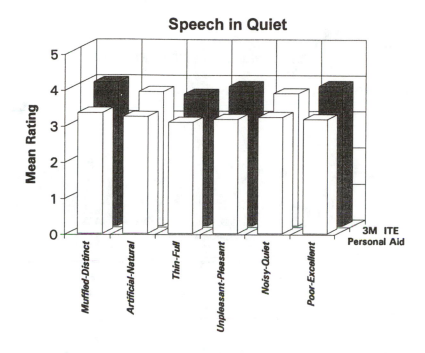

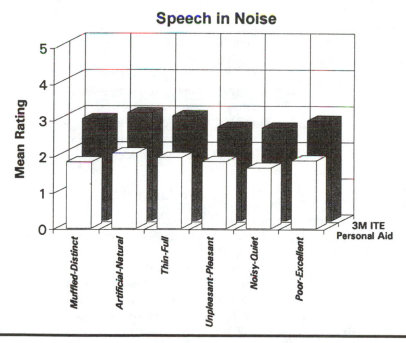

FIGURE 6.9.   Mean subjective ratings for the 3M ITE instrument and personal aids in different listening conditions. Shaded bars indicate categories where mean results are significantly different (p < 0.05, paired t-test, n = 34).

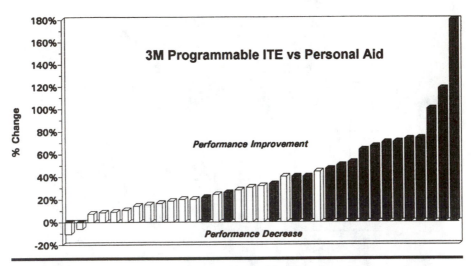

FIGURE 6.10. Speech recognition in noise results. Bars show the percentage change in score for each subject with the 3M ITE instrument compared to the personal aid score. Shaded bars indicate individuals whose scores are significantly different (p < 0.05) with the 3M instrument.

hearing aids adjusted to a comfortable volume for speech presented at 70 dB SPL, and the signal-to-noise ratio of the test stimuli (NU-6 monosyllables in multitalker babble) was adjusted for each individual in order to achieve approximately 50% correct recognition (Plomp and Mimpen, 1979). Each subject was then tested with the 3M instrument, using a program that produced a comfortable listening level, at the same S/N ratio arrived at for the personal aid. Almost all of the subjects (94%) showed some level of improvement with the 3M instrument. The shaded bars in this figure indicate individuals whose test scores were significantly different (p < 0.05) with the 3M instrument compared to the personal aid, based on a statistical analysis of the difference scores (Thornton and Raffin, 1978). The results of this more conservative analysis technique indicate that approximately one-half of the subjects (49%) achieved a significant measurable improvement in speech recognition in noise with the 3M instrument compared to their personal

aids, while none of the subjects had a score that represented a significant decrease in performance. Very similar results were obtained by Soli et al. (1990) in a study evaluating the 3M programmable BTE instrument where, using the same statistical criteria, 64% of the study subjects demonstrated improved speech intelligibility in noise with the 3M instrument compared to their personal aids fitted to a matching NAL prescription.

FUTURE DIRECTIONS

Programmable hearing instruments appear to have been readily accepted by the audiologic community and clearly represent the future direction of hearing instrument technology. Fully digital signal processing instruments remain on the horizon; however, a number of hurdles must be cleared before they become commonplace in clinical practice. The marriage of analog and digital technology in hearing instruments offers a new level of fitting flexibility to the clinician and creates significant new opportunities, but not without some cost. In many ways, programmable instruments have shifted the burden of hearing aid fitting squarely into the lap of the providers (rather than the manufacturers) and have exercised the dispenser's fitting skills beyond those required for conventional instruments. Because of the flexibility that programmables, and particularly the 3M instruments, offer the clinician, the potential for immediate advances in the area of fitting strategies seems great. As mentioned earlier, the concept and clinical practice of hearing aid fitting must extend beyond the frequency domain to encompass also the time-intensity domain of sound.

Research in the field of auditory physiology over the past decade has provided new insights into the function of the normal ear and how this function is altered by varying degrees of hearing loss. Many of the clinical observations regarding the auditory capabilities of individuals with different degrees of hearing loss can now be understood from an underlying physiological basis. It is naive to believe that one prescriptive formula for frequency response or one approach to signal processing will optimally correct these varying degrees of lost function. Clinical research examining different fitting strategies for different degrees of hearing loss is an obvious area of needed investigation.

Improvements in fitting strategies will ultimately benefit both the providers and the users of amplification and will continue to be a focus with the 3M programmable instruments. Because the 3M fitting system is software based, it is readily possible to incorporate new findings into clinically useful algorithms in a relatively short period of time. Next-generation fitting algorithms will go beyond standard audiometric results and prescriptive targets by considering the different requirements dictated by varying degrees of hearing loss when prescribing signal processing parameters for different listening situations. Combining the strengths of real-ear-based fitting with user-interactive fitting methodologies onto a single PC platform will also help to improve both clinical results and user satisfaction. Artificial intelligence (i.e., the ability of computers to "learn" based on performance feedback) is also a likely candidate to improve fitting procedures by "teaching" the fitting system what strategies are the most successful. 3M plans to continue to be a leader in the development of programmable instrument technology, fitting systems, and future technologies, such as fully digital systems, through continued innovation in the hearing health care field.

REFERENCES

Byrne, D., and Dillon, H. (1986). The National Acoustic Laboratories' (NAL) new procedure for selecting the gain and frequency response of a hearing aid. *Ear and Hearing* 7:257–265.

Cox, R.M., and Alexander, G.C. (1991). Preferred hearing aid gain in everyday environments. *Ear and Hearing* 12:123–26.

Engebretsen, A.M., Morley, R.E., and Popelka, G.R. (1987). Development of an ear-level digital aid and computer assisted fitting procedure: An interim report. *Journal of Rehabilitation Research and Development* 24(4):55–64.

Fabry, D.A. (1991). Programmable and automatic noise reduction in existing hearing aids. In: G.A. Studebaker, F.H. Bess, and L.B. Beck (eds.), *The Vanderbilt Hearing Aid Report II*. Parkton, MD: York Press.

Fabry, D.A., and Stypulkowski, P.H. (1992). Evaluation of hearing aid fitting procedures for multiple-memory programmable hearing aids. Annual Meeting of the American Academy of Audiology, Nashville, TN.

Franks, J.R. (1982). Judgments of hearing aid processed music. *Ear and Hearing* 3(1):18–23.

Freyman, R., and Nerbonne, G. (1989). The importance of consonant-vowel intensity ratio in the intelligibility of voiceless consonants. *Journal of Speech and Hearing Research* 32:524–525.

Gabrielsson, A., Schenkman, B.N., and Hagerman, B. (1988). The effects of different frequency responses on sound quality judgments and speech intelligibility. *Journal of Speech and Hearing Research* 31:166–177.

Goldstein, D., Shields, A., and Sandlin, R. (1991). A multiple-memory, digitally-controlled hearing instrument. *Hearing Instruments* 42(1):18–21.

Gordon-Salant, S. (1987). Effects of acoustic modification on consonant recognition in elderly hearing impaired subjects. *Journal of the Acoustical Society of America* 81(4):1199–1202.

Harford, E., and Fox, J. (1978). The use of high-pass amplification for broad-frequency sensorineural hearing loss. *Audiology* 12:10–26.

Johnson, J.S., Kirby, V.M., Hodgson, W.A., and Johnson, L.J. (1988). Clinical study of a programmable, multiple memory hearing instrument. *Hearing Instruments* 39:44–47.

Kates, J.M. (1991). The problem of feedback in hearing aids. *Journal of Communication Disorders* 24:223–235.

Killion, M.C. (1990). A high fidelity hearing aid. *Hearing Instruments* 41(8):38–39.

Killion, M.C., Staab, W.J., and Preves, D.A. (1990). Classifying automatic signal processors. *Hearing Instruments* 41(8):24–26.

Kuk, F.K. (1992). Evaluation of the efficacy of a multimemory hearing aid. *Journal of the American Academy of Audiology* 3:338–348.

Leijon, A., Eriksson-Mangold, M., and Bech-Karlsen, A. (1984). Preferred hearing aid gain and bass cut in relation to prescriptive fitting. *Scandinavian Audiology.* 13:157–161.

Levitt, H. (1991). Future directions in signal processing hearing aids. *Ear and Hearing* 12(suppl. 6):125–130.

Mangold, S. (1982). Programmable hearing aid. In: J. Raviv (ed.), *Use of Computers in Aiding the Disabled* (pp. 135–146). Amsterdam: North-Holland Publishing.

Mangold, S., Eriksson-Mangold, M., Israelsson, B., Leijon, A., and Ringdahl, A. (1990). Multi-programmable hearing aid. *Acta Otolaryngologica* (Suppl. 469):70–75.

Mangold, S., and Leijon, A. (1979). A programmable hearing aid with multi-channel compression. *Scandinavian Audiology* 12:121–126.

Mangold, S., and Leijon, A. (1981). Multichannel compression in a portable programmable hearing aid. *Hearing Aid Journal* 34(6):29–32.

Martin, M.C. (1973). Hearing aid gain requirements in sensorineural hearing loss. *British Journal of Audiology* 7:21–24.

Montgomery, A., and Edge, R. (1988). Evaluation of two speech enhancement techniques to improve intelligibility for hearing impaired adults. *Journal of Speech and Hearing Research* 31:386–393.

Moore, B.C., and Glasberg, B. (1986). A comparison of two-channel and single-channel compression hearing aids. *Audiology* 25:210–226.

Moore, B.C. (1987). Design and evaluation of a two-channel compression hearing aid. *Journal of Rehabilitation Research and Development* 24(4): 181–192.

Plomp, R., and Mimpen, A.M. (1979). Improving the reliability of testing the speech reception threshold for sentences. *Audiology* 18:43.

Preves, D.A., Fortune, T.W., Woodruff, B., and Newton, J. (1991). Strategies for enhancing the consonant to vowel intensity ratio with in the ear hearing aids. *Ear and Hearing* 12(suppl. 6):139–153.

Ringdahl, A., Eriksson-Mangold, M., Israelsson, B., Lindkvist, A., and Mangold, S. (1990). Clinical trials with a programmable hearing aid set for various listening environments. *British Journal of Audiology* 24:235–242.

Soli, S., Allsman, C., Eisenberg, L., et al. (1990). Hearing aid performance in noise: Laboratory and field evaluations of the Nicolet Prism, the Ensoniq Sound Selector, and the 3M MemoryMate hearing aid systems. House Ear Institute Technical Report.

Sullivan, J.A., Levitt, H., Hwang, J.Y., and Hennessey, A.M. (1988). An experimental comparison of four hearing aid prescription methods. *Ear and Hearing* 9:22–32.

Stypulkowski, P.H., Hodgson, W.A., and Raskind, L.A. (1992a) Clinical evaluation of a new programmable multiple memory ITE. *Hearing Instruments* 43(6):25–29.

Stypulkowski, P.H., Raskind, L.A., and Hodgson,

W.A. (1992b). 3M programmable instruments and fitting systems. *Seminars in Hearing* 13(2):135–142.

Thornton, A.R., and Raffin, M.J.M. (1978). Speech discrimination scores modeled as a binomial variable. *Journal of Speech and Hearing Research* 21:507–518.

Van Tasell, D.J., Larsen, S.Y., and Fabry, D.A. (1988). Effects of an adaptive filter hearing aid on speech recognition in noise by hearing-impaired subjects. *Ear and Hearing* 9:15–21.

CHAPTER 7

PROJECT PHOENIX, INC., 1984–1989: THE DEVELOPMENT OF A WEARABLE DIGITAL SIGNAL PROCESSING HEARING AID

Veronica H. Heide

Project Phoenix of Madison, Inc. (1984), named after a Phoenix Arizona meeting at which the project was approved, was a joint venture among the University of Wisconsin, the Wisconsin Alumni Research Foundation, and Nicolet Instrument Corporation to research and bring to market a digital signal processing hearing aid. The project also received additional support from the Technology Development Fund administered by the Wisconsin Department of Development. The magnitude of this venture cannot be overstated. It meant compromises on the part of all involved to accommodate different policies and procedures, as well as different styles of doing research, development, and manufacturing.

The first nine months of the project were devoted to the development of resources. In addition to researchers, clinical subjects were recruited from local communities, and software and hardware were acquired in preparation for data collection. The next six months were devoted to research toward the development of specific signal processing algorithms. Eighty-nine protocols, including pilot studies, were completed. The experiments fell into the categories of behavioral research, speech science, electrophysiologic research, mathematical modeling, and nonlinear systems analysis, and looked at the topics of external auditory canal acoustics, temporal resolution, profile discrimination, speech perception in noise, frequency resolution, masking effects, and auditory adaptation.

The term *individual* is perhaps the key word in the story of Project Phoenix. The participants believed that there were individual differences in auditory perception and that these individual differences were not easily measured by conventional testing (Hecox and Miller, 1987). Digital signal processing had the potential to provide new solutions for speech enhancement for the hearing impaired that were simply not possible to achieve using analog technology.

Since Project Phoenix ended, many people have asked, "If you had it to do all over again, knowing now what the end would be, would you?" The answer would be an unqualified "Absolutely!" Project Phoenix was people. It brought together audiologists, engineers, speech scientists, manufacturing specialists,

Unless otherwise noted, figures and photographs in this chapter are reprinted with permission of Nicolet Instrument Corporation, 5225 Verona Road, Madison, WI.

Nicolet Phoenix®, Aurora®, and FLEXSYS® are registered trademarks of Nicolet Instrument Corporation.

and managers. It brought together a university, a private company, and a not-for-profit corporation. Most of all, it brought hearing-impaired individuals into the product development cycle. This chapter highlights some of the significant technical accomplishments of the project. Some of these were products that were brought to market, others were not, but each played a significant role in the development of the world's first digital hearing aid, the Nicolet Phoenix.

WHAT WAS THE NICOLET PHOENIX?

The Nicolet Phoenix was the first wearable digital signal processing hearing aid available to the consumer. The two-piece device consisted of an analog front end in the form of a behind-the-ear hearing aid connected to a pocket computer with a cord. Sound was picked up by the microphone at ear level, pre-amplified, and fed to the pocket computer. Inside the pocket processor the continuously varying analog signal was converted into numbers, transformed through mathematical manipulation, and then returned to an analog signal that was sent through a receiver to the listener's ear (see Figure 7.1). This meant that the performance of the Phoenix was based not only on good analog engineering, but also on the skills of the mathematicians who wrote the programs that manipulated the numbers inside the processor.

The Nicolet Phoenix differed from digitally controlled analog devices in the way it processed sound. It also differed from other hearing aids in the philosophy and integration of the product's design, development, and fitting. Engineering and marketing worked side by side with the human factors group, consumers, and customer support, documentation, and training to make sure that they were all unified in their vision of what was important to the hearing-impaired

consumer. The device, the fitting system, the product development team, the audiologists involved in fitting the Phoenix, and the hearing-impaired users were linked together by a common desire to find new solutions to the many problems hearing-impaired consumers faced. The initial problems that the Phoenix addressed included hearing with fidelity for different configurations of hearing loss, hearing with minimal interference from background noise, and hearing without annoying acoustic feedback.

Inherent in the development of the digital hearing aid was the belief that the development of a method of fitting these digital hearing aids was just as important as the device itself (Miller, 1988; Hecox and Punch, 1988). This drove the development of the Aurora, a computer-based digital signal processing audiodiagnostic and hearing aid fitting system. Because of this fitting strategy, engineering and research staff for the Aurora and Phoenix worked closely together.

In this chapter we will talk about the development of the Phoenix as a project and as a device. We will discuss three significant technological achievements of the project: the development of the Portable Processing Unit, the Hearing Aid Listening system, and the Aurora (audiodiagnostic and hearing aid fitting system) Hearing Aid Fitting module. Finally, in the last section we will discuss the Nicolet Phoenix device. These projects are all landmark achievements in the areas of instrumentation for hearing evaluation, hearing aid evaluation, and hearing aid fitting.

THE PPU

Three areas were identified for initial product development of the digital hearing aid: frequency shaping, noise reduction, and loudness discomfort. These areas were chosen based on surveys of the industry and the con-

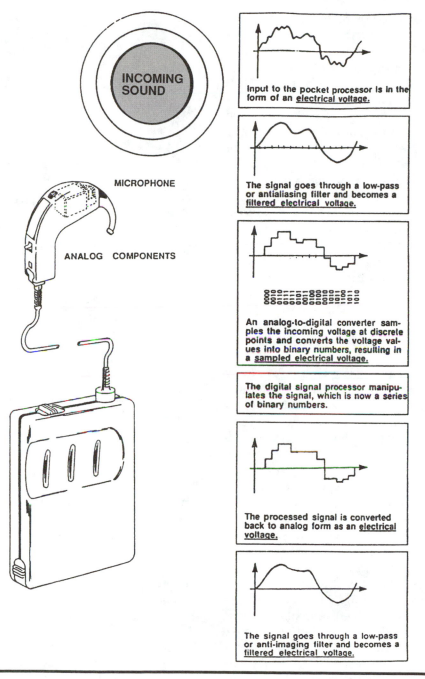

FIGURE 7.1.   The Nicolet Phoenix® and its signal path.

sumer. We felt that there was still much we needed to understand about the ear with sensorineural loss and felt that basic research as well as product development would be imperative to the successful development of new types of digital signal processing strategies. We also realized the need to characterize and evaluate the factors that contributed to individuals' preferences for sound processing as well as factors that improved some measurable aspect of performance, such as speech discrimination or matching a target gain rule.

Laboratory experiments were conducted in the areas of evoked potentials, real-ear measurement, and speech perception. It soon became apparent that, although laboratories were ideal for controlling a number of acoustic and research variables, it was essential to couple the laboratory data with real-world data. Thus was born our first portable digital hearing aid, the Portable Processing Unit (Figure 7.2) (Cummins and Hecox, 1987).

The Portable Processing Unit (PPU) was a battery-powered digital signal processing system measuring 8″ × 5″ × 3″ and weighing about 6 lbs. Four alkaline batteries powered the unit for about seven hours. A separate preamplifier box connected the wideband hearing aid microphone and receiver housed in the behind-the-ear case to the processing unit.

Incoming sound was received by the microphone of the behind-the-ear unit, conditioned by the preamplifier, and sent to the processor. Two separate channels were available, which provided the ability to evaluate binaural amplification strategies and two-channel noise canceling. The input channels contained low-pass filters (anti-aliasing) and were multiplexed into a single 12-bit analog-to-digital converter (ADC). The number of bits in the ADC is related to the accuracy with which a signal can be represented by the microprocessor. The PPU and the Phoenix used a CMOS TMS320C10 DSP chip as the microprocessor. This chip was the brain behind the

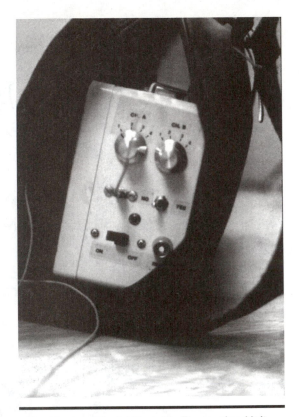

FIGURE 7.2.   Nicolet Portable Processing Unit (PPU).

box. The processor changed the signal according to the instructions in the program. The two output channels from the processing unit also contained a 12-bit digital-to-analog converter (DAC) followed by a 2-pole low-pass filter. The signal was sent back through the preamplifier and then to the hearing aid (Palmer et al., 1987).

The PPU had different modes of operation that were determined by the position of a 4-bit DIP switch mounted on the processor board. The operating modes included a self-diagnostics mode, monitor mode, and up to 14 other DSP applications modes. In the monitor mode, the PPU could communicate with another computer through an RS232 port to inspect memory, modify memory, download programs, upload programs, or reset the system. In the self-diagnostics mode, the two four-position switches were used to test gain, analog bandwidth, DAC linearity, and the overall system status. The 14 DSP applications were EPROM resident. Each of the fourteen application programs used up to 4k words of program memory and contained information about the program, the parameters set during the fitting process, and the data collected during a given experiment (Cummins and Hecox, 1987).

The PPU was invaluable for field research. Statistical data from the PPU's timeline log were recorded and analyzed. The PPU could record the acoustic level in the environment at sampling intervals of 1 to 15 seconds. A minimum and maximum sound pressure level was also recorded for each sample. In addition, a record was kept of the typical distribution of switch selections. A toggle switch was used as an event marker in the time line. This was typically used by the participants in our studies to mark the perception of something they perceived, such as the presence of a sound that was uncomfortably loud. This meant that we had a record of the actual sound level experienced by the participant in the field, as well as an indication of the *perception* of that loud sound on the part of the participant.

The PPU required cooperative efforts on the part of engineering and the human factors groups to define the complexity and number of algorithms to be tested, define the protocol, and decide how best to implement the protocol in the PPU. For example, it very quickly became apparent that although it would be nice to evaluate 16 algorithms in the field simultaneously, our subjects could realistically only evaluate three or four in one experiment without getting them mixed up. The use of the PPU required engineering support not only for the hardware and DSP program de-

velopment, but also for the development of a software package that could be used for programming and fitting.

The PPU protocols primarily involved comparisons between various digital algorithms such as multiband versus single-band compression, various strategies for noise reduction, loudness control, and speech enhancement. In one study, we wanted to find out if laboratory methods of prescribing gain were indicative of the gain level preferred by the subject in the real world.

Most comfortable loudness (MCL) levels were established in the laboratory to connected discourse. The PPU was programmed so that the subject was able to increase and decrease the volume in 4 dB steps. Their MCL served as the midpoint on the volume control. Timeline data from the PPU provided a record of the frequency with which various gain settings were selected.

The MCL data obtained in the field using the PPU were compared to the data collected in the laboratory. Of the 20 subjects tested, 10 left the volume at the prescribed setting; 7 used a gain setting 4 to 8 dB lower than the laboratory-preferred gain more than 50% of the time and 3 used a 4 dB higher gain setting than prescribed more than 50% of the time.

The results of this study and others using the PPU were important for the development of a fitting strategy for the Nicolet Phoenix and for the development of the software for the hearing aid fitting module of the Aurora audiodiagnostic workstation. If laboratory selection of the hearing aid fitting parameters had not been predictive of real-world success, then developing a hearing aid fitting module designed to be used in a sound-treated room using a nonportable computer would be inappropriate. We questioned, "Do we fit in a sound-treated room where we can control the environment, or do we fit in the real world where we have little control, but a more realistic acoustic space?" The final hearing aid fitting strategy used to fit the Phoenix incorporated both of these components and will be discussed in the final section of this chapter.

THE HEARING AID LISTENING SYSTEM: A SYSTEM FOR BEHAVIORAL COMPARISON OF MULTIPLE HEARING AIDS

Just as the field evaluations were greatly enhanced by the use of the PPU, we needed a device to facilitate rapid paired-comparison testing in the laboratory. We felt that paired-comparison testing was a valid method of evaluating client preference and relative intelligibility (Studebaker et al., 1982), yet we were not comfortable with the available clinical tools.

One method commonly used to perform paired-comparison testing in the clinic was to let a client listen to one hearing aid, take it off, fit the second hearing aid, and report which one was better. The disadvantage of this method was that in the time it took to take one aid off and put the second aid on and adjust it, the client had forgotten how the first aid sounded.

Master hearing aids were another clinically available tool used to incorporate client preference into the selection of amplification. The disadvantage of the conventional master hearing aid was that the examiner often introduced his/her own bias ("How about *this* one") into the selection process and that the components used in the master hearing aid circuit were different from the components used in the hearing aids that were actually received by the client.

Another method of implementing paired-comparison testing into the hearing aid selection process was to use a switch box or comparison box. Two hearing aids were attached to the comparison device using tubing (for BTE aids). The client listened through a hearing aid stethoscope or earphone to the aids, switching back and forth between them.

Although the comparison device offered the advantage of allowing fairly rapid switching between devices, the acoustical signal path was significantly altered by the device and the listening attachment (stethoscope).

In summary, traditional paired-comparison methods were too time consuming, introduced an examiner bias, used different circuitry than the aid the client ultimately received, and altered the acoustical signal path. The need for a device to facilitate rapid paired comparisons between hearing aids or between different DSP algorithms and different hearing aids was apparent.

The Hearing Aid Listening system (HAL) was designed as a multidevice comparison system for use in a controlled acoustic environment (Heide et al., 1987). The HAL system allowed the listener to switch rapidly and repeatedly among five hearing aids that were placed in the same sound field. The HAL system had the advantage over other comparative techniques of being able to switch rapidly between comparison hearing aids while also compensating for the change in the signal path so that the listener heard the device as if it were actually being worn.

Description of the HAL Hardware

The HAL system consisted of a PC with a signal processing coprocessor board, a black box containing five independent coupler/microphone amplifier channels that were fed into a channel selector whose output was sent to the listener's earmold through a receiver that was worn like a behind-the-ear (BTE) hearing aid (Figure 7.3). The five 2 cc acoustic couplers were arranged in a circle on top of the HAL. Each coupler was connected to a half-inch microphone, the gain of which was adjusted in three 20 dB steps according to the maximum power output of the corresponding hearing aid.

During a study, the BTE hearing aids to be

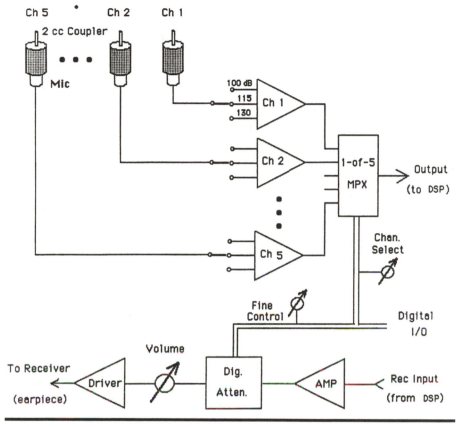

FIGURE 7.3. Hearing Aid Listening System (HAL).

evaluated were connected to the couplers with one inch of #13 standard walled tubing. The channel selection, which determined which hearing aid the listener heard, could be controlled remotely by the PC or by a selection knob on the front panel of the HAL. The selected output was externally processed and then passed through an attenuator and a potentiometer. The attenuator had a 0–46.5 dB range in 1.5 dB steps and could be controlled remotely by the PC or by a knob on the front panel of HAL. Finally, the signal was delivered to the HAL receiver, which was worn behind the listeners' ears and connected to their custom earmolds. Binaural studies were only possible using two HALs.

The parallel I/O interface card (Metrabyte PIO12) in the PC was used to determine whether the digital attenuator and microphone multiplexer were controlled remotely from the PC or by the listener from the front panel knobs. The signal processing was performed by a coprocessor board that plugged into the PC. Both ARIEL DSP-16 and ASPI PC/320 boards were used in different generations of the HAL. Both of these boards had an analog-to-digital converter (ADC), a digital-to-analog (DAC) converter, and a Texas Instruments 320 family DSP chip. The PC and DSP processors ran in parallel and were able to communicate back and forth. The sampling rate of the ADC and DAC was 16 kHz. The input and output were sent through anti-aliasing and anti-imaging filters (Krohn-Hite model 3343 filter containing 8th-order Butterworth low-pass filters) with cutoff frequencies of 7 kHz.

The use of a remote computer interface allowed flexibility in protocol development. Changes in the software could be made to modify existing protocols or create new protocols. The use of a remote computer interface also allowed the examiner to blind the subject as to which aids were being compared. The ability to perform such blinded studies made the HAL system not only a useful tool for comparing hearing aids, but also an invaluable tool for researching and developing new hearing aids and signal processing algorithms.

Digital Signal Processing in the HAL

The HAL receiver, earhook, tubing, and coupler introduced changes in the frequency response of the hearing aid at the listener's ear. DSP techniques were used to compensate for these changes so that the signal delivered to

the listener's ear was the same as if he or she were wearing the hearing aid (Figure 7.4). This was accomplished mathematically by subtracting the effects of these changes before the sound was presented to the listener. Technically, this was done by calculating inverse filters of the added path for each channel.

The acoustic properties of the HAL receiver, earhook, tubing, and coupler were modeled as linear shift invariant (LSI) systems. (A linear system is one in which the output can be modeled as the weighted sum of the inputs. Time or shift invariant means that a shift in time in the input only causes a shift in time in the output.) The filtering due to these volumes occurred at different places in the signal path, but according to the rules of LSI systems, the cascaded effect could be characterized by the impulse response of the coupled volumes. An inverse filter of these components was computed from the impulse response and introduced into the signal path. Since the inverse was also LSI, the position of the compensation filters in the signal path was not important.

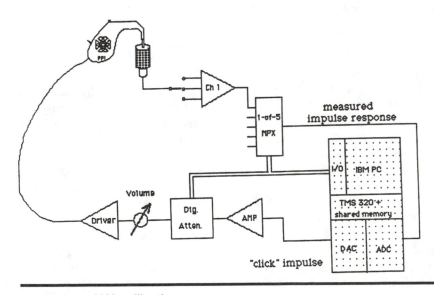

FIGURE 7.4.   HAL calibration.

The compensation filters were computed periodically using a calibration procedure in which the HAL receiver was connected to the 2 cc coupler. A series of impulses was generated by the DSP board. The impulses were presented through the HAL receiver, exciting the coupled volumes of the earhook, tubing, and coupler. The response of these volumes to an impulse was recorded by the microphone and sent back to the DSP board. The DSP board generated 100 impulses and averaged the responses. This averaging greatly reduced the effects of any environmental noise that might have been present. The DSP board then sent the impulse response, 120 samples or 7.5 msec in length, to the PC. An inverse filter to the averaged impulse response was computed by the PC using a constrained recursive least-squares deconvolution method. The compensation filter was a 50-tap Finite Impulse Response (FIR) filter.

The bandwidth of interest was limited by the anti-aliasing and anti-imaging filters, which had cutoff frequencies of 7 kHz. This bandwidth was sufficient to represent the bandwidth of the hearing aids. Because of this, the bandwidth of the inverse filter was also limited by putting a constraint on the first derivative of the solution to the deconvolution process. Intuitively, this means telling the inversion algorithm not to spend all its effort trying to compensate for frequencies above the range of interest.

Measurements of the compensated and uncompensated signal path were made with a Hewlett-Packard 3561A signal analyzer. Figure 7.5 shows the frequency response of the HAL without the external signal processing, or the uncompensated response, while Figure 7.6 shows the compensated response of the HAL. Note the rapid roll-off of the high-frequency response in the uncompensated response (Figure 7.5). In the compensated response in Figure 7.6, note that the system is flat out to 7 kHz. The sharp fall-off after 7 kHz

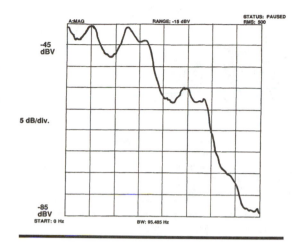

FIGURE 7.5. Uncompensated frequency response of HAL.

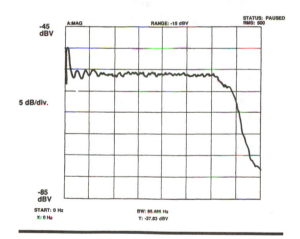

FIGURE 7.6. Compensated frequency response of HAL.

is due to the anti-aliasing and anti-imaging filters associated with digitization.

Use of the HAL for Laboratory Testing

The HAL system and listener were placed in a sound-treated booth that had been acoustically treated with Sonex acoustical foam, while the PC with the parallel I/O and DSP

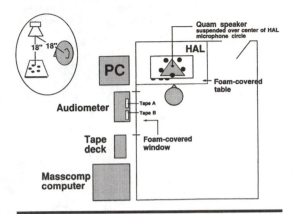

FIGURE 7.7.   Equipment configuration for HAL studies.

boards were outside the booth (Figure 7.7). A loudspeaker was positioned either above the circle of 2 cc couplers or at grazing incidence to the microphones of the BTE hearing aids to be evaluated. The acoustic environment in which HAL was placed was carefully controlled to insure that each of the five coupler/microphone/amplifier input channels received the same spectral shape and sound pressure level inputs. Measurements made of the acoustical environment insured that each hearing aid received the same spectral shape and sound level input within 3 dB.

The listener could be positioned inside the booth with HAL or inside another sound-treated booth. This allowed for flexibility in signal presentation. When the listener was positioned inside the same booth as the HAL, the subject received not only the output of the HAL, but also the direct field effect from the loudspeaker. The listener could also be isolated from the direct field effect of the loudspeaker by positioning him/her inside another sound-treated booth.

Evaluation of Loudness-Limiting Circuits of Hearing Aids

One of the basic goals in selecting a hearing aid is to find an instrument that provides ad-

equate gain without exceeding the listener's tolerance levels. The fitting goal is to maintain the speech input, but limit the output for loud, nonspeech input. This fitting goal is often difficult to achieve because the gain setting that is comfortable for a hearing aid user in a quiet room is typically not the preferred gain setting in a noisy environment.

Specifications for loudness-limiting capabilities of hearing aids have been defined by ANSI for steady-state sounds. However, ANSI specifications do not address impulse sounds. Transient sounds are insidious because most hearing aid limiting circuits do not react fast enough to completely limit the transient, and because of the fast nature of the transient, the listener may not perceive the sound to be uncomfortably loud.

A study was designed to look at how hearing aid users perceived the abilities of various hearing aids to limit loud sounds. The aids were an automatic signal processing aid, a hybrid-chip noise reduction aid, an AGC aid, a compression aid with a variable release time, and a digital hearing aid. The aids had been set according to the following criteria:

1. Knees of the AGC aids were set to their lowest settings.
2. Tone controls were adjusted to provide equivalent frequency response curves for a 50 dB SPL input (below the threshold of compression), as illustrated in Figure 7.8.

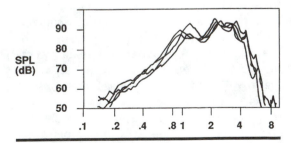

FIGURE 7.8.   Composite frequency response curves of hearing aids used in HAL study (50 dB input).

3. Gain for a 50 dB speech-noise input was set to provide 35 dB of gain.
4. Output controls of the aids were set to provide a maximum output of 120 dB at 2000 Hz. Peak output of the aids did not exceed 120 dB SPL, according to ANSI specs.
5. Peak and transient peak outputs were measured through a Zwislocki coupler. Input/output curves for rms versus crest factor

measurements were plotted for all test aids (Figure 7.9).

Three kinds of measures were performed on the hearing aids selected for inclusion in the study:

1. *ANSI standard curves.* Hearing aids were evaluated according to the ANSI standard (S-3.22, 1987) method of measurement. Curves

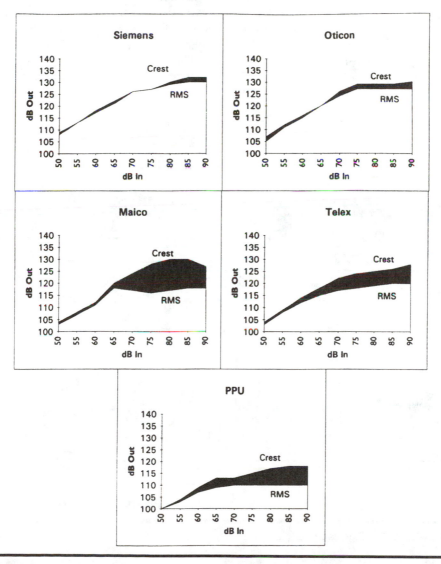

FIGURE 7.9.   Comparison of crest to RMS SPL of hearing aids used in HAL study.

included frequency response curves, full-on gain curves with 90 dB input, and so forth. All hearing aids used in the study met current manufacturer's specifications.

2. *AGC crest factor measurement.* The AGC crest factor was defined as the dB difference between the steady-state peak output of the aid for a test level and the peak output for a 25 dB transition from a conditioning level to the test level.

3. *Input dynamic range measurement.* The input dynamic range measure was meant to reflect the usable input dynamic range (in dB)—that is, the range of sound intensities that were bracketed by the individual's abil-

ity to hear just barely and the input level at which sound becomes uncomfortably loud.

Use of the HAL for Physical Measurements

The loudness-limiting circuits of hearing aids can be characterized with physical acoustic measurements, as well as psychoacoustic measurements of the hearing aids. The first part of the study used HAL to obtain physical measurements to ensure that the characterization reflected the same acoustic environment that would be encountered in the behavioral studies.

The responses of the five hearing aids to four types of impulsive sounds were recorded

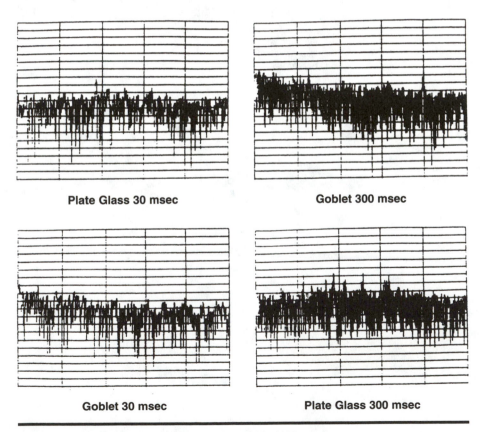

Plate Glass 30 msec

Goblet 300 msec

Goblet 30 msec

Plate Glass 300 msec

FIGURE 7.10.   Digitized sound samples used in HAL study.

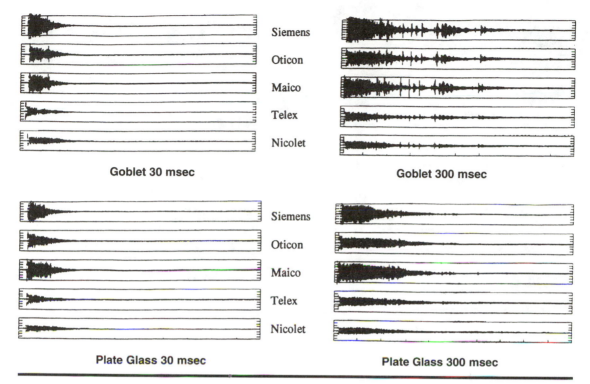

Goblet 30 msec

Goblet 300 msec

Plate Glass 30 msec

Plate Glass 300 msec

FIGURE 7.11.   Digitized recordings of responses of hearing aids to transient stimuli at 97 dB.

with the HAL system. The impulsive sounds used as stimuli were stylized from two recorded sound effects: a breaking goblet (GBL) and a breaking plate glass (PLT). This material was chosen based on differing spectral characteristics and short temporal rise times .

Stimulus Generation.   The sound effects were shaped with an exponential window with several different time constants. The two time constants chosen for the experiments were 30 msec and 300 msec. Figure 7.10 illustrates the two sound effects windowed with the two exponentials. The rise time of the impulse is 0.3 msec. The frequency response of the stimulus is also shown.

Response Recording. The two sound effects, a plate glass breaking and a goblet breaking, were presented at 97 dB SPL and 115 dB SPL to the five hearing aids. The responses of each of the hearing aids to the single presentation of each of the four stimuli were sampled, digitized, and stored. The responses of the five hearing aids were sampled at 20 kHz with a Masscomp 5500 with 12-bit resolution. The signal was anti-alias filtered to 10 kHz. The digitized recordings were then edited and displayed on a single page to allow visual comparison of the time series waveform (Figures 7.11 and 7.12).

The effect of position was found to cause at most a 3 dB difference in the output levels

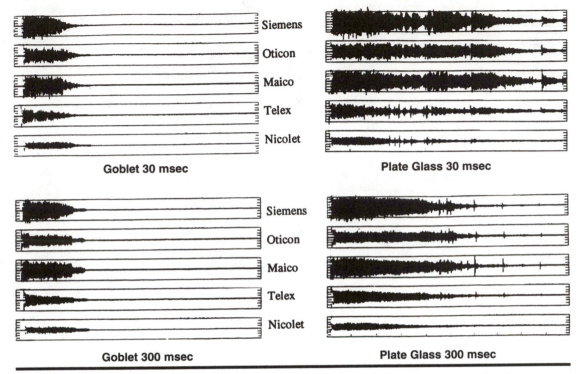

FIGURE 7.12.   Digitized recordings of responses of hearing aids to transient stimuli at 115 dB.

through the hearing aids; typically, the positions caused a difference of no more than 1 dB. This was acceptable for the purposes of our measurements.

Quantitative Analysis.   The amount of energy computed for a given integration period (500 msec) was chosen as a quantitative metric to compare the impulsive nature of the responses. Although crest factor measurements have been traditionally used to describe the relationship between peak amplitude and rms, Erdreich (1986) pointed out: "A single crest factor cannot be representative of a multiple peak, nonstationary waveform." He used a calculation of *kurtosis*, the same approach used to characterize impulsive helicopter noise by the ISO, to represent the peakedness of the amplitude distribution.

This approach was compelling to us as well. We felt that crest factor measurement presented a static measurement of a dynamic event. We decided to characterize the impulsiveness of a sound through various hearing aids by calculating kurtosis (the 4th moment of the amplitude distribution). The rms (dB) and kurtosis are plotted in Figure 7.13 as a function of the 40 response recordings. Note that Telex and the Phoenix have approximately the same rms levels, but differ remarkably in the shape of their amplitude distribution. The Telex has a greater computed kurtosis, indicating a more impulsive sound.

Use of the HAL for Behavioral Studies

The HAL made possible studies that involved rapid paired comparisons between

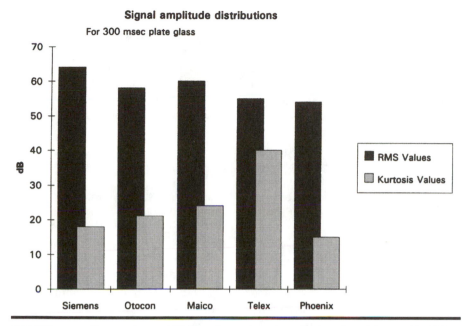

FIGURE 7.13. Comparison of RMS to kurtosis values for hearing aids used in HAL study.

devices. Although the previous physical measurements through the HAL had shown that the Nicolet Phoenix provided improved loudness-limiting capabilities, we had no evidence that this improvement was perceptually significant for the hearing-impaired individuals for whom it was designed.

Following the physical characterization of these impulsive sounds, three behavioral studies were performed in which various aspects of the output-limiting circuitry of the hearing aids were evaluated:

1. Loudness limiting of transients
2. Dynamic range for continuous discourse
3. Sound quality for different input intensities

Loudness Limiting of Transients. The participants' earmolds were connected to the HAL receiver earpiece. The participants wore the receiver connected to a custom earmold and were asked to adjust the volume of the HAL to their most comfortable level (a level that was neither too soft nor too loud). Transient digitized recordings of four impulsive environmental sounds were presented at 97 dB peak SPL with the continuous discourse in the background (50 dB HL). The participants were allowed to listen to the transient through pairs of hearing aids until they decided which aid limited the loudness of the transient most effectively. This typically required three to four presentations. The digital aid was compared with each of the four analog aids. Each comparison was presented to the participant three times for each of the four transient sounds.

Participants controlled the presentation of the transients using a three-button mouse. The far left button was pressed to switch between the comparison aids and the far right button was used to vote for their preferred aid. A total of 60 comparisons were made across participants (5 participants × 12 comparisons). The results showed that the digital aid was perceived to limit transients better than any of the other four aids 97% of the time.

Dynamic Range for Continuous Discourse. In the second study, participants were asked to listen to samples of continuous discourse presented through the loudspeaker to the HAL and to decide if the sample was acceptably loud or intolerably loud. The input intensities ranged from 63 to 93 dB SPL. The presentation level and order of hearing aid presentation were randomized. The speech samples were never presented at levels above those indicated to be too loud by the participant.

The results showed that all but one participant were able to tolerate louder speech with the digital aid than with the analog aids used in the study. The one participant who did not show a preference for the digital aid tolerated the same level of loud speech for all aids compared.

Sound Quality. In the third study, the same five participants were asked to judge the quality of a woman's voice at several intensities ranging from comfortable (63 dB SPL) to loud (93 dB SPL). The participants used the three-button mouse to switch between the comparisons and to vote for their preference. The digital aid was judged as having higher sound quality at higher intensity levels 98% of the time.

The HAL enabled us to demonstrate that the digital signal processing used to control loud noise in the PPU was significantly better than the loudness-limiting circuitry available in analog hearing aids. Even though we could prove this by using an oscilloscope, we were compelled by the mission statement of our project to demonstrate that this was a change that was perceptually significant for the hearing-impaired individuals for whom it was designed. It is altogether too easy to fall into the specification-sheet game of comparing

hearing aids. The true test of significant accomplishment lies in its benefit to the hearing-impaired individuals. The next time a representative from a hearing aid manufacturer comes knocking at your door with a specification sheet in hand, read it carefully and then ask, "Show me the data that describe the benefit for the hearing aid user."

Summary

The HAL system was used to investigate frequency shaping, noise reduction, and bandwidth-limiting studies. We felt that the use of the HAL facilitated timely data acquisition and allowed rapid device comparisons in acoustically characterized environments. This allowed us to obtain efficient, reliable behavioral data to corroborate laboratory studies.

The Hearing Aid Listening (HAL) system's ability to switch between hearing aids rapidly means that comparative studies such as these are possible for the following reasons:

1. The time it takes to switch between devices is fast enough that the participant can still remember what the first device sounded like. Although participants in traditional hearing aid comparison situations often have difficulty deciding which aid they prefer, this was not a problem in the HAL study.

2. The switching can be controlled manually inside the booth or remotely by computer. This allows for effective blinding of the participants if this is desired in a study.

3. The use of the HAL for physical acoustic measurements allows the characterization of the responses of the hearing aids under investigation in the same signal path and acoustic space as in the behavioral study.

The HAL system was used in our internal clinical trials of the digital aid, as well as in the above studies. The use of the HAL system facilitated the acquisition of laboratory data in a timely manner. It allowed us to evaluate hearing-impaired listeners' perceptions of sound quality, loudness limiting, and dynamic range characteristics of hearing aids, as well as obtain speech discrimination measurements through multiple hearing aids in a timely manner. The HAL was invaluable in comparing the performance of various algorithms under consideration for use in the Nicolet Phoenix, as well as for comparing various generations of the Nicolet Phoenix during the course of its development.

THE IMPORTANCE OF FITTING

It would be impossible to discuss the Nicolet Phoenix without mentioning the Nicolet Aurora. The Aurora was the first commercially available computer-based audiodiagnostic workstation. It provided full integration of test data between its modules. The Aurora modules included Audiometer, Real Ear, Hearing Aid Analyzer, Hearing Aid Fitting, Database, and a utilities module that included a sound level meter, as well as the routine for digital calibration of the earphones and loudspeakers. A personal computer module allowed access to DOS and DOS applications. An optional external PC-based middle ear analyzer was able to transfer its data to the Aurora data base through a serial data cable.

The Aurora was developed because of the Phoenix (PPI, 1987). The philosophy of Project Phoenix was that the fitting of this new technology was going to be just as important to the success of the device as the digital aid itself. Traditionally, hearing aid manufacturers had left the fitting of the device up to the dispenser. Nicolet chose to tackle it head on. Coming to consensus about the optimum fitting strategy was not an easy task, especially since development work on the Nicolet Phoenix was proceeding in parallel with the work on the Aurora.

Exhaustive literature reviews that would

be worthy of any doctoral dissertation were performed and summarized in short order. Experts were consulted. Phone calls were made to key researchers in the area of hearing aid selection. We quickly came to the conclusion that there are many different ways to fit hearing aids.

Since we were not sure which method or combination of methods would ultimately prove to be successful, we incorporated the ability to perform functional gain, speech discrimination, real-ear analysis, and hearing aid analysis into the modules of the Aurora. Digital signal processing was used in the Aurora to generate accurate test signals and to analyze test data rapidly. The multitasking nature of the Vertx operating system of the Aurora allowed for the possible future development of software that would provide the flexibility to perform multiple tasks simultaneously; for example, the potential to analyze a hearing aid in the background while performing a hearing evaluation in the audiometer mode.

Using Real Ear to fit the hearing aid to the client's target gain rule was one strategy that was evaluated. The Aurora Real Ear module was one of our customers' favorite modules and the mother of another Nicolet product, the FLEXSYS. It incorporated digitally generated wideband noise and pure tone test signals with signal averaging (Punch, Chi, and Allan, 1990) and a patented algorithm that allowed the examiner to determine how far the probe microphone was from the eardrum (Chan and Geisler, 1990). In addition, the color-coded curves and separate screens for the calculated insertion loss/gain and in situ loss/gain measurements made it a terrific teaching tool by which to learn real-ear measurements (Heide, 1991).

The Real Ear module also incorporated a new measurement called the *real ear-coupler difference* measurement, which provided a way to obtain the difference between in situ gain (aided response of the hearing aid in the client's ear) and the 2 cc coupler response of a hearing aid. From this measurement a target 2 cc coupler response could be obtained. The target coupler response was then used as a template to find the 2 cc coupler response from manufacturers' specification books that would meet the target gain rule the examiner had selected (Punch et al., 1990).

Project Phoenix was founded on the premise that there were individual differences in hearing losses that could not be characterized by conventional measurements. Real-ear measurements were helpful in understanding what was going on in the ear canal, but did not incorporate client preference as a criterion for successful fitting.

Gilbert and Sullivan may have had the answer when they said, "Let the punishment fit the crime." We felt that it was time that certain aspects of the hearing aid fitting be moved into a real-world environment. Background noises for hearing aid fitting should be selected based on the environments where the individual is experiencing difficulty, rather than the carefully modulated and manufactured multi-talker noise so often used in diagnostic testing. This meant that clients were encouraged to make tape recordings of their office noise or kitchen noise and bring it in for the hearing aid fitting. We asked spouses to read from *Reader's Digest* or other periodicals during the fitting, if these voices were difficult for the hearing-impaired person to hear. We wanted to recreate the situations where the hearing-impaired listener was having difficulty. We encouraged examiners to bring music with a wide dynamic range into their fittings and to use material that was relevant to the client and representative of the types of sounds that they would encounter in the real world.

Revised Simplex Method

The first hearing aid fitting strategy incorporating client preference was developed for the Nicolet Aurora to select the programs for

frequency shaping and noise reduction in the Nicolet Phoenix. This method was based on a modified simplex method of adaptive paired-comparison testing (Levitt, 1978). The work of Neuman et al. (1987) on adaptive hearing aid selection strategies was compelling to us because it showed that hearing-impaired subjects could reliably and efficiently converge on a preference for sound processing.

Levitt et al. (1987) describe the simplex method as "... statistically more efficient than the other two procedures (round robin and tournament paired comparison methods), but requires a computer for rapid selection and control of the experimental conditions." The Aurora hearing aid fitting procedure was designed:

1. To provide a method of individualizing the electroacoustic characteristics of the hearing aid.
2. To have an efficient and reliable method of evaluating client preference.
3. To insure that the acoustic experience of the hearing impaired during the fitting was a valid predictor of their preference in the real world.
4. To insure that the signal path used in the fitting was the same as that used in the digital hearing aid.

The Revised Simplex Test in the hearing aid fitting module of the Aurora implemented the rules of the simplex method based on the responses of the client. This adaptive paired-comparison test was used to determine a client's preference for the digital algorithms that were to be programmed into the Nicolet Phoenix. The first two algorithms that were developed were those for frequency shaping and noise reduction.

In the Revised Simplex Test on the Aurora, a two-dimensional matrix (Figure 7.14) was constructed for each of the test conditions. These conditions included determining the client's preference for frequency response,

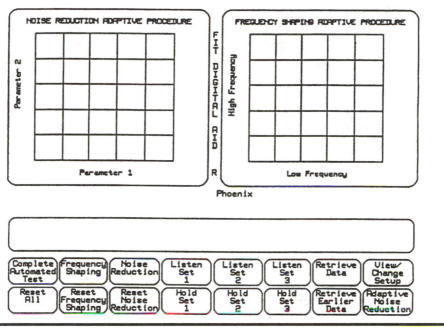

FIGURE 7.14. Revised Simplex Test matrix.

frequency response in noise, and noise reduction. In the frequency-shaping matrix, the rows corresponded to changes in low-frequency gain and the columns corresponded to changes in high-frequency gain. Each cell represented a possible frequency shape that the client could choose.

The digital filters in the Nicolet Phoenix were set so that their center frequencies corresponded to the audiometric frequencies of 250, 500, 1000, 2000, and 4000 Hz. The frequency response for the starting center cell was selected based on the client's audiometric thresholds and the examiner-selected target gain rule. The New NAL (Byrne and Dillon, 1986) rule was the default rule. The amount of gain at 1000 Hz was fixed. Changes in gain in the high frequencies and low frequencies above and below 1000 Hz were always made in equal amounts of 6 or 12 dB. For example, if clients listened to the center cell and the cell immediately to the right, they would be comparing the target gain rule-based response to one that had 6 dB added to both 250 and 500 Hz.

One of the features and ultimate drawbacks to our implementation of the Revised Simplex Method was that the choice of cells to be compared was always based on the previous winner. This meant that if the client moved in the wrong direction either accidentally or on a whim, it was very difficult for him to find his way back to an area of preference. That is why this method took the client about an hour to an hour and a half to complete the selection of the three algorithms. If this hour of fitting time had resulted in algorithm selection that compared favorably with client preference and performance in the real world, then certainly it would have been time well spent. The feedback that we received from our human factors group and from our protocol participants was that it was tedious and time consuming, but most of all it was not meeting our criteria of providing a valid indicator of preference in the real world.

The Sliding Scale Test

The Sliding Scale (Figure 7.15) was developed by our human factors group. It provided a fast and reliable method of accurately determining client preference. The average time it took to complete selection of all three algorithms using the Sliding Scale Test was 30 minutes. The Sliding Scale provided eleven choices of algorithms. The client could slide up or down the scale centered around a rule-based algorithm. For example, in selecting the frequency response, the center of the scale was the New NAL target rule. Each step up or down the scale changed the slope by 3 dB. The Sliding Scale allowed the examiner to select the midpoint of the scale from a variety of target gain rules, including a hand-made rule. This gave the examiner control over the target, and still provided a means of finding out client preference.

A hand-held client response box was used to control the selection process. The response box incorporated three buttons (Figure 7.16). The client pressed the top red button to add high-frequency emphasis to the response and pressed the lower blue button to add low-frequency emphasis to the response. The client pressed the round green button to vote for his or her preferred response. The examiner could also control the selections from the keyboard on the Aurora.

The Sliding Scale Method of hearing aid fitting provided a hearing aid fitting procedure that met our criteria for reliability, validity, and speed. It provided a method of determining client preference for frequency shaping that could be used to fit not only the Nicolet Phoenix, but any hearing aid. The Sliding Scale test could be used to find the client's preferences for frequency shaping using the Hearing Aid Fitting module. After the selection was made, the examiner obtained a 2 cc coupler response of his/her preference. This was used as a template from which to set the analog hearing aid. The examiners could

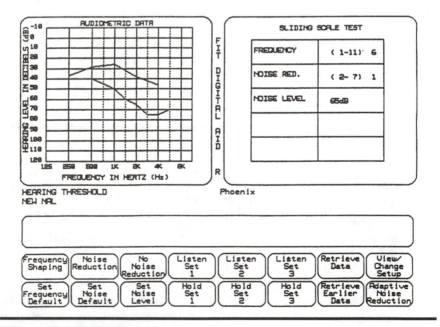

FIGURE 7.15. Sliding Scale Test screen.

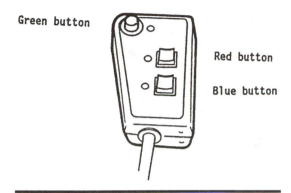

Green button

Red button

Blue button

FIGURE 7.16. Aurora® patient response button.

also evaluate the effects of various frequency responses on speech discrimination by going into the Audiometer mode with their preferred response or any response that they were interested in evaluating.

The Sliding Scale Test and the Revised Simplex Test provided objective measurements of client preference. The Hearing Aid Fitting module was the ultimate master hearing aid because it used the computer to keep track of the client's responses, removed the examiner bias often found in the use of a conventional master hearing aid, and preserved the accuracy of the signal path by having the client make his selections while wearing the Phoenix earpiece.

Summary of Hearing Aid Fitting Procedure

In summary, the hearing aid fitting procedure provided the dispenser of the Nicolet Phoenix with a reliable and valid method of determining client preference for frequency shaping and noise reduction. The system and the procedure were flexible enough to allow the hearing aid fitting to be performed inside or outside a sound-treated booth. This represented a "coming out" party for the field of audiology since hearing aid evaluation and

fitting were traditionally performed inside a sound booth.

The hearing aid dispensers were charged with the responsibility of finding out where clients were having difficulty and then setting up the fitting environment to recreate the situations where the client was having difficulty. Telemarketers were totally confused because all of a sudden the top ten audio cassette tapes purchased by audiologists included Julie Harris reading *Out of Africa*, cocktail party noise, airplane noise, and office noise, in addition to NU-6 and W-22. Hearing aid dispensers started reading and quoting from magazines such as *Digital Audio*, *Stereo Review*, and *PC Magazine*. They started getting out of their offices and into the situations where their clients were having trouble: the real world.

The Aurora/Phoenix hearing aid fitting strategy brought a new dimension into hearing aid selection procedures in addition to traditional measurements of speech discrimination, speech reception thresholds, functional gain, and real-ear measurements. The material used for the hearing aid selection process *purposefully* had a wide dynamic range to allow the client to experience the behavior of the hearing aid in multiple sound environments as part of the selection process. This was a departure from the typical types of test materials used for clinical evaluation. The client was an integral part of the hearing aid selection process, and if the data collected using the Sliding Scale Hearing Aid Fitting method is any indication, hearing-impaired individuals *can* give us reliable and valid indications of their preferences for sound processing.

In summary, the Aurora Hearing Aid Fitting module provided hearing aid dispensers with an efficient, reliable, and valid indicator of client preferences for sound processing. This module could be used to select the program for frequency shaping and noise reduction for the Nicolet Phoenix or to select the frequency response for an analog hearing aid. It helped us understand that hearing-impaired individuals are able to hear differences between hearing aid characteristics if they are given the right tools.

THE NICOLET PHOENIX

The Nicolet Phoenix was introduced in July of 1988 (Figure 7.17). The first version was a two-piece device consisting of a pocket-sized computer connected to an analog hearing aid designed specifically for the digital interface. One of the hardest obstacles to overcome was the configuration. It was difficult to explain that this technology was a giant step forward rather than a giant step backward by just looking at the device. The microphone and all of the traditional analog components of a hearing aid were located in the behind-the-

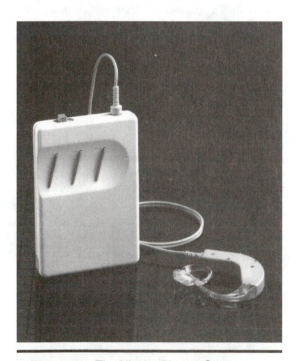

FIGURE 7.17.   The Nicolet Phoenix®.

ear piece. This connected to the pocket processor with a cable.

We were often asked why we did not get rid of the cable. The answer was simple. The cable transmitted information two ways: The analog signal from the earpiece went to the processor to be converted into a digital signal, was manipulated and converted back to an analog signal, and then traveled back to the earpiece. (See Hussung and Hammill, 1990, for an introduction to digital terminology and concepts.). The cable was the only way that we could be sure of the integrity of the signal transmission in both directions. FM, infrared, and ultrasonic transmitters were considered, but never used due to the potential compromise in performance.

The Phoenix had three buttons that could be programmed to perform in different ways. For example, in its simplest configuration each button contained one program. In the Variable Phoenix program, the same processor was programmed to behave entirely differently. Five programs for frequency response (typically centered around the clients' preferences) were programmed into button 1, and five programs for noise reduction were programmed for button 2. Each press of the button advanced the clients to the next program within that button. The third button allowed the clients to reverse the direction of progression on the button they were using.

One of the many challenges we faced as a project team was trying to educate dispensers about the electroacoustics of this new technology using references that were familiar. From the hearing aid dispenser's point of view, the most familiar reference for discussing the electroacoustics of a hearing aid was the ANSI S3.22-1987 standard. Dispensers were accustomed to comparing numbers and curves from the ANSI test battery to make a decision about the appropriateness of a certain hearing aid for their clients. However, this standard was never intended as a design standard. In the forward to the standard, the ANSI Standards Committee on Bioacoustics S3 made it quite clear that the purpose of developing the standard was to give manufacturers a measurement standard to determine if the product they had made met their design specifications.

The Nicolet Phoenix broke all the rules when it came to using the curves and values from the ANSI test to look at performance. In this section we will talk about some of these considerations because they apply not only to the Nicolet Phoenix, but also to the evaluation and fitting of other nonlinear hearing aids.

Frequency Shaping

If frequency shaping flexibility was important to the client, the Nicolet Phoenix provided thousands of frequency shapes by reprogramming the hearing aid. Five frequency bands centered around the audiometric test frequencies of 250, 500, 1000, 2000, and 4000 Hz were used to set the five digital filters in the Pocket Processor. In addition to flex-

ibility of the shape of the response, the client could have as many as ten different responses in one hearing aid.

In 1987 the concept of reprogramming a hearing aid rather than returning an aid to the manufacturer was new. Because it was a new concept, dispensers were unsure what to do with the flexibility that they had. We were trying to find creative ways to convey the idea that the possibilities were essentially endless. How do you provide one frequency response that shows all the options? Of course, you cannot. We chose instead to provide the dispenser with examples of some of the creative responses to convey the message that almost anything was possible (Figure 7.18).

The digital signal processing in the Nicolet Phoenix resulted in frequency responses that were adaptive (according to the program) as a function of time and intensity. The frequency response that one saw on paper changed depending on level of input and whether or not one used a pure tone sweep or speech noise (Figure 7.19).

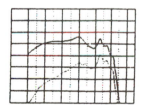
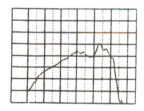
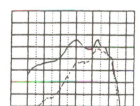
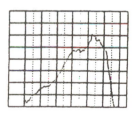

(a) Moderately sloping, high-frequency emphasis   **(b) Steeply sloping, high-frequency emphasis**

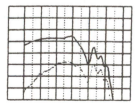
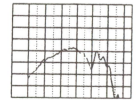

(c) Low-frequency emphasis

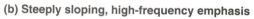

FIGURE 7.18.   Sample frequency responses for the Nicolet Phoenix®.

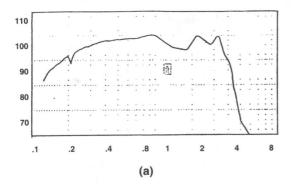

(a)

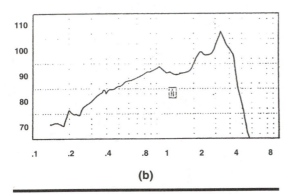

(b)

FIGURE 7.19. Frequency response of Nicolet Phoenix® to pure tone sweep (top) and complex noise (bottom).

The long time constants on the analog AGC in the front end caused a ballooning or blooming effect in the low frequencies at high intensity levels. Also, when inputs of high intensity and high frequency were used, they caused the receiver impedance to go up (current went down) and depressed the high-frequency response. As a manufacturer we were required to use pure tone response curves to ship with our hearing aids. This accounted for more than one phone call to customer support because as soon as the dispenser saw the 90 dB input curves he/she would call and report a hearing aid that was not programmed properly. So, based on input from our customers, we started to ship all our aids with an additional set of curves called a Level Composite, which

showed a series of frequency response curves to speech noise at levels ranging from 50 to 90 dB in 10 dB increments.

Equivalent Input Noise (EIN) Level

The purpose of obtaining an EIN measurement is to try and find out how noisy the circuit of the hearing aid is. To obtain the EIN value, SPL measurements of the hearing aid in the coupler are made with and without input signals presented to the hearing aid. For example, in an AGC hearing aid the average SPL in the coupler using an input level of 50 dB SPL over the three frequencies of 1000, 1600, and 2500 Hz is measured. The input level of 50 dB is subtracted from this average value. The 50 dB input signals are then taken away and a measurement is made without any input to the hearing aid. Although this measurement strategy using a 60 dB input works fine for linear hearing aids, there are several factors described in the ANSI standard that may be responsible for obtaining a high EIN value in the face of a very quiet AGC hearing aid circuit:

1. The hearing aid may have a kneepoint below 50 dB.
2. The bandwidth of the hearing aid may be too narrow.
3. There may be a high level of ambient noise in the room where the aid is being tested.
4. The amount of time between the measurements with and without input to the hearing aid may be too short for AGC aids with long time constants to react. This will result in a high EIN measurement value because the AGC circuit has not sufficiently recovered before the next measurement is made. The Hearing Aid Analyzer software in the Aurora took this into account.

In the case of the Nicolet Phoenix all of these conditions were met, plus we added the variable of new processing. EIN measurements made while the hearing aid was in a noise reduction program appeared high, not because the circuit was noisy, but because of the type of sound processing that was being performed (proprietary).

Control Of Loud and Soft Sounds

The Nicolet Phoenix used different processing strategies to keep speech comfortable and keep loud sounds from becoming uncomfortable. Digital signal processing was used to limit transients while the front-end AGC in the hearing aid earpiece kept speech audible. The client could control the gain for speech by varying the volume of the hearing aid, much like an input compression hearing aid. The analog AGC had an attack time of 250 msec and a release time of 3 seconds. This minimized the pumping effects found in conventional one-circuit-does-all AGC hearing aids. The digital processing was responsible for capturing transients. It made adjustments to the signal on a millisecond-by-millisecond basis. A third and final peak-clipping circuit was included for added loudness-limiting protection. This symbiotic relationship of the various components of the hearing aid benefited the hearing-impaired client because speech was maintained at a comfortable level, and transients were audible, but not uncomfortable, and did not cause the front-end AGC to compress speech.

ANSI defines attack time as the *time* between the abrupt increase from 55 to 80 dB and the point where the level has stabilized to within 2 dB of the steady value for the 80 dB input sound pressure level. The release time is defined as the interval between the abrupt drop from 80 to 55 dB and the point where the signal has stabilized to within 2 dB of the steady state value for the 55 dB input sound pressure level. The direction of each of the levels shall be sufficiently long (at least five times the longest attack or release time) so as

not to influence the measured attack and release time.

The calculation of attack and release times for the Nicolet Phoenix were accurate so long as the dispenser used the Aurora Hearing Aid Analyzer. We found, however, that other hearing aid analyzers gave dispensers erroneous attack and release times because they did not allow enough time between the presentation of the 55 and 80 dB levels used in this measurement for the AGC to recover (5×3 seconds).

In evaluating new processing schemes, it is very important to characterize the behavior of the hearing aid over frequency, intensity, time, and duration of the stimulus. Two new special tests were developed for the Aurora Hearing Aid Analyzer that allowed us to characterize the behavior of the Phoenix and other hearing aids (Figure 7.20). The first new test was called the Linearity Analysis Test and allowed the examiner to obtain the frequency response to two different intensity levels of speech-shaped noise that were modulated every 250 msec on a square wave. Since all the other ANSI tests were static tests of hearing aid behavior, they did not characterize the behavior of a hearing aid in a dynamic environment where the levels of speech and background noise are fluctuating.

The second new test developed for the Aurora Hearing Aid Analyzer was the Maximum Output Limit Test. A 6.5 msec duration impulse was used to measure the peak maximum output of a hearing aid to an impulse signal. The resulting peak output in millivolts and dB was reported, as well as the latency (amount of time it took for the sound to travel from the loudspeaker, through the box, through the hearing aid circuit, and reach the coupler microphone), and the signal peak (3 dB higher than the rms value). In addition to providing a way of testing our new digital signal processing algorithms, these two tests also provided a new manufacturing standard for new product evaluation prior to shipment.

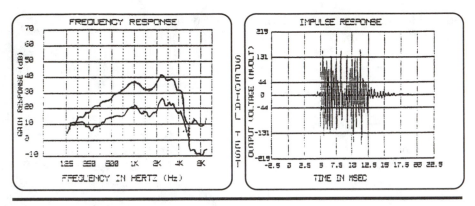

FIGURE 7.20.   Nicolet Aurora® special tests for hearing aid analysis: Linearity Analysis Test (left) and Maximum Output Limit Test (right).

New Sound Processing Strategies

In addition to algorithms for frequency shaping and noise reduction, the Nicolet Phoenix Project was working on algorithms for speech enhancement and feedback reduction. Loudness control and increased dynamic range were features of the Phoenix. The digital loudness limiting with its fast time constants captured transients and benefited clients by making loud sounds comfortable. The analog AGC in the behind-the-ear unit had long attack and release times that benefited the clients by keeping the long term speech signal at a comfortable level and making soft sounds audible. Because of the digital signal processing and analog conditioning, the dynamic range of the hearing-impaired individuals who wore the Phoenix was increased. The benefit to the hearing-impaired clients was an increase in the fidelity of the music.

Some examples of unique applications of DSP in the Nicolet Phoenix used by Nicolet Phoenix dispensers included the use of digital filtering to minimize a frequency-specific sound. This was particularly helpful for a dentist who wanted to filter out the sound of the high-speed drill he used. Another creative audiologist went for a ride in her client's motor home and did a third-octave band filter analysis of the noise in the van, recorded the van noise on tape, then programmed a frequency shape and noise-reduction program to limit the amplification of background noise and improve speech intelligibility for her client in that situation.

Digital signal processing provides the flexibility in signal processing to benefit the unique and personal characteristics of individual hearing deficits. Williamson and Punch (1990) have discussed some of the issues in developing new speech enhancement techniques. Their point of involving engineers, researchers, and audiologists in the development cycle is significant. The task of algorithm development involves an exchange of information between the field and the laboratory. Project Phoenix created such an environment. The result was an open line of communication among all those involved with the project.

CLOSING REMARKS

You will find many opinions as to why Project Phoenix folded. The following reasons are some that we believe contributed to the lack of success of the project. We believe that they are extremely important lessons for the hearing health care industry to learn and that they hold severe implications for the success or failure of future new products, the health of the industry, the access of consumers to new technologies, and ultimately the ability of our profession to thrive.

1. A distribution network was lacking. It is hard to launch a national advertising campaign with only 100 dispensers in the country and without representation in all 50 states.

2. The educational mission was too ambitious. The technology and interface were new to hearing health care providers as well as to consumers.

3. The impact of the cost of new technology on the price of the device was not well accepted. In 1989 the suggested retail price for the Phoenix was $1995. Portable laptop computers were just becoming available on the market at a cost of over $6000, and for those in the computer industry at the time, the response to the price was positive. However, the response from many (not all) of the hearing health care providers was not.

4. Was the instrument rejected based on the client's perception of its size, power consumption of the processor, or performance; or was it based on the dispenser's expectations for size, power consumption, and time involved in fitting the Phoenix? We could not explain the high success rate in some offices compared to the high return rate in other offices based solely on the performance of the Phoenix. There were many expectations to meet on the part of the consumer, dispenser, and manufacturer. The interdependency of all of us on one another cannot be emphasized enough.

5. In 1987, when the first Aurora shipped, very few offices had computers. The Aurora/ Phoenix Project attracted the exceptional audiologists or dispensers who saw the potential for improving their practice and the quality of sound processing for the hearing-impaired individuals they served.

6. In 1987, the rumors that we were going out of business were rampant within the industry. Some of the stories about what was *supposedly* happening to the Aurora and Phoenix were quite incredible, and in time, some of the rumors became a self-fulfilling prophecy. Many doors and minds were closed to the technology and its benefits as people listened to well-known experts within the field who spoke with great authority and misinformation about the limitations of the Aurora or Phoenix. People believed these "experts" without trying to find out if what they had heard was based on fact or supposition.

7. Another problem was the failure to find a joint venture partner to provide monies to bring the behind-the-ear digital aid to market quickly.

We can also look at some of the more positive aspects of Project Phoenix. It served as the impetus for the development of individualized hearing aid fitting strategies, programmable hearing aids, and for further research and development into the application of digital signal processing techniques for speech enhancement for the hearing impaired. It prompted other hearing aid manufacturers to start pursuing performance options as well as size options for consumers. It brought audiologists out of the sound booth for hearing aid evaluation and fitting. It was the first hearing aid on the market for consumers to incorporate true digital signal processing. It was the first to provide dispensers with a fitting method as well as a device. The project represented the hearing aid industry at its best in terms of its level of involvement in education, research, engineering, basic science, and cooperation among the top professionals of the day.

ACKNOWLEDGMENTS

The author acknowledges the contributions of Rita Palmer Hussung and Ken Cummins

(PPU), Tom Worrall (HAL hardware), and Rick Jenison (hearing aid characterization using HAL), and Bill Balmer (electroacoustics) in the writing of these sections of this chapter. Special thanks to Eric Miller, Product Manager for the Nicolet Phoenix, for his enthusiasm in the face of all odds.

The author also acknowledges the men and women of Project Phoenix, the hearing-impaired individuals who participated in the research, the audiologists and dispensers who saw the light and had the vision to see the future, and the hearing-impaired individuals who ultimately benefited and continue to use the technology in the Nicolet Phoenix. Finally, thanks to Kurt Hecox, whose vision made a dream into reality.

REFERENCES

Byrne, D., and Dillon, H. (1986). The National Acoustic Laboratories' (NAL) new procedure for selecting the gain and frequency response of a hearing aid. *Ear and Hearing* 7:257–265.

Cummins, Kennith L., and Hecox, Kurt E. (1987). Ambulatory testing of digital hearing aid algorithms. RESNA 10th Annual Conference, San Jose, CA.

Chan, J.C.K., and Geisler, D. (1990). Estimation of eardrum acoustic pressure and of ear canal length from remote points in the canal. *Journal of the Acoustical Society of America* 79(4):990–998.

Erdreich, J. (1986). A distribution based definition of impulse noise. *Journal of the Acoustical Society of America* 79(4):990–998.

Hecox, K.E., and Miller, E. (1987). Foundations for the introduction of new hearing instrument technologies. *Hearing Instruments* 38(11).

Hecox, K.E., and Punch, Jerry L. (1988). The impact of digital technology on the selection and fitting of hearing aids. *American Journal of Otology* 9 (Suppl.).

Heide, V.H. (1991). Variables in real ear measurement. *Hearing Instruments* 42(3).

Heide, V.H., Balmer, W.F., Cummins, K.L., Worrall, T., and Zhu, X. (1987). A laboratory system for behavioral comparison of multiple hearing aids. Presented at ASHA, November 9.

Hussung, R.A., and Hamill, T.A. (1990). Recent advances in hearing aid technology: An introduction to digital terminology and concepts. In: C. Sammeth (ed.), Digital Hearing Aids. *Seminars in Hearing* 11(1).

Levitt, H. (1978). Adaptive testing in audiology. In: C. Ludvigsen and J. Barfod (eds.), Sensorineural hearing impairment and hearing aids. *Scandinavian Audiology* (Suppl. 6).

Levitt, H., Sullivan, J.A., Neuman, A., and Rubin-Spitz, J.A. (1987). Experiments with a programmable master hearing aid. *Journal of Rehabilitation Research and Development* 24(4):29–54.

Miller, E. (1988). Digital signal processing in hearing aids: Implications and applications. *The Hearing Journal*, April.

Neuman, A.C., Levitt, H., Mills, R., and Schwander, T. (1987). An evaluation of three adaptive hearing aid selection strategies. *Journal of the Acoustical Society of America* 82(6).

Palmer, R., Cummins, K., Heide, V., and Williamson, M. (1987). A portable unit for evaluating digital hearing aid algorithms. Presented at ASHA, November 8.

Project Phoenix, Inc. (PPI) (1987). A comprehensive instrument for clinical audiology and hearing aid fitting. *Hearing Instruments* 38(1).

Punch, J., Chi, C., and Allan, J. (1990). Signal averaging in real ear probe tube measurements. *Ear and Hearing* 11(5).

Punch, J., Chi, C., and Patterson, J. (1990). A recommended protocol for prescriptive use of target gain rules. *Hearing Instruments* 41(4):12, 14, 16, 18–19.

Sammeth, C. (ed.) (1990). Digital hearing aids. *Seminars in Hearing* 11(1).

Studebaker, G.A., et al. (1982). Paired comparison judgments of relative intelligibility in noise. *Journal of the Acoustical Society of America*. 72:80–92.

Texas Instruments Inc., (1988). TMS320: Helping the deaf hear. *Details on Signal Processing* 15.

Williamson, M.J., and Punch, J.L. (1990). Speech enhancement in digital hearing aids. In: C. Sammeth (ed.), Digital hearing aids. *Seminars in Hearing* 11(1).

CHAPTER 8

THE APPLICATION OF DIGITAL TECHNOLOGY TO COCHLEAR IMPLANTS

Judith A. Brimacombe and Anne L. Beiter

Cochlear implants are biomedical devices that electrically stimulate remaining auditory nerve fibers to produce hearing percepts in individuals who are profoundly deaf and obtain minimal information from amplified sound. Over the past 15 to 20 years, cochlear implant systems have evolved from single-channel to more complex multichannel systems. A number of investigators have reviewed the historical development of different single-channel and multichannel cochlear implant systems (Luxford and Brackmann, 1985; Staller, 1985; Shallop and Mecklenburg, 1987; Mecklenburg and Shallop, 1988; Tyler and Tye-Murray, 1991; and Mecklenburg and Lehnhardt, 1991).

While current systems differ from each other in fundamental ways, there are also some commonalities among them. Figure 8.1 illustrates in general how a cochlear implant works. All cochlear implant systems begin with the output from a microphone, which is an analog electrical signal. The signals from the microphone are sent to an externally worn processor where they are analyzed before being delivered to the electrodes implanted within or in close proximity to the cochlea. The type of processing that is carried out by the external unit differs across systems and may

include digital, analog, or a combination of digital and analog processing. In systems that utilize digital technology, the ongoing variations in the electrical analog of the acoustic signal are defined by a set of discrete numerical values. The resulting output from the processor, be it analog or digital, is then sent to the implanted portion of the system.

The stimulation delivered to the electrodes is in either an analog or pulsatile form. Analog electrical stimulation implies that a continuously varying electrical voltage or current is applied to the electrodes. On the other hand, pulsatile stimulation, as used in digital systems, is discrete, and the electrical stimulation pulses are defined by their duration and amplitude. In either case, the application of an electrical stimulus to the electrode-tissue interface results in activation of auditory neurons. The resulting electrical discharge travels through the central auditory pathways and is interpreted by the brain as sound.

The best example of the application of digital technology to cochlear implants is found in the Nucleus 22 Channel Cochlear Implant System. This cochlear prosthesis is the result of two decades of research and ongoing collaboration between the University

Unless otherwise noted, figures and photographs in this chapter are reprinted with permission of Cochlear Corporation, 61 Inverness Drive East, Englewood, CO.

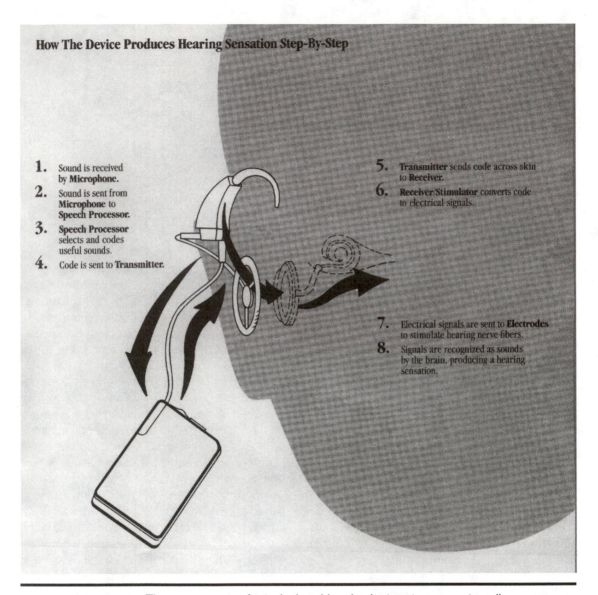

How The Device Produces Hearing Sensation Step-By-Step

1. Sound is received by **Microphone.**

2. Sound is sent from **Microphone** to **Speech Processor.**

3. **Speech Processor** selects and codes useful sounds.

4. Code is sent to **Transmitter.**

5. **Transmitter** sends code across skin to **Receiver.**

6. **Receiver/Stimulator** converts code to electrical signals.

7. Electrical signals are sent to **Electrodes** to stimulate hearing nerve fibers.

8. Signals are recognized as sounds by the brain, producing a hearing sensation.

FIGURE 8.1.   The components of a typical cochlear implant system: an externally worn microphone, speech processor and transmitter, and an implantable receiver/ stimulator and electrode array.

of Melbourne, Melbourne, Australia, and Cochlear Proprietary Limited, Sydney, Australia. A review of the historical development of this multichannel cochlear implant can be found in Clark et al., 1987.

The Nucleus 22 Channel Cochlear Implant System, illustrated in Figure 8.2, consists of the implantable receiver/stimulator and electrode array, a body-worn speech processor, and an ear-level, directional, electret micro-

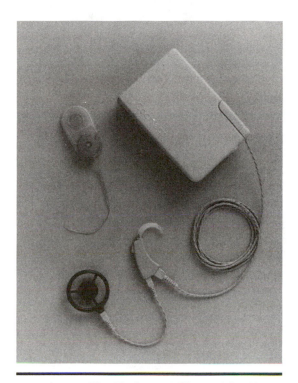

FIGURE 8.2. The Nucleus 22 Channel Cochlear Implant System.

tracts and encodes specific parameters of the signal and sends the resulting digital code to the externally worn transmitting coil. The speech processor is programmed individually for each patient using an IBM PC-compatible computer, interface, and customized software. The programming system allows the clinician to determine electrical current thresholds and maximum comfort levels for electrical stimulation of each electrode pair. These measurements will vary from patient to patient and within a given patient across time. These psychophysical data are digitized and stored in a random-access memory (RAM) in the speech processor. This information forms part of the digital instruction code that is transmitted to the cochlear implant. The stream of digital information is sent across the skin via a radio frequency (RF) carrier and is picked up by the internal receiving coil of the cochlear implant. The receiver/stimulator decodes the digital information and delivers charge-balanced biphasic pulsatile electrical stimulation to selected electrode pairs within the cochlea (see Figure 8.3).

phone and transmitting coil. Digital technology is an integral part of the system's internal and external components.

To summarize how this particular system works, incoming acoustic signals are picked up and transduced by the microphone and sent to the speech processor. The processor is essentially a personal microcomputer. It digitally ex-

DESCRIPTION OF THE COCHLEAR IMPLANT

The cochlear implant includes the receiver/ stimulator and attached to it, a banded electrode array. The array is made up of 32 evenly spaced platinum bands supported on a flexible silicone rubber carrier. The most proxi-

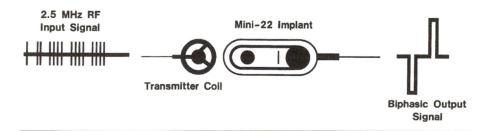

FIGURE 8.3. Digital information path.

mal 10 bands provide additional mechanical stiffness to the array, but are not connected to the receiver/stimulator. The remaining distal 22 bands are active electrodes; each one is attached to the receiver/stimulator by an individually insulated platinum-iridium wire. These insulated wires course through the molded silicone rubber carrier so that the array is smooth for easy insertion into the scala tympani. The electrode array tapers from a diameter of 0.6 to 0.4 millimeters at its tip.

The receiver/stimulator is an electronic device that is designed to stimulate pairs of electrodes with charge-balanced biphasic current pulses. It is powered and controlled by the signals received from the external speech processor. The receiver/stimulator is composed of power supply components and a custom-made integrated circuit. The power necessary to run the circuit is supplied by the battery in the speech processor. The power is transmitted across the skin as a part of the specific string of digital information that also specifies which electrode pairs should be stimulated at any point in time. Therefore, power consumption is minimized as power is available only when it is needed for electrical stimulation. The integrated circuit controls stimulation to the electrodes by decoding the digital information and generating the appropriate biphasic stimulation pulses that are delivered to the electrode pairs.

The electronics are encased in a hermetically sealed titanium and ceramic package and embedded in a biocompatible, medical-grade silicone rubber. Ceramic feedthroughs within the hermetically sealed capsule allow connection of the electrode array to the electronics. The platinum receiving coil and a rare-earth magnet are also part of the receiver/stimulator. These components are outside the hermetic package. The internal magnet provides the attraction to keep the external transmitting coil, which includes a companion adjustable magnet, in place over the site of the implant.

The power for the integrated circuit and the data that define the electrical stimulation parameters to the electrode pairs are transmitted electromagnetically on a 2.5 MHz carrier frequency across the two closely spaced coils. Electromagnetic induction is the most reliable and efficient method of transmitting signals across the skin (Clark et al., 1987). These signals can be transmitted over a distance of approximately 8.5 mm between the transmitting and receiving coils. The information and power are transmitted on the RF carrier on a stimulus-by-stimulus basis.

Transmission of data to the implanted receiver/stimulator is by a series of discrete data bursts that represent the chosen electrode(s), the distance between stimulating electrodes (referred to as stimulation mode), the stimulating current, and amplitude and duration of the biphasic current pulse. Each time a stimulus is delivered, a data frame comprising six bursts of pulses at a rate of 2.5 MHz is transmitted to the receiver/stimulator as shown in Figure 8.4. The first pulse is the sync burst, which resets the system before transmission of the remainder of the data stream. Next, the active electrode is selected by the number decoded from the second burst. The number decoded from the third burst defines the reference electrode for electrical stimulation (Crosby et al., 1985). For bipolar stimulation, the reference electrode is adjacent to the active electrode. The reference electrode chosen may be farther from the active electrode, as shown by the bipolar +1 and bipolar +2 stimulation modes in Figure 8.5. Note that the reference electrode is always distal to the active electrode—that is, more apically placed along the array.

The fourth, fifth, and sixth bursts define the amplitude of the stimulating current and the duration of the negative and positive phases of the biphasic current pulse delivered to the electrode pair (see lower portion of Figure 8.4) (Crosby et al., 1985). Nominally,

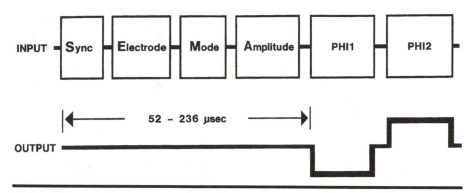

FIGURE 8.4.   The format of the six data pulses that are transmitted to the receiver/stimulator package for each biphasic charge-balanced current pulse delivered to an electrode pair.

the range of current output is from 25 microamperes (μA) to 1.5 milliamperes (mA). This large current range is reduced to a manageable number of steps by using a logarithmic transformation of voltage [similar to the decibel (dB) scale]. Each step represents approximately a 2.5% increase in actual charge delivered to the electrode pair.

Charge is the product of current amplitude and pulse width and is directly related to the loudness percept generated. Charge density is defined as the charge delivered divided by the surface area of the electrode. Charge density correlates with electrochemical, histological,

and physiological tissue changes as a neural system is electrically stimulated over time (Brummer and Turner, 1975; Walsh and Leake-Jones, 1982; Shepherd, Clark, and Black, 1983; Webb et al., 1988; Shepherd, Franz, and Clark, 1990).

There are a number of advantages to the digital transmission of signals for a cochlear implant. First, the ongoing acoustic signal is coded as a series of numbers, and that information is used to stimulate more than one electrode pair. Because the information is in a digital as opposed to an analog form, only a single RF transmission path is required. Sec-

FIGURE 8.5.   The stimulation mode refers to the location of the indifferent, or reference electrode relative to the stimulating, or active electrode. In the bipolar configuration, the reference electrode is located next to the active electrode, in the apical direction, thereby making 21 electrode pairs available for stimulation on the electrode array. In the bipolar +1 mode, the electrode adjacent to the active is skipped and the reference electrode becomes the next more apical electrode. In this mode, 20 electrode pairs are available for stimulation. Reprinted with permission from Patrick and Clark, 1991. Copyright © by Williams & Wilkins, 1991.

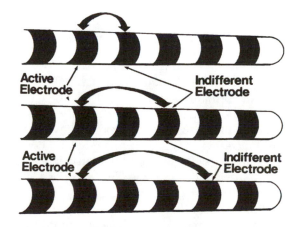

ond, the probability of the stimulator becoming operational in response to interference from other RF signals is extremely rare. This is because the stimulator portion of the implant will not receive power and generate electrical stimuli unless the correct data sequence is received. In addition, the use of a relatively high-frequency carrier makes the system impervious to contamination from low-frequency signals. Finally, because the current source for stimulation is controlled digitally, the stimuli sent to each electrode pair are well-defined—that is, the amplitude, width, and rate of the biphasic current pulses are specified digitally.

The receiver/stimulator is placed under the skin, in a surgically created depression in the mastoid bone, and the electrode array is placed into the scala tympani through an opening made in or near the round window. Detailed information on the surgical technique, as well as any special considerations, may be found in Clark et al., 1987; Webb et al., 1990; Clark et al., 1991; and Clark, Cohen, and Shepherd, 1991.

WEARABLE SPEECH PROCESSOR

F0/F2 and F0/F1/F2 Coding Strategies

The first wearable speech processor (WSP) used with the Nucleus 22 Channel Cochlear Implant System encoded estimates of three parameters of speech that had been shown to be important for speech recognition. These parameters were the amplitude of the speech envelope, fundamental frequency (F0), and second formant frequency (F2) (Tong et al., 1979; Tong et al., 1980; Tong et al., 1982). Development of this speech processor, with its F0/F2 coding strategy, commenced in 1981, and laboratory tests were completed in 1982. Continued research at the University of Melbourne in 1984 demonstrated that a speech coding strategy that included estimates of the first formant frequency (F1) and amplitude, in

addition to the three parameters listed above, enhanced speech understanding (Dowell et al., 1987; Blamey et al., 1987a; Blamey et al., 1987b; Blamey and Clark, 1990). This strategy, referred to as F0/F1/F2, presented two spectral components to different sites within the cochlea. The peak of spectral energy of the first formant in the frequency range of 280 to 1000 Hz was extracted, processed, and presented to a more apical electrode pair within the cochlea, while the second formant information in the frequency range of 800 to 4000 Hz was sent to a more basal electrode pair. Electrical stimuli representing the amplitudes of F1 and F2 were delivered sequentially to the electrode pairs as two charge-balanced current pulses separated in time by 0.8 msec. As with the earlier F0/F2 coding strategy, the rate of electrical stimulation was proportional to the fundamental frequency of the voice. An illustration of the temporal characteristics of the F0/F1/F2 coding strategy is presented in Figure 8.6. For this example, the rate of stimulation is 250 Hz.

The F0/F2 and F0/F1/F2 speech processors incorporate both analog and digital circuitry. Analog circuits are used to measure the speech parameters described above. Each of these parameters is represented by a voltage level. These levels are converted to a digital format. Mathematical look-up tables are used to convert the formant frequency information to electrode number and the amplitude information to current output (Patrick et al., 1990). A simplified block diagram of the F0/F1/F2 processor can be found in Figure 8.7.

At the front end of the WSP, the microphone preamplifier is controlled by an automatic gain control (AGC) circuit. The AGC amplifier reduces the range of amplitude values of incoming speech signals to be processed by the device. It limits the peaks of the output amplitude to a level that is acceptable for subsequent signal processing and yet comfortable for the user, as the acoustic input amplitude varies over a much wider range (Clark and

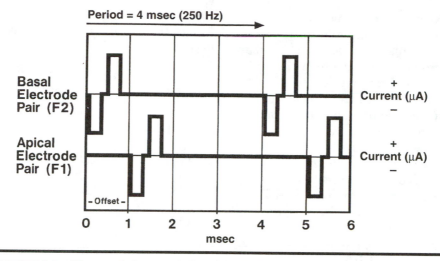

FIGURE 8.6.   Temporal characteristics of the F0/F1/F2 speech feature extraction coding strategy. In this example, the rate of electrical stimulation is 250 Hz.

Tong, 1985). The AGC circuit produces a signal with a fixed peak value and a dynamic range of approximately 30 dB below that value. A sensitivity control allows the user to control the maximum gain of the AGC in five discrete steps: 32, 56, 66, 74, and 80 dB (Blamey et al., 1987a).

The fundamental frequency of voiced phonemes within the range of 50 to 300 Hz is derived from the zero crossings of the low-pass

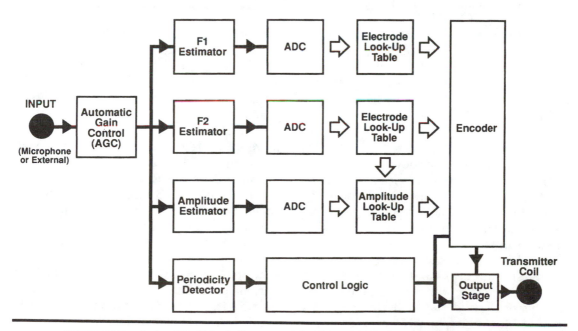

FIGURE 8.7.   A simplified block diagram of the Wearable Speech Processor (WSP).

filtered envelope of the waveform and converted into electric pulse rate to determine the rate of stimulation to a given electrode pair. Because very little low-frequency periodicity is detected for voiceless sounds, the extracted pulse rate is random in nature. This results in a stimulation rate that is random, around 100 Hz, producing a noise-like percept (Blamey et al., 1987a).

The first and second formants of speech are characterized by a concentration of energy within the range of approximately 250 to 1000 Hz and 800 to 3200 Hz, respectively (Peterson and Barney, 1952). Analog circuitry within the speech processor extracts peaks of energy in the range of 280 to 1000 Hz for the estimate of F1, and in the range of 800 to 4000 Hz for the estimate of F2. The output of these filters is routed to a zero crossings counter. A voltage is produced that is proportional to the estimated formant frequency. This voltage is sampled by the analog-to-digital (A-D) converter, and the electrode number that corresponds to the estimated formant frequency is read from a mathematical look-up table that is stored in the digital memory of the speech processor (Clark and Tong, 1985). This memory is an erasable, programmable, read-only memory (EPROM) chip.

The primary function of the look-up table is to translate the frequency of the dominant spectral peaks (F1 and F2) to electrode position within the cochlea. To perform this function the electrodes are numbered sequentially starting at the round window. Electrode 1 is the most basal electrode and electrode 22 is the most apical along the array. Stimulation of different electrodes normally results in pitch perceptions that reflect the tonotopic organization of the cochlea.

To allocate the frequency range for the F1 and F2 spectral peaks to the total number of electrodes, an algorithm divides the total number of electrodes available for use into a ratio of 1:2. Approximately one-third of the

TABLE 8.1. Frequency boundary allocations for 20 electrodes in a bipolar +1 stimulation mode.

Electrode	Frequency Boundaries	
	Lower	Upper
20	280	400
19	400	500
18	500	600
17	600	700
16	700	800
15	800	900
14	900	1000
13	1000	1112
12	1112	1237
11	1237	1377
10	1377	1531
9	1531	1704
8	1704	1896
7	1896	2109
6	2109	2346
5	2346	2611
4	2611	2904
3	2904	3231
2	3231	3595
1	3595	4000

most apically placed electrodes are assigned to the F1 frequency range (280 to 1000 Hz). The remaining two-thirds of the electrodes are assigned to a bandwidth within the F2 range (800 to 4000 Hz). Table 8.1 provides an example of frequency-to-electrode mapping. Note that the frequency boundaries of the more apical electrodes (electrodes 20 through 14) cover the F1 range, and the bandwidths are all approximately 100 Hz wide. The frequency boundaries of electrodes 13 through 1 cover the F2 range and are divided into logrithmically equal bands.

The amplitudes of F1 and F2 are also sampled and converted to a number representing an electrical stimulation level. These current output levels represent a range of hearing from just detectable (threshold) to maximum acceptable loudness and are stored in a look-up table representing current amplitude. The psychophysical measures stored in the look-up table are patient specific and vary depending on electrode pairing and the number of remaining neural elements in the cochlea (Pfingst, Spelman, and Sutton, 1980). A number of other variables affect the psychophysical measures obtained. A thorough discussion of these factors can be found in Pfingst, 1990.

Figure 8.7 shows that in the final stages of signal processing, the data in the look-up tables are accessed by the speech processor's encoder chip to generate the pulse burst sequences that power up and control the implanted receiver/stimulator (see Figure 8.4). The pulse burst sequences are transmitted via the RF output stage to the implanted receiver/stimulator.

MINI SPEECH PROCESSOR

Preliminary research for a new speech processor began in early 1984 at the University of Melbourne (Dowell et al., 1990). This new speech processor, introduced in 1989, was designed to provide additional speech feature coding strategies. On the practical side, it was also necessary to reduce its size and weight for better use by pediatric cochlear implant recipients.

To allow enhanced speech processing, the mini speech processor (MSP) includes three high-frequency bandpass filters in addition to the F1 and F2 filters. The high-frequency filters are incorporated into an integrated circuit. In theory, the addition of more high-frequency information should provide better discrimination of phonemes with high-frequency spectral content (e.g., voiceless consonants). These filters provide energy estimates in three high-frequency bands: 2000 to 2800 Hz (band 3), 2800 to 4000 Hz (band 4), and 4000 to approximately 6000 Hz (band 5). The high-pass filter for band 5 is limited by the frequency response characteristics of the microphone. A block diagram of the MSP is shown in Figure 8.8.

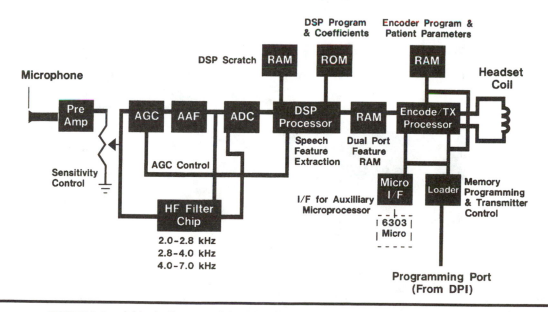

FIGURE 8.8.   A block diagram of the Mini Speech Processor (MSP).

The MSP uses a dedicated, custom-designed digital signal processor (DSP) for the extraction of F0, F1, and F2. The DSP also includes an analog preamplifier, A-D converter, and encoder. The preamplifier provides AGC to keep the signal within the computational range of the DSP (Patrick et al., 1990). Finally, because the DSP can extract many more features from the acoustic signal, it provides greater flexibility in coding strategy research development.

The function of the AGC circuit in the MSP is to maintain a 30 dB operating range. As in the WSP, it uses the most recent peak value in the signal to determine the gain and rapidly decreases the gain with the onset of a high-level signal. The patient-operated sensitivity control sets the maximum AGC gain of the microphone preamplifier and consequently determines when the AGC gain becomes active. The minimum input signal level required for stimulation is determined by the setting of the sensitivity control. Figure 8.9 illustrates that when the sensitivity control is set to maximum (number 8), sounds of approximately 45 dB sound pressure level (SPL) or higher result in stimulation at the patient's maximum comfort level; signal inputs of approximately 15 dB result in stimulation at the patient's threshold for hearing. Signal inputs less than 15 dB are not processed. As the end-user decreases the sensitivity control, greater input values are needed to result in stimulation. Note that a 30 dB operating range is always maintained, while the sensitivity control is continuously variable over a 45 dB range.

After the AGC circuit, a low-pass filter conditions the signal so that it can be sampled by the A-D converter. The A-D conversion is performed at a sampling rate of 10 kHz.

In the final stage of processing, the output from the DSP is converted into a series of pulse bursts as described in the section entitled Description of the Cochlear Implant. These bursts are transmitted to the implanted receiver/stimulator. The pulse burst sequences are controlled by the end-user's program or MAP. The MAP consists of the frequency-to-electrode and amplitude-to-stimulation level look-up tables described

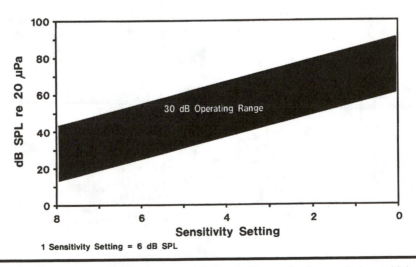

FIGURE 8.9.   Operating range of the AGC circuit. The patient-operated sensitivity control sets the maximum AGC gain of the microphone preamplifier and is continuously variable over a 45 dB range.

earlier. In the WSP, the MAP is stored in the EPROM. In the MSP, the MAP is stored in the random-access memory (RAM) of the MSP. The advantage of the RAM is that it can be instantaneously reprogrammed without the need for ultraviolet light erasure as is the case with an EPROM.

Multipeak Speech Coding Strategy

Several speech feature extraction coding strategies are available with the MSP. In addition to the F0/F2 and F0/F1/F2 strategies, the MSP utilizes the energy in the three high-frequency bands (bands 3, 4, and 5) to provide additional spectral information to the end-user. This coding strategy, referred to as the multipeak (MPEAK) scheme, extracts from the ongoing acoustic waveform the spectral peaks representing F1 and F2, as well as amplitude estimates from the three high-frequency bands. Frequency boundaries for the electrodes assigned to represent F1 and F2 are identical to those used in the F0/F1/F2 coding strategy (refer to Table 8.1); however, bands 3, 4, and 5 are assigned to fixed basal electrodes. A typical electrode allocation for bands 3, 4, and 5 is provided in Table 8.2.

In the MPEAK strategy, for voiced phonemes and environmental sounds with a low-frequency periodic component, the stimulation rate to the electrodes is equal to the fundamental frequency. In addition, because these sounds contain very little energy above 4000 Hz, the fixed electrode representing band 5 is not stimulated. In contrast, for aperiodic sounds such as voiceless phonemes, the rate of stimulation typically is higher and is random between 200 and 300 Hz. Voiceless sounds contain little energy below 1000 Hz, thus the electrode that would represent F1 is not stimulated. When using the MPEAK coding strategy, four electrode pairs are always selected for stimulation regardless of whether the input is

TABLE 8.2. Electrode allocation for bands 3, 4, and 5 when using the MPEAK coding strategy.

280–1000 Hz	F1
800–4000 Hz	F2
2000–2800 Hz	Band 3–Electrode 7
2800–4000 Hz	Band 4–Electrode 4
4000 Hz and above	Band 5–Electrode 1

periodic or aperiodic. The determination of which electrodes are selected is dependent on the spectral content of the acoustic signal. The electrodes are stimulated in fast sequence from the basal to apical end of the electrode array. Figure 8.10 illustrates this sequential stimulation for voiced and voiceless sounds.

For any acoustic signal, the amount of current delivered to the electrodes selected for stimulation is proportional to the energy within the filter bands (F1, F2, and bands 3, 4, and 5). In addition, the amplitude of stimulation is always within the patient's measured dynamic range (i.e., threshold to maximum comfortable loudness) for each electrode. This assures that the electrical stimulation results in a perceptible yet comfortable hearing sensation.

PROGRAMMING THE SPEECH PROCESSOR

Following the surgical placement of the cochlear implant, there is typically a four-to-six week recuperative period prior to programming of the speech processor. Once the surgical incision has healed and swelling over the area of the receiver/stimulator has reduced, the cochlear implant recipient returns to the clinic for the fitting of the external equipment. The first step in the fitting process is to program the speech processor. To carry out this task, an IBM PC-compatible computer, a custom-designed interface unit, and special-purpose software are used.

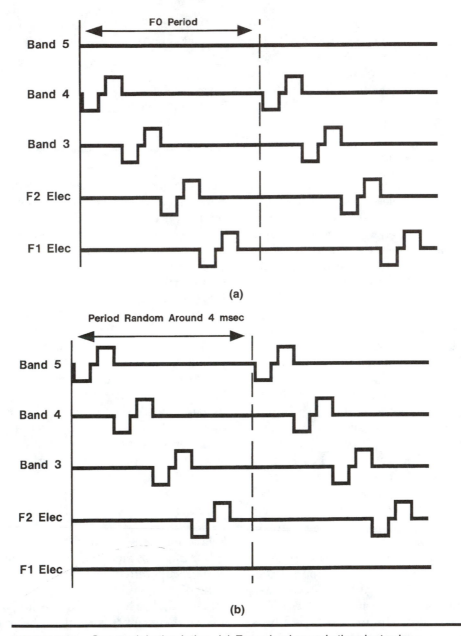

(a)

(b)

FIGURE 8.10.   Sequential stimulation. (a) For voiced sounds the electrodes representing F1, F2, and bands 3 and 4 are utilized. The electrode assigned to band 5 is not stimulated. (b) For voiceless sounds, the F1 electrode is not used and electrodes representing F2 and bands 3, 4, and 5 are stimulated. Reprinted with permission from Patrick and Clark, 1991. Copyright © by Williams & Wilkins, 1991.

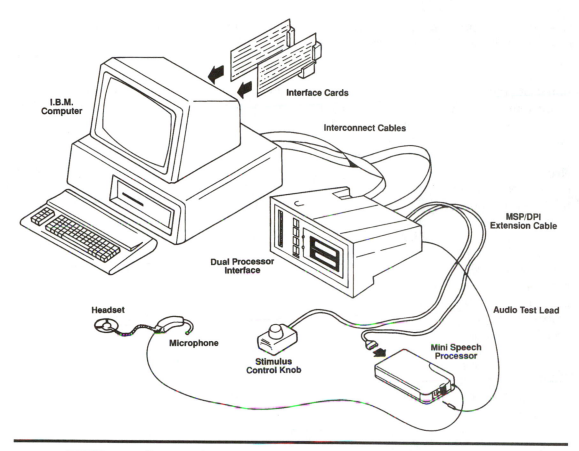

FIGURE 8.11. Programming system hardware. Reprinted with permission from Beiter and Brimacombe, 1993. Copyright © by Williams & Wilkins, 1993.

The programming system is illustrated in Figure 8.11. The hardware consists of an IBM PC-compatible computer, two multibit interface cards that are placed into the computer, and an interface unit that holds the speech processor. The two interface cards and unit are designed to physically and electrically connect the speech processor to the computer. This allows the computer to control the electrical stimulation that is delivered by the speech processor. Much of the circuitry for controlling the speech processor is contained on the two interface cards that reside in the computer. One of the cards controls the WSP. It contains a RAM, referred to as a shadow RAM, which "shadows" the data in the WSP's EPROM by disabling it and connecting the RAM to the speech processor's signal lines (address, data, and control buses). The interface card can change the contents of the shadow RAM quickly and thereby control the operation of the speech processor on a stimulus-to-stimulus basis. The second interface card controls the MSP. It uses a serial link to communicate directly with the RAM in the MSP. The interface unit has a display containing 22 light-emitting diodes (LEDs) that indicatates which electrode is being stimulated during psychophysical testing. In addition to the mechanical housing for the two types of speech processors, the interface unit contains an ultraviolet light source for erasing the WSP's EPROM. The speech processor and headset can be checked for proper operation using the programming equipment.

Customized software is used to perform specific psychophysical tests. Based on the patient's responses, a program or MAP is configured that defines the parameters of electrical stimulation for that patient. The most important psychophysical measure is the determination of the patient's dynamic range for each electrode pair to be used in the final MAP. This is accomplished by establishing the threshold and maximum acceptable loudness for each electrode pair. These loudness measures are stored on line for later use in configuring the speech processor's MAP. Once dynamic ranges have been established, each electrode pair is loudness balanced at the maximum acceptable loudness level. This procedure assures a more natural sounding quality to the speech signal. Then electrode pairs are stimulated in rapid succession from base to apex or apex to base to verify appropriate place-pitch ordering. Any electrode pairs eliciting nonauditory sensations (e.g., facial nerve stimulation) are eliminated from the program. As the cochlear implant recipient becomes more accustomed to the sound received through the cochlear implant, refinements to the speech processor's MAP are made. This flexibility is especially important when programming young children (Beiter, Staller, and Dowell, 1991). More information on speech processor programming can be found in Roberts (1991).

SUMMARY OF SPEECH CODING STRATEGIES

The Nucleus multichannel cochlear implant system utilizes a speech processing design that incorporates the extraction of key speech features from the acoustic signal, codes these

electrically, and presents them in the form of pulsatile stimulation to the electrode array. Specifically, the intensity of the acoustic signal is directly proportional to the delivered amplitude of the electrical current. The overall pitch of sound (F0) is related to the rate of pulsatile stimulation at the stimulating electrode pair; and peaks of energy (F1, F2, and bands 3, 4 and 5) in the frequency spectrum associated with specific phonemes are correlated with selective stimulation at different locations within the cochlea. The speech feature extraction strategies have evolved from the fairly simple single-formant tracker (F0/F2) to a two-formant tracker (F0/F1/F2) and, finally, to the MPEAK strategy, which encodes additional important high-frequency information. Although the ability of individual cochlear implant recipients to use this coded information for the understanding of speech varies greatly, improvements in the hardware to perform feature extraction, as well as the addition of more speech information, have generally resulted in significant improvements in patient performance.

SPEECH PERCEPTION RESULTS

F0/F2 versus F0/F1/F2

To date, over 5000 profoundly deafened adults and children have been implanted with the Nucleus multichannel cochlear implant worldwide. Numerous investigators have reported the results obtained on a variety of speech perception measures with adult patients who have used one or more of the speech coding strategies (Dowell, Mecklenburg, and Clark, 1986; Blamey et al., 1987b; Dowell et al., 1987; Gantz et al., 1987; Gantz et al., 1988; Tyler, Moore, and Kuk, 1989; Dowell et al., 1990; Spivak and Waltzman, 1990; Tye-Murray, Lowder, and Tyler, 1990; Skinner et al., 1991). In general, almost all patients demonstrate improvements in their speechreading abilities in the bimodal condition (vision plus audition) compared to the vision-alone condition. On the other hand, the auditory-only abilities of recipients vary considerably, from those who score significantly better postoperatively on closed-set tests but do not demonstrate open-set word recognition abilities to those who recognize many words and sentences presented in an open-set format.

A number of studies have been undertaken to determine if changes in speech coding strategies are associated with speech perception performance changes. Dowell et al. (1987) evaluated two different groups of subjects; one group used the original F0/F2 strategy, and the other the F0/F1/F2 coding scheme. The two groups were not significantly different from each other with respect to age at onset and duration of profound deafness. The results indicated that the subjects using the F0/F1/F2 strategy performed significantly better, especially on the more difficult auditory-only, open-set recognition tests. The mean score on the Central Institute for the Deaf (CID) Sentences of Everyday Speech test (Davis and Silverman, 1978) more than doubled with the newer scheme (mean score of 35.4% for subjects using the F0/F1/F2 strategy compared to a mean score of 15.9% for those using the original F0/F2 coding scheme). In addition, subjects using this strategy showed less degradation in performance when tested in a competing noise background.

Tye-Murray, Lowder, and Tyler (1990) tested five subjects, first using the F0/F2 and then the F0/F1/F2 strategy. These subjects also performed significantly better on difficult auditory-only, open-set word and sentence recognition measures with the F0/F1/F2 scheme. As in the Dowell et al. (1987) study, these subjects achieved better scores in the presence of background noise when using the strategy that included first formant in-

formation. These researchers also performed an information-transfer analysis (Miller and Nicely, 1955) on the consonant confusion matrices for the vision-alone and bimodal conditions. The results suggested that the addition of the first formant provided greater transmission of the features of voicing, duration, and overall envelope.

Brimacombe and Beiter (1992) compared postoperative performance on the open-set CID Sentences test for 71 patients using the original F0/F2 speech coding strategy to that of 232 patients who had used the F0/F1/F2 strategy exclusively. The mean postoperative open-set CID Sentences test scores for these two groups were 11% for those using the F0/F2 strategy and 32% for those using the F0/F1/F2 coding strategy. An analysis of variance revealed that patient performance with the F0/F1/F2 strategy was superior to performance with the F0/F2 strategy.

F0/F1/F2 versus MPEAK

Comparative performance of profoundly deafened adults using the FO/F1/F2 and MPEAK coding strategies has been studied by two groups of researchers. Dowell et al. (1990) compared the results for two groups of subjects: one group using the WSP and its F0/F1/F2 coding strategy and the other the MSP and its MPEAK coding scheme. The two groups, comprising four subjects each, were matched on age, cochlear implant experience, and postoperative speech perception results using the F0/F1/F2 coding strategy. The open-set stimuli consisted of the Bamford-Kowal-Bench (BKB) Sentences (Bench and Bamford, 1979) administered in the auditory-only condition in quiet and with competing noise [20, 15, and 10 dB signal-to-noise ratios (SNR)]. Results revealed a highly significant difference in performance between the two groups. Mean sentence scores in quiet were 54.8% for the F0/F1/F2 group and 88.0% for the MPEAK group. In competing noise, the MPEAK group maintained a significantly higher level of performance than the F0/F1/F2 group. Even in the most difficult listening condition (10 dB SNR), the MPEAK group achieved a mean score of 64.5%.

Skinner et al. (1991) studied the performance of a group of five subjects who first used the WSP with its F0/F1/F2 scheme, then the MSP with its MPEAK coding strategy. Again, BKB sentences were used to compare performance in quiet and noise (20, 15, and 10 dB SNR). Results revealed that on average, subjects using the MPEAK strategy scored significantly higher than when using the F0/F1/F2 strategy. Mean scores were 70% for the MPEAK scheme and 51% for the F0/F1/F2 strategy. Performance in noise for all SNRs was significantly better when using the MPEAK strategy. In the most unfavorable listening condition (10 dB SNR), average performance was 48% for the MPEAK condition and 20% for the F0/F1/F2 scheme.

Finally, Brimacombe and Beiter (1992) also compared postoperative performance on the open-set CID Sentences test for 232 patients using the F0/F1/F2 strategy and 64 patients using the MPEAK scheme. An analysis of variance revealed that patient performance with the MPEAK strategy was superior to performance with the F0/F1/F2 strategy.

Summary

As mentioned above, a number of investigators have demonstrated the benefits provided by multichannel cochlear implants for appropriately selected profoundly deafened individuals. It is interesting to note that as speech coding strategies become more complex, providing additional cues, adult subjects perform significantly better on difficult open-set speech tasks. Although speech perception abilities have improved with advances in

speech coding strategy research, on average, performance falls well below that of normal-hearing listeners. As technology improves, it is likely that performance will follow suit. The final section explores the future direction of speech coding strategy research for multichannel cochlear implants.

FUTURE DIRECTIONS

Research is currently under way at the University of Melbourne to determine whether speech perception abilities of 22 channel cochlear implant recipients can be improved using an experimental processor, referred to as the spectral maxima sound processor (SMSP). This experimental unit uses 16 bandpass filters to estimate the ongoing acoustic spectrum. The center frequencies of these filters range from 250 to 5400 Hz. The filters' frequency spacings are linear up to 1650 Hz and logarithmic beyond 1650 Hz. The signals are rectified and low-pass filtered, then estimates of the amplitudes of the 16 spectral components are converted to digital form for additional processing. The 16 most apical electrode pairs are used to track the 16 bandpass filters, with the lowest-frequency bandpass assigned to the most apical electrode pair. Progressively higher frequency bandpasses are assigned to more basally placed electrodes. The output from the six filters with the largest amplitudes is used to generate pulsatile electrical stimulation that is delivered to six electrode pairs in a rapid, sequential format. The rate of stimulation is fixed at 250 Hz (McKay et al., 1991).

This experimental processing strategy has been compared to the MPEAK scheme in the same group of four subjects. Subjects were tested with a variety of speech material, including closed-set vowel and consonant recognition tests and open-set monosyllabic words and sentences, in an auditory-only condition. Sentence material was presented in quiet and with competing noise (25, 20, 15, 10, and 5 dB SNR). Results revealed that all four subjects performed significantly better on sentence materials, as the listening condition became degraded when using the SMSP. For example, at a 10 dB SNR the mean sentence score was 50.0% for the MPEAK strategy and 78.7% for the SMSP. Using the experimental strategy, improved performance was also demonstrated for the most difficult test in the battery, that is, open-set monosyllabic words. Mean scores were 39.9% for the MPEAK scheme and 57.4% for the SMSP. It is interesting to note that three of the four subjects achieved mean open-set monosyllabic word scores ranging from 66% to 75% (McKay, McDermott et al., 1992). These scores are comparable to those expected for individuals with a moderate hearing handicap (Goetzinger, 1978).

Research is also under way at the Research Triangle Institute, through a National Institutes of Health grant, to study alternative speech processing strategies for cochlear implants. Wilson et al. (1991) have studied the speech perception abilities of seven users of the Ineraid multichannel cochlear implant with an experimental speech processing scheme that they refer to as the continuous interleaved sampling (CIS) strategy. These subjects are implanted with an array consisting of six intracochlear stimulating electrodes and a remote reference, which connect to a percutaneous pedestal (Dorman et al., 1988). The experimental speech processing strategy consists of trains of balanced biphasic pulses delivered to each of the six electrodes in a rapid, sequential fashion. The amplitudes of the pulses are determined from the envelopes of six bandpass filters. Then the envelopes are rectified and low-pass filtered. Finally, the amplitude of each stimulus pulse is deter-

mined by a power law transformation of the corresponding channel's envelope signal. This transformation compresses the signal into an appropriate dynamic range. A key feature of this experimental strategy is its relatively high rate of stimulation on each channel, usually above 800 Hz.

Seven subjects have used the CIS strategy in the laboratory. Results of open-set sentence testing revealed that the subjects scored significantly better when using the CIS strategy than with the Ineraid compressed analog (CA) speech processor. Mean sentence scores in quiet were 87% for the CA strategy and 99% for the CIS scheme. On the most difficult test in the battery, the open-set monosyllabic word test, mean scores improved from 43% for the CA strategy to 63% for the CIS scheme (Wilson et al., 1991). These scores obtained in quiet are remarkably similar to those reported by McKay et al. (1992).

The findings of these two groups of investigators are very encouraging. A growing body of evidence suggests that performance will continue to improve as more sophisticated signal processing schemes evolve. The use of a greater number of channels of electrical stimulation to provide more spectral information, higher stimulation rates to preserve the temporal fine structure of speech, digital signal processing to preserve important amplitude cues, and improved noise reduction techniques have improved speech recognition to levels never before imagined. It remains to be seen whether further advancements in technology will allow even greater improvements in the speech perception abilities of profoundly deafened individuals. As technology advances and our knowledge of the auditory system expands, it is likely that the long-term research objective will be the replacement of an essentially nonfunctional sensory system with a man-made prosthesis.

REFERENCES

Beiter, A.L., and Brimacombe, J.A. (1993). Cochlear implants. In: J.G. Alpiner and P.A. McCarthy (eds.), *Rehabilitative Audiology: Children and Adults*. Baltimore: Williams and Wilkins.

Beiter, A.L., Staller, S.J., and Dowell, R.C. (1991). Evaluation and device programming in children. In: S.J. Staller (ed.), Multichannel cochlear implants in children (pp. 25S–33S). Suppl to *Ear and Hearing*, 12, no. 4.

Bench, J., and Bamford, J. (1979). *Speech-Hearing Tests and the Spoken Language of Hearing-Impaired Children*. London: Academic Press.

Blamey, P.J., Dowell, R.C., Clark, G.M., and Seligman, P.M. (1987a). Acoustic parameters measured by a formant-estimating speech processor for a multiple-channel cochlear implant. *Journal of the Acoustical Society of America* 82:38–47.

Blamey, P.J., Dowell, R.C., Brown, A.M., Clark, G.M., and Seligman, P.M. (1987b). Vowel and consonant recognition of cochlear implant patients using formant-estimating speech processors. *Journal of the Acoustical Society of America* 82:48–57.

Blamey, P.J., and Clark, G.M. (1990). Place coding of vowel formants for cochlear implant patients. *Journal of the Acoustical Society of America* 88:667–673.

Brimacombe, J.A., and Beiter, A.L. (1992). Evolution of speech coding strategies for the Nucleus 22 Channel Cochlear Implant System. Presented at a Satellite Symposium following the XXI International Congress of Audiology, Tokyo, September.

Brummer, S.B., and Turner, M.J. (1975). Electrical stimulation of the nervous system: The principle of safe charge injection with noble metal electrodes. *Bio-electrochemistry and Bioenergetics* 2:13–25.

Clark, G.M., and Tong, Y.C. (1985). The engineering of future cochlear implants. In: R.F. Gray (ed.), *Cochlear Implants* (pp. 211–228). San Diego: College Hill Press.

Clark, G.M., Blamey, P.J., Brown, A.M., et al. (1987). In: C.R. Pfaltz (ed.), *Advances in Oto-Rhino-Laryngology*, *vol.38*. The University of Melbourne-Nucleus multi-electrode cochlear implant. Basel: Karger.

Clark, G.M., Cohen, N.L., and Shepherd, R.K. (1991). Surgical and safety considerations of multichannel cochlear implants in children. In: S.J. Staller (ed.), Multichannel cochlear implants in children (pp. 15S–24S). Suppl to *Ear and Hearing*, 12, no. 4.

Clark, G.M., Franz, B.K.-H., Pyman, B.C., and Webb, R.L. (1991). Surgery for multichannel cochlear implantation. In: H. Cooper (ed.), *Cochlear Implants: A Practical Guide* (pp. 169–200). London: Whurr Publishers.

Crosby, P.A., Daly, C.N., Money, D.K., Patrick, J.F., Seligman, P.M., and Kuzma, J.A. (1985). Cochlear implant system for an auditory prosthesis. United States Patent 4,532,930.

Davis, H., and Silverman, S. (1978). *Hearing and Deafness* (pp. 536-538). New York: Holt, Rinehart and Winston.

Dorman, M.F., Hannley, M.T., McCandless, G.A., and Smith, L.M. (1988). Auditory/phonetic categorization with the Symbion multichannel cochlear implant. *Journal of the Acoustical Society of America* 84:501–510.

Dowell, R.C., Mecklenburg, D.J., and Clark, G.M. (1986). Speech recognition for 40 patients receiving multichannel cochlear implants. *Archives of Otolaryngology* 112:1054–1059.

Dowell, R.C., Seligman, P.M., Blamey, P.J., and Clark, G.M. (1987). Speech perception using a two-formant 22-electrode cochlear prosthesis in quiet and in noise. *Acta Otolaryngologica* 104:439–446.

Dowell, R.C., Whitford, L.A., Seligman, P.M., Franz, B.K-H., and Clark, G.M. (1990). Preliminary results with a miniature speech processor for the 22-electrode Melbourne/Cochlear hearing prosthesis. *Otorhinolaryngology, Head & Neck Surgery* 1167–1173.

Gantz, B.J., McCabe, B.F., Tyler, R.S., and Preece, J.P. (1987). Evaluation of four cochlear implant designs. *Annals of Otology, Rhinology and Laryngology* 96(Suppl. 128):145–147.

Gantz, B.J., Tyler, R.S., Knutson, J.F., et al. (1988). Evaluation of five different cochlear implant designs: Audiologic assessment and predictors of performance. *Laryngoscope* 98:1100–1106.

Goetzinger, C.P. (1978) Word discrimination testing (1978). In: J. Katz (ed.), *Handbook of Clinical Audiology* (pp. 149–158). Baltimore: Williams & Wilkins.

Luxford, W.M., and Brackmann, D.E. (1985). The history of cochlear implants. In: R.F. Gray (ed.), *Cochlear Implants* (pp. 1–26). San Diego: College Hill Press.

McKay, C., McDermott, H., Vandali, A., and Clark, G.M. (1991). Preliminary results with a six spectral maxima sound processor for the University of Melbourne/Nucleus multiple-electrode cochlear implant. *Journal of the Otolaryngological Society of Australia* 6:354–359.

McKay, C.M., McDermott, H.J., Vandali, A.E., and Clark, G.M. (1992). A comparison of speech perception of cochlear implantees using the spectral maxima sound processor (SMSP) and the MSP (MULTIPEAK) processor. *Acta Otolaryngologica* 112:752–761.

Mecklenburg, D.J., and Shallop, J.K. (1988). Cochlear implants. In: N.J. Lass, L.V. McReynolds, J.L. Northern, and D. E. Yoder (eds.), *Handbook of Speech-Language Pathology and Audiology* (pp. 1355–1368). Toronto: B.C. Decker.

Mecklenburg, D.J., and Lehnhardt, E. (1991). The development of cochlear implants in Europe, Asia, and Australia. In: H. Cooper (ed.), *Cochlear Implants: A Practical Guide* (pp. 34–57). London: Whurr Publishers.

Miller, G.A., and Nicely, P.E. (1955). An analysis of perceptual confusions among some English consonants. *Journal of the Acoustical Society of America* 27:338–351.

Patrick, J.F., Seligman, P.M., Money, D.K., and Kuzma, J.A. (1990). Engineering. In: G.M. Clark, Y.C. Tong, and J.F. Patrick (eds.), *Cochlear Prostheses* (pp. 99–124). Edinburgh: Churchill Livingstone.

Patrick, J.F., and Clark, G.M. (1991). The Nucleus 22-channel cochlear implant system. In: S.J. Staller (ed.), Multichannel cochlear implants in children (pp. 3S–9S). Suppl to *Ear and Hearing*, 12, no. 4.

Peterson, G.E., and Barney, H.L. (1952). Control methods used in a study of the identification of vowels. *Journal of the Acoustical Society of America* 24:175–184.

Pfingst, B.E. (1990). Psychophysical constraints on biophysical/neural models of threshold. In:

J.M. Miller and F.A. Spelman (eds.), *Cochlear Implants: Models of the Electrically Stimulated Ear* (pp. 161–185). New York: Springer-Verlag.

Pfingst, B.E., Spelman, F.A., and Sutton, D. (1980). Operating ranges for cochlear implants. *Annals of Otology, Rhinology, and Laryngology* 89:1–4.

Roberts, S. (1991). Speech-processor fitting for cochlear implants. In: H. Cooper (ed.), *Cochlear Implants: A Practical Guide* (pp. 201–218). London: Whurr Publishers.

Shallop, J.K., and Mecklenburg, D.J. (1987). Technical aspects of cochlear implants. In: R.E. Sandlin (ed.), *Handbook of Hearing Aid Amplification* (pp. 265–280). San Diego: College Hill Press.

Shepherd, R.K, Clark, G.M., and Black, R.C. (1983). Chronic electrical stimulation of the auditory nerve in cats: Physiological and histopathological results. *Acta Otolaryngologica* 399 (Suppl.):19–31.

Shepherd, R.K., Franz, B.K.-H., and Clark, G.M. (1990). The biocompatibility and safety of cochlear prostheses. In: G.M. Clark, Y.C. Tong, and J.F. Patrick (eds.), *Cochlear Prostheses* (pp. 69–98). Edinburgh: Churchill Livingstone.

Skinner, M.W., Holden, L.K., Holden, T.A., et al. (1991). Performance of postlinguistically deaf adults with the Wearable Speech Processor (WSP III) and Mini Speech Processor (MSP) of the Nucleus multi-electrode cochlear implant. *Ear and Hearing* 12:3–22.

Spivak, L.G., and Waltzman, S.B., (1990). Performance of cochlear implant patients as a function of time. *Journal of Speech and Hearing Research* 33:511–519.

Staller, S.J. (1985). Cochlear implant characteristics: A review of current technology. In: G.A. McCandless (ed.), Cochlear Implants (pp. 23–32). *Seminars in Hearing*, New York: Thieme-Stratton.

Tong, Y.C., Black, R.C., Clark, G.M., et al. (1979). A preliminary report on a multiple-channel cochlear implant operation. *Journal of Laryngology and Otology* 93:679–695.

Tong, Y.C., Clark, G.M., Blamey, P.J., Busby, P.A., and Dowell, R.C. (1982). Psychophysical studies for two multiple-channel cochlear implant patients. *Journal of the Acoustical Society of America* 71:153–160.

Tong, Y.C., Millar, J.B., Clark G.M., Martin, L.F.,

Busby, P.A., and Patrick, J.F. (1980). Psychophysical and speech perception studies on two multiple channel cochlear implant patients. *Journal of Laryngology and Otology* 94: 1241–1256.

Tye-Murray, N., Lowder, M., and Tyler, R.S. (1990). Comparison of the F0F2 and F0F1F2 processing strategies for the Cochlear Corporation cochlear implant. *Ear and Hearing* 11:195–200.

Tyler, R.S., Moore, B.C.J., and Kuk, F.K. (1989). Performance of some better cochlear implant patients. *Journal of Speech and Hearing Research* 32:887–911.

Tyler, R.S., and Tye-Murray, N. (1991). Cochlear implant signal-processing strategies and patient perception of speech and environmental sounds. In: H. Cooper (ed.), *Cochlear Implants: A Practical Guide* (pp. 58–83). London: Whurr Publishers.

Walsh, S.M., and Leak-Jones, P.A. (1982). Chronic electrical stimulation of auditory nerve in cat: Physiological and histological results. *Hearing Research* 7:281–304.

Webb, R.L., Clark, G.M., Shepherd, R.K., Franz, B.K.-H., and Pyman, B.C. (1988). The biologic safety of the Cochlear Corporation multiple-electrode intracochlear implant. *American Journal of Otology* 9:8–13.

Webb, R.L., Pyman, B.C., Franz, B.K.-H., and Clark, G.M. (1990). The surgery of cochlear implantation. In: G.M. Clark, Y.C. Tong, and J.F. Patrick (eds.), *Cochlear Prostheses* (pp. 153–180). Edinburgh: Churchill Livingstone.

Wilson, B.S., Finley, C.C., Lawson, D.T., Wolford, R.D., Eddington, D.K., and Rabinowitz, W.M. (1991). Better speech recognition with cochlear implants. *Nature* 352:236–238.

CHAPTER 9

APPLICATION AND FITTING STRATEGIES FOR PROGRAMMABLE HEARING INSTRUMENTS

Robert W. Sweetow

The first eight chapters in this textbook present useful information about digital hearing systems in general, as well as a rather detailed overview of several commercially available digitally programmable hearing aids in particular. In Chapter 10, Valente compares selected digitally programmable systems and contrasts their advantages and limitations. He reviews clinical and electroacoustic factors that should be considered by dispensers and audiologists contemplating the selection and fitting of programmable hearing instruments.

In this chapter, emphasis will be placed on fitting and selection strategies that can be employed with digitally programmable hearing aids. Clearly, the flexibility afforded to the hearing health professional and the user of programmable aids provides a broader, and sometimes different, array of fitting strategies. Some of these methods are based on existing procedures employed for analog aids. Other fitting and selection procedures can be approached in a rather novel manner. It is not the intent of this chapter to find a "winner" among commercially available systems. Indeed, during the period of time it took to complete this chapter, several other programmable systems have been introduced. It is a near certainty that additional systems will be available before this book is published. In fact, an attempt to se-

lect a single winner among programmable hearing aids is ludicrous because one of the great advantages of programmable instruments is their flexibility. This is due to the fact that every hearing-impaired listener presents his or her own unique set of acoustic needs. Clinical determination regarding which adjustable parameters are applicable to a specific patient must be assessed on an individual basis. Since it would be extremely difficult to offer all of the potentially useful features in one programmable system, the array of individual demands underscores the need for the availability of several programmable systems from which the appropriate selection can be made.

Therefore, philosophies, strategies, and techniques discussed in this chapter will focus more on individual features of programmable systems, rather than on specific makes and models of the hearing instruments themselves. Only after ascertaining the necessary and desired acoustic response characteristics for a specific patient can the dispenser determine which programmable system best interfaces with need.

PATIENT CANDIDACY

Because of the flexibility characteristic of programmable hearing aids, there is probably an appropriate system that will provide a suitable fit for nearly every mild to severely hearing-impaired patient. However, this statement does not imply that all hearing aid candidates require a digitally programmable system. Since there may be a considerable expense in terms of monetary cost to the patient, as well as time spent by the dispenser, one must determine whether or not any given patient needs a programmable instrument. Unless the hearing health professional can present supporting clinical data that the most suitable aid for the patient is a programmable one, there may be little justification for its selection. If goals can be reached using conventional analog aids, it is the simplest, most

economical path. Nevertheless, there is an increasing number of reasons why digitally programmable systems may be more convenient and acoustically superior to conventional analog aids. Some of the issues dispensers should consider when making this determination are described in the following paragraphs.

Does the patient present an unusual audiometric configuration as characterized by frequency notches, reverse slopes, or multiple changes in slope magnitude, degree, or direction? Examples of these audiometric types are shown in Figures 9.1, 9.2, and 9.3. Notwithstanding attempts using special earhook cou-

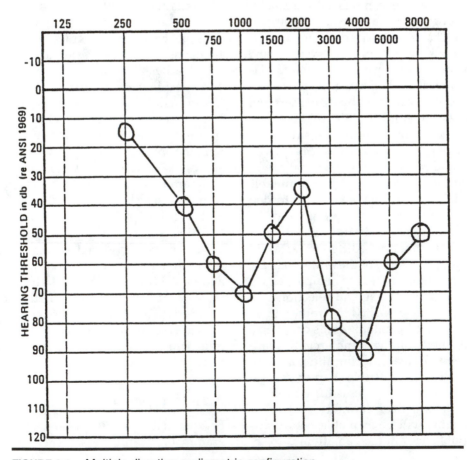

FIGURE 9.1.   Multiple direction audiometric configuration.

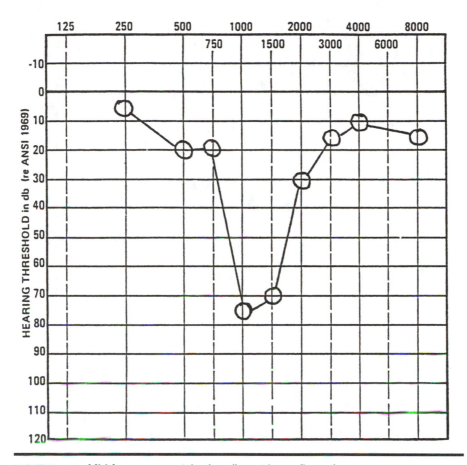

FIGURE 9.2. Mid-frequency notched audiometric configuration.

pler arrangements for postauricular aids (Killion, 1984; Schwartz, 1991), it is often a difficult clinical task to achieve an optimal fit for these audiometric configurations utilizing conventional hearing instruments. Furthermore, not all BTE aids are compatible with these hooks, and such acoustic modification technology is often not applicable to ITE or ITC aids. For these audiometric configurations, certain programmable aids can achieve extremely fine tuning and closely approximate recommended target gains. It is important to consider that the more unusual the fitting requirements, the closer the dispenser might come to meeting recommended targets with a programmable aid having multiple

frequency channels with adjustable crossover frequencies. Figure 9.3 depicts a reverse notched audiogram. An attempt to reach target gain with a single-channel versus a multiple-channel hearing aid for this aid is shown in Figure 9.4. Note that the target gain for this reverse notched audiogram was "overshot" when using a single-channel programmable analog aid [Figure 9.4(a)]. However, with a multichannel aid [Figure 9.4(b)] target gain was closely approximated.

Does the patient have fluctuating hearing? Conventional analog hearing aids have an average life expectancy of 3 to 5 years. It remains to be seen whether the life expectancy of pro-

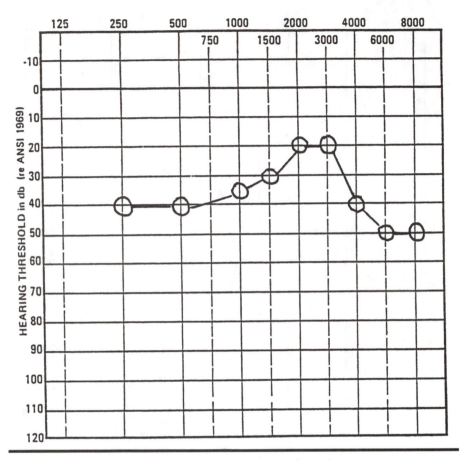

FIGURE 9.3. Reverse slope notched audiometric configuration.

grammable aids will be the same or longer. It is certain that if a patient's hearing fluctuates, even a well-functioning nonprogrammable aid will have to be replaced to maintain pace with significant changes in the patient's hearing level. Consider, for example, patients with Menière's syndrome, hormonal fluctuation, or progressive ototoxicity. Programmable aids can meet the changing amplification needs of these patients. Often the extent of necessary electroacoustic changes exceeds that obtainable even with conventional analog aids having active filtering potentiometers.

Figure 9.5(a) shows two extreme frequency responses obtainable with an analog BTE that has very active low-frequency cut filters. Figure 9.5(b) indicates the difference in dB between these two responses. Compare these two responses to that obtainable through a digitally programmable BTE shown in Figure 9.6. Not only can the dispenser produce dramatic changes such as these by reprogramming the instrument, but the use of hearing aids having multiple memories can assist the patient *and* the dispenser by allowing for programming of *anticipated* changes without necessitating frequent return visits for reprogramming procedures.

An additional advantage of programmable aids for fluctuating hearing can be

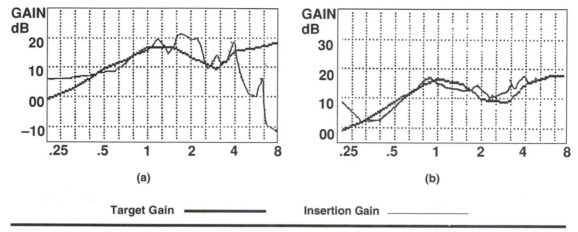

(a)

(b)

Target Gain ━━━━━━━━━   Insertion Gain ━━━━━━━━━

FIGURE 9.4. Target gain. (a) Target match achieved with a single-band programmable instrument. (b) Target match achieved with a multiple-band programmable instrument.

shown for patients reporting sudden hearing loss. For these patients there are often dramatic changes in sensitivity and audiometric configuration occurring within two months following onset. It is not clinically practical to change to another hearing aid while waiting for the hearing level to stabilize. For this reason, the application of programmable aids is apparent and defensible.

Is the dispenser uncertain of the most desirable acoustic and electroacoustic parameters for a given patient?   An example of a patient presenting incomplete information is a child unable to voluntarily provide sufficient audiological information necessary to make definitive decisions about amplification needs. Cognitively and centrally impaired adults are additional examples. As more clinical infor-

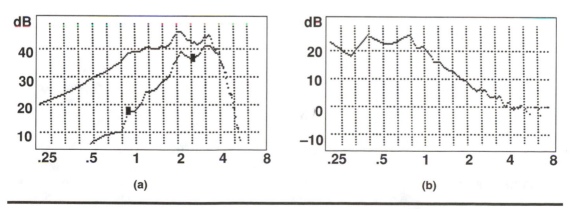

(a)

(b)

FIGURE 9.5.   (a) The two extreme low-frequency responses measured from a conventional instrument containing very active filtering potentiometers. (b) The difference (in dB) between the two curves shown in (a).

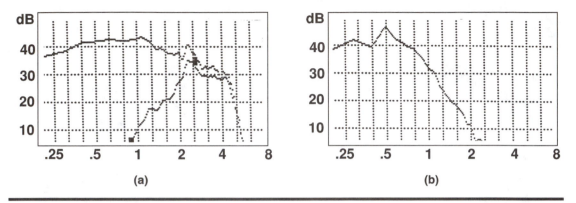

FIGURE 9.6. (a) Two low-frequency responses measured from a programmable instrument. (b) The difference (in dB) between the two curves shown in (a).

mation becomes available, the more informed the dispenser becomes, allowing for appropriate settings of the aids. Most hearing health professionals, using conventional analog aids, fit children with instruments that provide maximum flexibility via potentiometer adjustments. As shown above, the amount of flexibility available to the dispenser is much greater with digitally programmable systems. In addition, some of the technological features available in these systems, such as advanced compression and programmability of the telecoil response, may be very useful.

Do the patient's listening environments place a variety of electroacoustic demands on the hearing aid? Would the patient function better in different environments if he/she had more than one hearing aid response to choose from? Libby and Sweetow (1987) observed that a linear, nonprogrammable hearing aid set for one acoustic environment may not be appropriate for other environments in which listening takes place. If patients routinely experience a variety of acoustic environments, even an automatically adaptable, conventional hearing aid may not be as suitable as one having several different acoustic programs immediately accessible to the user. Prior to the

introduction of multimemory programmable aids, the best attempt at meeting the demands of a changing acoustic environment came from so-called ASP (automatic signal processor) instruments. These hearing aids are characterized by the ability to adapt to the environment by altering electroacoustic parameters as a function of the input signal. Specifically, most ASP hearing aids reduce low-frequency gain when the input signal at the microphone exceeds a certain dB level. In some cases, the input signal sensor operates at a fixed frequency. If, for example, the signal input at the microphone exceeds 70 dB at 200 Hz, the amount of low-frequency gain is reduced by increasing the frequency response slope (or raising the low-pass filter cutoff frequency). In other cases, the hearing aid may perform either a spectral or temporal analysis of the incoming signal and reduce gain at those frequencies comprising the offending noise.

There are certain limitations inherent in either of these tactics. The major problem is that a portion of the acoustic energy of the noise also contains frequencies critical to speech understanding. Therefore, an alteration of the noise spectra can affect the intelligibility of the speech signal. In either case, there are time constraints involved that might disrupt speech perception, particularly if the frequency response is changing in the presence of a rapidly fluctuating background noise. This may be particularly deleterious for listeners relying mainly on temporal cues, such as those with severe or profound losses (Boothroyd et al., 1988)

Several studies have produced conflicting results regarding whether or not ASP hearing aids provide substantial improvement in speech perception and discrimination (Tyler and Kuk, 1989; Van Tassel, Larsen, and Fabry, 1989). For programmable aids featuring user-controlled multiple memories, some of the pitfalls inherent in automatically adaptable responses can be avoided by selecting the memories that best enhance speech for that acoustic environment for that particular listener.

Does the patient have difficulty obtaining adequate gain without the production of acoustic feedback?   Feedback is usually caused by leakage of amplified acoustic energy from the ear canal back into the microphone of the hearing aid (Lybarger, 1982). It is intuitively obvious that to prevent feedback, one should strive to acheive a more complete acoustic seal of the external auditory meatus. Unfortunately, improving the acoustic seal may magnify the occlusion effect, increasing the tactile sensation intrameatal pressure, and, in some cases, even producing greater insertion loss. Venting the earmold or ITE shell may reduce these unwanted effects, but at the same time increase the probability of acoustic feedback.

If one cannot reduce feedback via acoustic modification, another tactic often employed is electroacoustic modification. Many hearing aids have feedback reduction potentiometers. Typically, these operate by one of two schemes. Either they shift the peak away from the feedback-producing frequency, or they reduce the high-frequency gain. In either case, feedback may be minimized at the expense of rendering certain high-frequency speech sounds inaudible.

Some multichannel programmable hearing aids allow for a reduction of a fairly narrow band of frequencies from which feedback is arising so that intelligibility is not sacrificed. Furthermore, the use of real-ear probe microphone measures permits the dispenser to determine precisely the frequency and intensity of audible and incipient feedback so that appropriate adjustments can be made.

Does the patient require compression in more than one channel?   The majority of patients fitted with hearing aid devices have sensorineural hearing loss. Moreover, the majority of patients with sensorineural hearing losses suffer from loudness recruitment. Some form of loudness control should be present in the instrument response to prevent damage to the ear and to maintain sound at an intensity level below that which is uncomfortable to the patient.

Considering the known effects of distortion that can be produced by hearing aids governed by peak clipping, it is surprising to note that over 80% of the hearing aids currently sold in the United States are linear instruments (Hawkins, personal communication, 1992). To minimize this distortion, which is particularly devastating to the sensorineural-impaired listener in noisy environments, many instruments utilize one or more forms of compression or automatic gain control (AGC). Single-band AGC operates by reducing the overall gain level across the frequency range when a certain SPL is exceeded (either at the input or output stage, depending on the type of AGC). One problem with this method is that a reduction of high-frequency gain, resulting from an excessive low-frequency noise input, can reduce the intelligibility of consonant sounds. In addition, since loudness perception does not grow uniformly across frequencies, there is no reason to impose the same compression parameters (knee, ratio, and temporal factors) across all frequencies. Hearing aids that contain multiband compression offer significant benefits over single-channel compression instruments. These benefits were described by Pluvinage in Chapter 2 and will be discussed later.

Do patients reject analog hearing aids because of perceived poor quality of sound? Evidence suggests that hearing aids containing irregular frequency responses (numerous peaks and valleys) may not sound as good to sensorineural-impaired listeners and may force them to lower the volume to the point of rendering important sounds inaudible (Bornstein and Randolph, 1983). Some programmable systems permit the dispenser to smooth peaks in selected frequency regions, while others have inherently smoother responses.

For each of the examples presented above, electroacoustic performance characteristics vital to improved hearing of these individuals are easily accessible with programmable aids. If the patient requires any of these features, these instruments should be considered. Having decided that such aids are to be tried, one must next tackle the difficult task of determining which of the available instruments to evaluate.

RATIONALE FOR PROGRAMMABLE HEARING AID SELECTION

It is essential to establish which programmable features are applicable for a specific patient. These features must be assessed on an individual basis and cannot be assumed entirely on the basis of hearing impairment classification only. Each hearing deficit will likely require its own fitting algorithm. No single signal processing approach will work for the

majority of patients (Hecox, 1988). Thus, *versatility* is the key word. Effectively utilizing the versatility inherent in programmable hearing aids depends on the dispenser's knowledge of the interaction between the hearing aid's available features and the accurate measurement of the perceptual and psychoacoustic needs of the patient. Significant improvement is needed in the clinical evaluation of perceptual and psychoacoustic deficits as well as the strengths of hearing-impaired listeners in order to improve algorithms. In keeping with the concept of flexibility, however, one must recognize that algorithms presented by even the most sophisticated computer should be viewed only as starting points in the final tuning of the hearing aid response.

Needs Assessment

The needs assessment of a hearing-impaired individual must encompass both *subjective* (obtained via the case history) and *objective* (obtained via the clinical testing) data collection. At the minimum, the following questions should be asked during the subjective evaluation.

What does the patient hope and expect to gain from amplification? Because of the relatively high cost of digitally programmable hearing aids, many patients expect miracles. Some potential users have been misled, either by other satisfied users or by overly enthusiastic advertisements that suggest that these "high-tech" aids are capable of eliminating background noise. Features unique to programmable systems, such as multiple memories, multiband compression, and adjustable release time can, in fact, improve the patient's perception in noisy listening environments. However, realistic expectations must be conveyed to the listener. These aids do not eliminate background noise. It should be pointed out to the prospective user that elimination of background noise is neither realistic nor necessarily advisable. A world void of background is analogous to a world limited to black and white. Normal listeners experience background noise; they simply are better able to extract the primary acoustic message and place it "in front." This, not the elimination of background noise, should be the goal.

How often is the patient exposed to noisy environments? How do these environmental noises affect the patient's performance? The patient who is rarely subjected to environmental noise may not require an amplification system having multiple memories. If so, it may be more important to concentrate on other features, such as additional flexibility in frequency shaping provided by multiple channels or increasing the sensitivity of the telecoil. Patients not adversely affected by noise may prefer the sound quality of a wide-frequency-band system appropriate for his/her type and magnitude of hearing loss. There may be no need to markedly reduce low-frequency amplification if a patient with a relatively flat audiometric configuration seldom converses in a communicative environment in which noise is present. It may be more important to concentrate on the patient's perception of his or her own voice.

How loud or disturbing are these changing environmental conditions? How large are the rooms in which listening takes place? How far away are the speakers? Are the rooms highly reverberant? The dispenser should obtain a description of the most difficult listening environments. Tape recordings may augment the patient's verbal description. The answers to these questions can be primary indicators of the need for certain features, such as full dynamic range compression, directional microphones, or adjustable release times. These features are available in some, though not all, of the current systems.

How do various noise environments affect the patient's performance? What can the patient do to control listening situations? It is clinically astute to ascertain which background noise environments create problems for the patient. If there are a number of them, establish priorities that can be incorporated into the programming strategy. Determination of what, if any, attempts are made by the patient to improve his listening situations will assist the dispenser in subsequent counseling and in the determination of a prognosis. The user willing to adopt listening strategies providing assistance beyond that provided by the hearing aids themselves is more likely to succeed.

Is the patient's primary complaint one of having difficulty understanding the speech of certain individuals? Some patients indicate experiencing difficulty only when listening to certain voices, such as those of children or females. Obtain an accurate description of these speakers' voices. If a variety of voices elicit descriptions of different problems for the hearing-impaired listener, multimemory systems may be appropriate. The author has used multimemory aids with particular effectiveness for some professional counselors who report major difficulty in their ability to understand certain male versus female patients.

Does the patient have difficulty understanding conversation over the telephone? How important is telephone use for the patient? Does, or will, the patient utilize assistive listening devices requiring telecoils? The telecoil sensitivity listed by manufacturers of digitally programmable systems covers a rather broad performance range. Some systems have no telecoil at all. If the patient is to rely on the microphone input only from the amplification system, consider whether an ITE might be more susceptible to feedback. If so, it may be necessary to utilize a multi-memory system that has one memory dedicated to telephone use by modifying the frequency response to roll off the frequencies above 2500 Hz. Also, implementation of the new American with Disabilities Act may make the availability of assistive listening devices so much more accessible that telecoil usage may become indispensable.

How are significant others affected by the patient's hearing problem?   The advisability of involving significant others in the aural rehabilitation process is not limited to programmable systems only. They should be involved in the rehabilitation process regardless of the hearing instrument type selected. However, the increased flexibility provided by programmable systems allows for even greater incorporation of additional information provided by significant others. These significant others often recognize negative situations that otherwise may go unreported, or even undetected. An example of this is the presence of acoustic feedback, which the listener does not hear because of a high-frequency hearing loss.

Does the patient have tinnitus? If so, does it present a significant problem?   An effective management method for patients suffering from intractable tinnitus is the use of hearing aid amplification (Surr, Montgomery, and Mueller, 1985). It is unclear whether amplification is helpful because (a) it produces direct stimulation of the basilar membrane at a specific frequency range coinciding with the perceived pitch of the ongoing tinnitus; (b) it creates an upward spread of masking caused by background noise amplified by the hearing aid; (c) it arises from the internal noise produced by the hearing aid itself; or (d) it diminishes the perception of tinnitus by introducing an acoustic distraction (Sweetow, Cato, and Levy, 1991).

Because of this lack of understanding (or the individuality displayed by each tinnitus sufferer), matching the pitch of the patient's perceived tinnitus does not yet provide the dispenser with sufficient information to know how to program the hearing instruments to best accommodate the need for adequate amplification and/or masking of the tinnitus. Thus, programmable aids, allowing for rapid user comparisons among acoustic parameters, can be useful for these kinds of patients in settling on compromises. Multi-memory aids permit dedicating one program for normal listening purposes and another program for effective masking of tinnitus.

Has the patient had previous experience with hearing aids? Was the patient satisfied with the particular aid previously tried? If not, why not? Was the previous hearing aid a linear aid?   If the patient was a satisfied user of linear hearing aids, the introduction of programmable systems having significant compression may be initially unacceptable. This is a common occurrence because the patient was accustomed to consistently greater acoustic gain. Counseling may resolve the issue, or it may be useful to utilize multi-memories with similar frequency responses but different compression (versus linear) characteristics. Severity of the compression ratio and/or kneepoint may need to be introduced or altered gradually. The dispenser must also accept the fact that some, though in this author's experience, few, users never accept compression. As stated earlier, this may be particularly true for listeners with severe or profound losses.

In addition, the dispenser should explore the features of hearing aids previously rejected by the dissatisfied patient and use that information in selecting alternative amplification systems. For example, if the patient was unable to adapt to the occlusion effect, it would be useful to select a system in which earmold or shell acoustics can be altered. This might not be physically possible with certain programmable ITE aids because of their physical size. This does not preclude attempts with electroacoustic modification of programmable aids, however.

Does the patient's profile dictate specific physical characteristics of the hearing aid? Does the patient's vanity preclude certain sizes or styles? Is battery size and need for more frequent battery replacement in many programmable systems an issue? As with conventional instruments, the selection of a programmable instrument must take into consideration issues related to the physical properties of the hearing aid system itself. Approximately 80% of hearing aids dispensed are of the ITE type (Mahon, 1989). At the time of this writing, only a couple of programmable systems are available in an ITC model, though more will certainly be introduced.

Comfort and cosmetic factors are matters of personal taste. (The author considers a mini BTE coupled to a nonoccluding retainer mold to be less visible than most ITE and some ITC aids). Even so, there are acoustic advantages and limitations to ITE and ITC aids that should not be overlooked. Because of the resonance effect dictated by the concha, there is a 4–6 dB enhancement between 2500 and 6000 Hz (a less than 2 dB advantage below 2000 Hz) at the microphone location of an ITE compared to a BTE (Gartrell and Church, 1990; Lybarger and Teder, 1986; Cox and Risberg, 1986).

Conversely, ITE instruments may limit the amount of gain they can provide without generating feedback. Erickson and Van Tasell (1991) demonstrated that ITE devices can produce a maximum peak insertion gain of 41–58 dB. If 10 dB reserve gain is allowed, the range of estimated peak-use gain from adequately fitted power ITE instruments is only

31–48 dB. An even lower amount of gain is available for ITC aids. The maximum values will be affected by frequency response, presence of feedback, and size and shape of the ear canal.

There is another major advantage to BTE programmable aids that should be taken into account. That advantage is the additional acoustic flexibility offered by earmold modifications. The ability to modify an earmold, or use a no-mold (or retainer) type of fitting, allows for significantly reduced insertion loss and a reduction in the occlusion effect. Figure 9.7 illustrates the dramatic difference produced by an occluding earmold versus a nonoccluding one. This reduction of loss of the patient's natural real-ear unaided response (REUR) means that despite the potential increase in feedback from a nonoccluding fit, many hearing loss patients can be fitted successfully with less gain. Curran (1991) reports that the maximum insertion gain obtainable with open-mold fittings is 25–30 dB. Because the REUR is not lost, this means that a significantly reduced volume-control setting may meet the patient's acoustic gain needs.

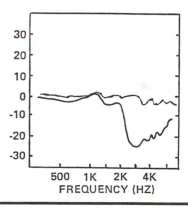

FIGURE 9.7. Loss of the REUR produced by a completely nonoccluding earmold (upper curve) and that produced by a closed-shell earmold (lower curve).

Is the patient's manual dexterity such that a remote control is easier or more difficult to manipulate than ear-level controls? Is the addition of another physical component to the system likely to increase the possibility that the patient might misplace part of the system? For some individuals who either object to or display difficulty manipulating controls at ear level, the larger controls on a remote control may be ideal, provided, of course, that the controls on the remote unit are large and easy to operate. Most remote controls allow the user to make instantaneous changes in volume and/or program (in multimemory systems). The remotes differ, however, in terms of their size, shape, and signal transmission characteristics (i.e., FM versus ultrasound). A drawback to those remote controls utilizing ultrasound transmission is that they require a line of sight and operate most effectively when the remote control is positioned 18–24 inches away from the hearing aid. The orientation of the remote to the sensor within the hearing aid might be critical. The author's clinical experience suggests that there may be more transmission problems for ultrasonic transmission than for FM transmission when certain spatial conditions exist (enclosed space, e.g., in an automobile). Also, there can be interference from security systems that operate at similar carrier frequencies.

Certain remote-controlled systems have no volume control on the aids themselves. This means that if the user accidentally misplaces the remote control, it may be impossible to vary the volume control settings. Some manufacturers produce programmable systems that allow for manual adjustment of the volume in lieu of the remote control.

Another important issue is that some of the early versions of remote-controlled systems forced the user into total dependency on the remote. For these systems, the user had no ear-level controls and had to rely on the remote control to change from one program to another or to adjust the volume control. In addition, if the battery contact was interrupted (e.g., when changing the battery), the remote control was required simply to turn the hearing aid back on. This can present a real problem to the individual who misplaces or forgets the remote unit. Certainly if this type of aid is selected, patients should be encouraged to change batteries on a regular basis at home. They also should be encouraged to purchase a spare remote control. Fortunately, an updated version of this particular hearing aid now provides the option of ear-level memory so that the aid can be turned on without the remote (though there still is no provision for volume or program changes without the remote).

For those programmable aids that do not utilize remote controls, there are also certain considerations. At least one system has no volume control, per se, but instead has two separate push buttons that switch the aid into its various programs. For some users, this physical arrangement is easier to control than a rotary volume wheel. However, for others it is confusing because the user cannot determine visually or tactually which program he/she is in. Some remote controls that offer LCDs (liquid crystal displays) are helpful because they allow the patient to make rapid visual determinations of which program the aid is operating in and at what particular gain setting. For others, this determination is not important. There also may be a momentary pause or audible signal present whenever the program is changed that can be displeasing to some users.

How much of a consideration is the monetary cost of programmable hearing aids? Might the increased cost force the patient to try monaural, rather than binaural, programmable instruments? Programmable aids are more expensive than most conventional hearing aid devices. The cost of two programmable instruments may exceed the budget for some individuals. One might

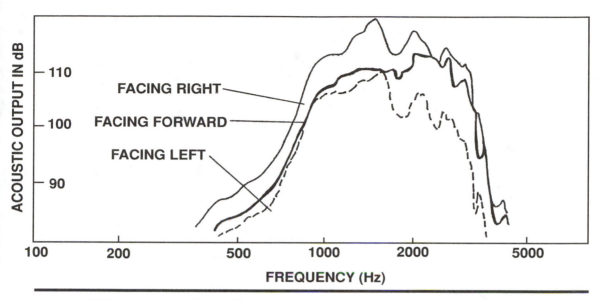

FIGURE 9.8.   Intensity reaching the ear as a function of speaker azimuth. The loudspeaker was located at a 90-degree azimuth facing the listener's right ear. The head shadow effect is the difference between the curves labeled "facing right" and "facing left."

question whether a patient is better served with two conventional hearing aids or with one programmable hearing aid. There are no overwhelming data collected regarding this question, but the same binaural advantages apply to digitally programmable hearing aids as to conventional analog systems. For example, binaural amplification is important in minimizing the effects of the head shadow that are present in at least 30% of listening environments. Placing the aided ear in a position allowing an advantageous azimuth can alter SPL by as much as 17 dB from 2–5 kHz (Figure 9.8). With proper positioning in an acoustic environment, binaural loudness summation advantage is 2–3 dB. In noise, binaural hearing permits the listener to take advantage of interaural phase differences, such as masking level differences. Reports by Silman, Gelfand, and Silverman (1984) and Silverman and Silman (1990) raise the possibility that auditory deprivation effects of the unaided ear may occur.

Thus, whenever feasible, hearing aid candidates for programmable and nonprogrammable hearing aids should be encouraged to evaluate binaural amplification unless contraindicated. If the cost of programmable aids prevents patients from being fitted binaurally, one must seriously weigh the advantages of improved acoustic performance obtainable with programmables versus the improved performance obtainable with binaural fittings, be they conventional or programmable. There are instances in which the binaural fitting of hearing aids with slightly inferior sound quality may be preferable to fitting a programmable instrument monaurally.

Objective Needs Assessment

The psychoacoustic or objective needs assessment requires tests that define suprathreshold perceptual attributes such as loudness growth, loudness discomfort, spectral resolution, temporal resolution, masking functions, word recognition skills based on continuous discourse tracking, and so forth. All of these tests are available in a laboratory, though some need to be revised and shortened to make them clinically suitable for hearing aid fitting applications. There are other psychoacoustic tests (for example, the Loudness Growth by Octave Band procedure explained by Pluvinage in Chapter 2) that are closely linked with the fitting strategies for certain programmable systems. As will be discussed later in this chapter, these tests should not be considered unique to any single system, but are applicable to a variety of digitally programmable aids.

GENERAL FITTING CONSIDERATIONS

Regardless of whether one uses conventional analog or digitally programmable hybrid systems, there are three criteria that must be satisfied in the successful fitting of hearing aids.

1. *The effectiveness of any hearing aid fitting strategy is greatly diminished unless audibility is established for specific frequency regions.* The significance of audibility has been recognized for decades. It has been addressed theoretically by the Articulation Index (AI) concepts introduced by French and Steinberg (1947) and later refined by Pavlovic (1989). In a recent publication, Humes and Roberts (1990) demonstrated how the AI can predict patient performance. They also used a modified version of the AI (Speech Transmission Index) to account for room reverberation and other acoustic factors. They demonstrated that signal audibility is the single most important ingredient for auditory performance. Establishing audibility across the speech spectrum is at the very core of fitting strategies put forth by Seewald (1988), Skinner et al. (1982), Hawkins et al. (1989), Cox (1983), and Loven (1991). Programmable aids, through flexible frequency shaping, can be of great assistance in providing a wide range of gain as a function of frequency.

2. *The amount of speech energy necessary for ensuring audibility must not exceed the patient's uncomfortable, or loudness discomfort, level at any frequency.* Otherwise, the patient will reduce the volume control setting, thus rendering certain speech sounds inaudible when they are presented at normal conversational levels. The hearing health professional must remember that both of these criteria must be satisfied to obtain an optimal fit. The interrelationship between these two requirements is essential and must be incorporated into programming strategies. Although the optimal hearing aid fitting goal might be to enhance speech intelligibility, patient comfort is a prerequisite. Madell et al. (1991) reported that 32% of patients who returned hearing aids did so because of loudness discomfort. It is not an easy task to maintain audibility while ensuring comfort for the wide range of intensities generated by speech. This is particularly true for certain fixed-response, linear instruments. Programmable aids allow the dispenser great flexibility in establishing those parameters needed to ensure satisfaction of both criteria.

3. *The patient's perception of his own voice must be acceptable.* For many years, hearing health professionals ignored or discounted the importance of the patient's report of how his own voice sounds. Patients were often erroneously informed that they would become accustomed to their own, newly amplified vocal production. The highest speech-signal intensity reaching the ear is usually the patient's own voice. Instantaneous peaks of 90–95 dB SPL occur regularly. Some conversational levels can produce peaks of 105 dB SPL. Tyler and Kuk (1989) reported that sensorineural-impaired listeners prefer less low-frequency gain for their own voices, but more low-frequency gain when listening to others. Clinical procedures to ensure comfort when the patient is speaking include the use of deep canal fittings (Killion, Wilbur, and Gudmundsen, 1988) and attempts to reduce the occlusion effect via tube fittings, low-frequency gain adjustments, and so forth.

PRESCRIPTIVE APPROACHES

Dispensers fitting programmable hearing instruments must establish realistic objectives and develop methods to verify that electroacoustic goals are attained. The question is, how can the dispenser incorporate increased flexibility, inherent in certain programmable hearing aids, into a well-structured fitting strategy? To answer this question, one must achieve the three critical criteria discussed in the previous section. Current technology employing real-ear measures and prescriptive formulas (with their associated ear-to-coupler conversions) provides a means by which one can accomplish these goals.

It was stated previously that the flexibility of digitally programmable hearing aids allows the hearing health professional to achieve remarkably close target gains. There are important issues regarding target gains and prescriptive formulas, however, that must be recognized.

1. *No one prescriptive formula is correct for all individuals.* Figure 9.9 shows differences in insertion gain prescribed by various fitting formulas. Note that the target gain prescribed by POGO or the Berger method may be the desired prescriptive approach for providing audibility for a patient with a severe or profound loss, but the NAL II formula may be more appropriate for ensuring both audibility and comfort for those with a mild or moderate loss. Similarly, the optimal formula for a mildly sloping loss may not be the same as the optimal formula for a sharply sloping loss. In fact, there are numerous fitting ap-

proaches that can be employed to help determine whether audibility has been achieved without exceeding comfort levels (Skinner et al., 1982; Seewald and Spiro, 1985; Hawkins et al., 1989; Cox, 1983; Loven, 1991) For example, Seewald's Desired Sensation Level approach plots unaided and aided thresholds and tolerance levels in the individual's ear canal (in SPL). These data are then compared to the desired amplified speech spectrum level. Figures 9.10 and 9.11 illustrate how this approach can be used to determine whether sufficient gain is present to ensure audibility without exceeding tolerance. In Figure 9.10, note that when sufficient gain is present, the desired SSPL 90 is exceeded by the real-ear saturation response. As a result, the patient would lower the volume, subsequently producing insufficient gain. In Figure 9.11, SSPL 90 has been reduced. Now the patient can raise the gain to a suitable level, simultaneously ensuring audibility without exceeding tolerance levels. Another advantage of plotting aided responses in this manner is that it allows the dispenser to determine whether there is adequate headroom (Preves, 1990). Some programmable systems have built-in mechanisms to ensure that adequate headroom is maintained so that distortion products are minimized.

2. *Optimum frequency response changes as a function of the signal input level.* Ideally, recommended target gains should restore audibility *and* comfort for soft, moderate, and loud acoustic signals. Unfortunately, most fitting formulas are applicable only to linear aids (Neuman and Levitt, 1990) and are based on threshold data rather than on direct measures of comfort, as suggested by Skinner (1979) or Cox (1983). In this author's opinion, enhanced nonlinear capabilities of digitally programmable aids, particularly those with multiple bands, represent the greatest advantage of these systems. It seems imperative, therefore, to consider these factors in the

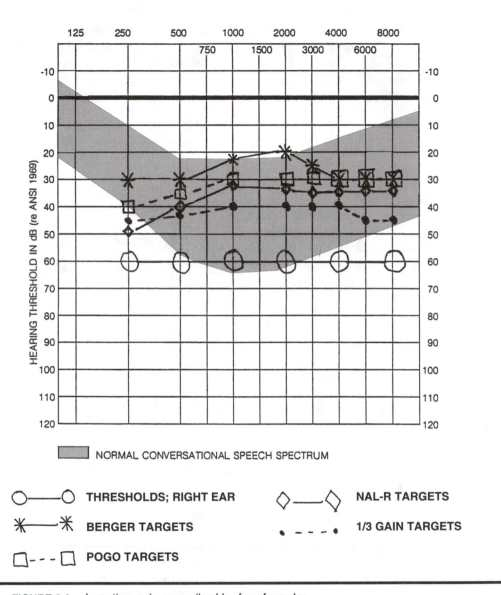

NORMAL CONVERSATIONAL SPEECH SPECTRUM

○——○ **THRESHOLDS; RIGHT EAR**

✳——✳ **BERGER TARGETS**

◻- - -◻ **POGO TARGETS**

◇——◇ **NAL-R TARGETS**

• - - - • **1/3 GAIN TARGETS**

FIGURE 9.9. Insertion gain prescribed by four formulas.

proper programming of these hearing aids. It is recommended that real-ear insertion responses be measured with a 50, 70, and 90 dB SPL input and that the target match be based on a 50 dB input.

3. *Matching a target gain recommended by a prescriptive formula or computer-specified algorithm is only the initial step in the fitting process.* Fine-tuning beyond the specified target is essential if the user's acoustic needs are to be met.

4. *One must guard against creating a false feeling of security encouraged by prescriptive formulas.* Despite the use of the term "expert fitting systems" by one manufacturer of digitally pro-

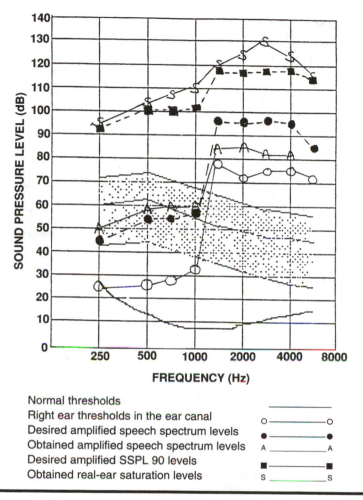

FIGURE 9.10. Initial worksheet illustrating the Desired Sensation Level approach. Desired amplified speech spectrum levels were not obtained because the patient lowered the volume control setting due to excessive SSPL 90 settings.

grammable aids, there is no assurance that the dispenser is an expert or has done an expert job. It is imperative that one does not get so enamored of sophisticated technology that the critical role of realistic patient counseling (Downs, 1991) in conjunction with all hearing aid fittings is overlooked.

There is no doubt that the interfacing of probe microphone real-ear measures with programmable hearing aid response greatly

enhances the fitting procedure (Sweetow and Mueller, 1991). If the dispenser does not have access to a real-ear system, however, reasonably simple conversions can be made (Hawkins, Cooper, and Thompson, 1990) so that functional gain and 2 cc coupler targets are based on the average real-ear characteristics. Although less ideal than using the individual's real ear, additional modifications can be made on the basis of certain assumptions regarding resonance differences

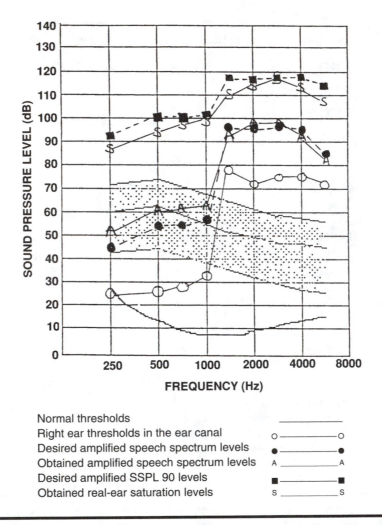

Normal thresholds
Right ear thresholds in the ear canal   o————o
Desired amplified speech spectrum levels   ●————●
Obtained amplified speech spectrum levels   A————A
Desired amplified SSPL 90 levels   ■————■
Obtained real-ear saturation levels   s————s

FIGURE 9.11. Revised worksheet illustrating the Desired Sensation Level approach. Desired amplified speech spectrum levels were obtained following a reduction of SSPL 90 settings, a slight change in the tone control, and an enlarging of the vent.

and real-ear-to-coupler differences (especially important when comparing an adult's ear to a child's ear). Then, functional gain can be plotted against a normal conversational speech spectrum (Figure 9.12).

Having expressed all of these caveats regarding real-ear measures, attention is now directed to the fact that programmable aids can achieve most target gain requirements with remarkable accuracy. Mueller and Jons (1989) studied deviations from NAL targets for more than 500 nonprogrammable in-the-ear hearing aids after a real-ear insertion gain (REIG) target match was achieved at 2000 Hz. Scattergrams of their data are shown in Figure 9.13. Note that target gain at 4000 Hz was

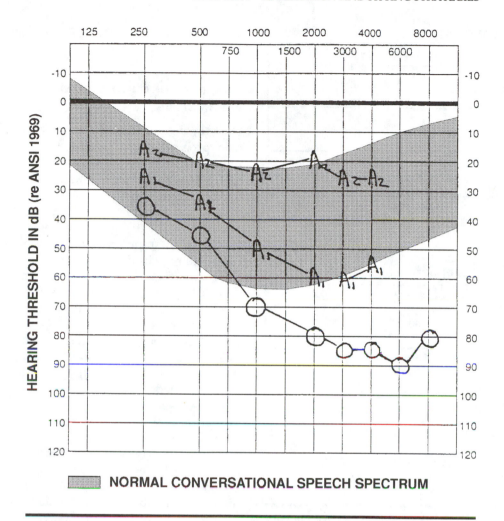

FIGURE 9.12. Two sets of aided thresholds demonstrating functional gain on an audiogram illustrating conversational speech range. Note that instrument A₁ will leave many consonants inaudible.

rarely achieved. It was usually missed at 3000 Hz, as well. They found that the amount of deviation from target gain falling within the 90th percentile was 8 dB at 1500 Hz, 9 dB at 3000 Hz, and 13 dB at 4000 Hz. The deviation from target gain that fell within the 70th percentile was 4 dB at 1500 Hz, 6 dB at 3000 Hz, and 9 dB at 4000 Hz. Sweetow and Mueller (1991) examined target gain matches using a single-channel programmable BTE hearing aid. They found that REIG deviated from target gain by no more than 6 dB at any frequency for high-frequency and gradually sloping losses, and by no more than 8 dB at any frequency for the more difficult to match reverse slope notch and cookie bite audiometric configurations. One must be cautious in making direct comparisons between these

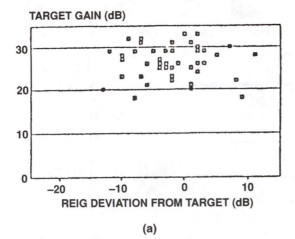

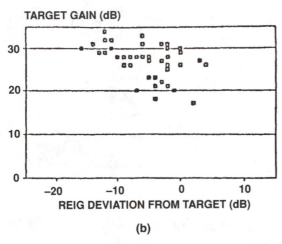

FIGURE 9.13. REIG deviations from NAL targets. Values are plotted as a function of target gain for 3000 Hz (a) and 4000 Hz (b). REIG was initially set to achieve target at 2000 Hz. Reprinted with permission from Mueller and Jons, 1989.

two sets of findings. In addition to the limited sample size of the Sweetow and Mueller data, there is an inherently greater versatility in available acoustic coupling modifications when using BTE aids. Theoretically, however, the individually programmed target gain match should be no worse than the best case achievable by fitting a nonprogrammable instrument.

PROGRAMMING INDIVIDUAL PARAMETERS

Once the decision has been made to try a specific programmable system, the dispenser must next attend to the actual process of programming the hearing aid. Rather than focusing on programming strategies for specific makes and models of digitally programmable instruments, overall strategies related to clinical manipulation of adjustable features will now be discussed.

Programming the instrument and the patient's assessment of its performance must incorporate analysis of perceptual attributes. Emphasis must be placed on the individual's prioritized weighting of the importance of these attributes. These priorities should have been established during the subjective and objective needs assessment. It is essential to prioritize issues, recognizing that certain compromises (noise reduction versus speech intelligibility, intelligibility versus tinny speech quality, gain versus loudness comfort, feedback versus high-frequency gain, etc.) may be inevitable. Having established priorities, the dispenser can begin consideration of programming the various features available with digitally programmable systems.

Frequency Shaping with Single-Channel Systems

Frequency shaping affects both audibility and hearing instrument comfort. Programmable systems allow for extreme modification of frequency response. Some systems use a single band and allow for changes in gain, slope, or output. If the dispenser selects a programmable system that utilizes a single band, there are certain issues that should be considered when adjusting the slope response.

Often one adjusts the frequency response based on the assumption that too much low-frequency amplification produces an upward spread of masking, in addition to overamplifying background noise (Martin and Pickett, 1970; Sweetow, 1977). As a result, low-frequency gain is often reduced. However, narrowing the bandwidth can adversely affect intelligibility. According to the classic French and Steinberg study, as bandwidth decreases it is necessary to increase the overall intensity in order to maintain a constant level of speech intelligibility. For example, to maintain a 60% discrimination score for a system passing acoustic energy contained between 850 Hz and 1700 Hz, the intensity must be increased by 25 dB compared to a wide-band presentation.

Staab (1988) hypothesized that low-frequency suppression may not be in the best interest of the patient. He reported that 70% of speech intelligibility and 38% of the power is contained within the 500–2000 Hz range. Critical information regarding the second formant and formant transitions can be reduced when the frequency slope is adjusted to reduce the low-frequency gain. Staab states that high-quality amplification of the midfrequencies may be more important than high-frequency emphasis achieved by lowering low-frequency gain.

Rosen and Fourcin (1986) presented data that they obtained during feature extraction experiments illustrating the important contribution to speechreading made by low-frequency information. Similar data reported by Punch and Beck (1986) and Sung and Sung (1984) indicate enhancement of word recognition when low-frequency amplification is combined with emphasis of the high frequencies (as is available with programmable aids).

Despite studies advocating or condemning low-frequency amplification on the basis of enhanced or diminished speech intelligibility scores, the fact remains that listener preference (both to other voices and their own) may represent the highest order of sensitivity. It certainly represents the most critical factor in getting a patient to use a hearing aid. The needs and preferences of the individual take precedence over any single assumption based on research data. In setting low-frequency slope, both subjective (the patient's description of his acoustic environments) and objective (upward spread of masking and other masking functions) information is essential. Priorities must be established regarding the need for low-frequency reduction (perhaps to minimize certain background noises) versus the need for second formant and formant transition information.

Keep in mind when reading the manufacturers' specifications as to the versatility obtainable through their aids that the use of certain coupling systems will reduce the range in the absolute extremes. Table 9.1 shows data collected by Sweetow and Mueller (1991) indicating that an 11–15 dB range (400–500 Hz) was obtained between the highest and lowest programmable gain for a certain aid in the 2 cc coupler for a closed-mold fitting. There was no gain change at these frequencies when an open mold was utilized. Therefore, the fitter should be aware that the amount of change will be affected by the coupling system.

Frequency Shaping with Multichannel Systems

To obtain more specific frequency tuning, (e.g., for unusual audiometric configurations), the dispenser may want to consider those programmable systems that incorporate relatively independent multiple channels. Systems are currently available that incorporate two and three, and one system even has 13 bands. Flexibility is enhanced by these systems since the dispenser has the power to manipulate cutoff frequencies in order to obtain a reduction in a narrower

TABLE 9.1.   Range of responses (in dB) at extreme filter settings.

	Frequency									
	400	*500*	*800*	*1000*	*1250*	*1600*	*2000*	*2500*	*3200*	*4000*
2 cc	25	24	21	18	15	12	7	7	9	11
Closed	10	18	22	21	16	9	9	8	6	9
Open	0	0	8	14	11	10	2	2	1	6

band (i.e., the low frequencies) without deleteriously affecting the adjacent band (i.e., the midfrequencies). Keep in mind, however, that not all multichannel systems have absolutely independent channels. The use of multimemory systems further renders the initial setting of the low-frequency slope less important because the patient can select the program that best suits the environment.

Setting High-Frequency Gain

Since it is rather difficult (using *any* of the prescriptive formulas) to obtain a target match in the 3000–4000 Hz region, and since audibility at this region is so important to speech discrimination, it is advisable to program the hearing aid, initially, to obtain target gain at 3000 and 4000 Hz. The primary reason it is so difficult to obtain adequate high-frequency gain is due to the loss of the REUR caused by the coupling of the aid to the external auditory meatus. It is at this initial stage of programming that decisions regarding earmold or shell configuration need to be made. Thus, whenever possible, it is wise to attempt to use the most open coupling system possible, without producing feedback.

If feedback is produced, (remember to check for feedback generated by jaw movements), one should identify the frequency region of the feedback via real-ear measurements and either reduce gain at that frequency or shift the peak frequency. The narrower the

bandwidth required to reduce or eliminate feedback the better. Multiple-channel systems, particularly the 13-band system) come to mind for resolving this problem.

Setting Low-Frequency Gain

Once the desired high-frequency gain has been achieved, programming concerns can shift to the lower frequency range. It is relatively easy to set the low-frequency gain according to prescriptive formulas. Nonetheless, consideration must be given to whether a single-memory or multiple-memory system should be chosen. If a single-memory instrument has been selected, the information obtained during counseling regarding the patient's acoustic environments and needs must be appraised carefully. A compromise may need to be reached between optimal sound quality for quiet environments and optimal quality for noisier environments. Additionally, the patient's own voice must receive a high priority. Compromises may have to be made to ensure patient satisfaction. Contrary to conventional wisdom, the author has found that by raising rather than lowering low-frequency gain, one can reduce the occlusion effect for some patients wearing certain high-fidelity instruments. Because of the fitting flexibility afforded by these systems, additional considerations can be made that significantly alter the fitting recommendations prescribed either by formulas or by the algorithms specified by the system's programming unit.

Figure 9.14 shows the audiogram of a patient fitted with a two-channel programmable hearing aid. The algorithm calculated by the programming unit called for a low-input, low-frequency gain of 8 dB and low-input, high-frequency gain of 20 dB (crossover frequency of 2000 Hz) with approximately a 2:1 compression ratio for both low-band and high-band channels. The patient reported the sound quality to be excellent when he was in adverse environments, but in fairly quiet rooms, the aid sounded too noisy. After a short reprogramming session, it was determined that the patient was reacting to noise he was hearing due to his normal hearing sensitivity for the very high frequencies. The program was changed to provide 16 dB gain for the low-frequency channel and only 6 dB gain for the high frequencies, with the crossover frequency moved up to 2800 Hz, a 3:2 compression ratio for the low-frequency channel, and a 1:1 compression ratio (fixed knee at 45 dB) for the high-frequency channel.

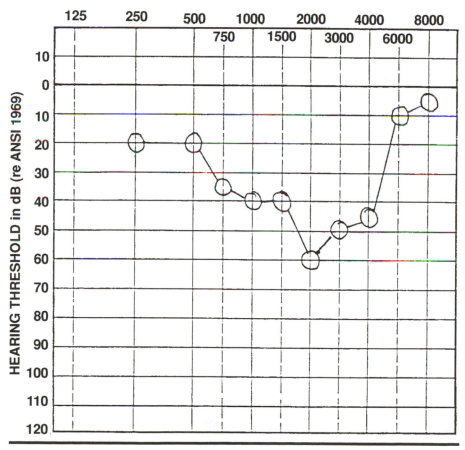

FIGURE 9.14.   Audiogram for a patient reporting that the programmable aid was too noisy.

Smoothing of Acoustic Peaks

Figure 9.15 shows frequency responses of an older and a new hearing aid. It was anticipated, based on target gain data, that the patient would prefer the instrument with the primary peak at 2700 Hz. Instead, she preferred her old conventional hearing aid with the peak at 1800 Hz. She admitted that in certain environments, she did not like her own aid. The patient was provided with a multi-memory aid with program 1 set to provide a frequency response similar to her old aid and program 2 to provide a smoother mid-frequency response with the 1800 Hz peak smoothed. The patient gradually became accustomed to and, indeed, preferred the program with the higher primary peak. When this occurred, the aid was reprogrammed so that the first program was that specified by the NAL prescription, and program 2 was reset to better meet the patient's needs in noisy environments.

Fitting Multimemory Instruments to Match Environmental Needs

One of the most useful features available in some digitally programmable hearing aids is the capacity to utilize multiple memories. No one hearing aid seems to be optimal for all listening environments. Therefore, why not offer the patient choices of acoustic response to interface best with the environment in which listening is taking place? This concept is not entirely new. For years, some conventional analog hearing aids have offered user-manipulated tone-control switches.

The optimal number of multiple memories to meet listening needs is unknown. There are no research data to support the concept that the more memory choices the better. It is possible that too many choices might confuse the user and create difficulty in rapidly selecting the "right" program choice. Even so, the psychological advantage of offering the patient some control over the listening environment is significant. The number of available program choices for listeners varies from two to as many as eight. Systems with multiple memories can be used effectively for aural rehabilitation and hearing aid orientation purposes.

Consider the following report cited by Sweetow and Mueller (1991).

This individual had normal hearing through 1500 Hz and was seen in conjunction with the fitting of binaural hearing aids. His primary hearing difficulty occurred during group meetings in which he was frequently involved. At the time of the fitting, target gain was calculated and the instrument was programmed. This response is shown as response A of Figure 9.16. The patient, however, objected to this response saying that it sounded "tinny" and did not think the use of the hearing aid made a significant difference in his hearing ability. By manipulating the low-cut and slope adjustment features, they provided responses B, C, and D in the remaining three memory locations of the instrument. The patient now had the option of adding 15 dB of gain at 1000 Hz (response D), even though most research conclusions suggest that this response would be a poor choice for this patient, relative to

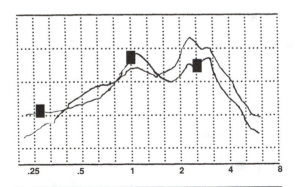

FIGURE 9.15.   Frequency responses for a multimemory aid programmed to provide a response with an 1800 Hz primary peak, and another response with a 2700 Hz primary peak.

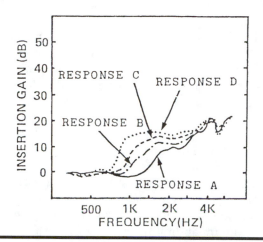

FIGURE 9.16. Four frequency responses from a multimemory aid set to assist the patient in gradually progressing from response D to response A. Reprinted with permission from Sweetow and Mueller, 1991.

understanding speech in noise. . . . As the patient becomes accustomed to programmable hearing aid use, he will gradually increase his use of response A by progressing through responses C and B. The flexibility of providing four different settings could lead to amplification acceptance that may not have occurred had he been offered only the amplification response shown in response A.

All procedures for programming multimemory aids are based on subjective information gathered during the interview of the patient. In addition, fitting strategies should take into account the patient's audiometric configuration and the coupling configuration utilized. The author often reserves one program for telephone use. The astute dispenser will obtain the relevant information from the patient to ascertain just how many listening environments require a separate program of their own.

The use of the data-accessing and data-logging features available in some systems can provide the dispenser with information relating to how frequently the user is select-

ing certain memories. The fitter may want to consider changing the acoustic responses of those memories seldom used.

Setting Maximum Output

The importance of setting this parameter to ensure that the maximum output is below the patient's LDL has ben stressed in this chapter. There are a variety of approaches (Cox, 1983; Hawkins et al., 1987) available to help select SSPL 90 characteristics. As stated earlier, it is essential to establish the real-ear saturation response (RESR) using both complex noise inputs (to assimilate speech) and a swept pure-tone input (Revit, 1991). If real-ear measures are not available, certain software versions offer tables to convert earphone-derived LDLs to 2 cc coupler responses (Hawkins, Cooper, and Thompson (1990).

Setting Compression Characteristics

While it is a reasonably safe assumption that a sensorineural-impaired individual will have some degree of loudness recruitment, there is no way, short of clinical assessment, to determine at which frequencies and to what degree recruitment is occurring. Two patients having identical audiograms often present significantly different loudness growth patterns. The *compression ratio* is extremely vital and should be determined by the results of a loudness growth test. While the Loudness Growth by Octave Band (LGOB) test was specifically designed for one programmable system, it can be used to determine certain desired compression parameters for nearly all of the programmable systems. The use of multiple channels provides the fitter with the ability to be precise in specifying which frequencies should have certain compression kneepoints and compression ratios. Having the ability to provide linear amplification for one channel, a 3:1 ratio for another channel, and perhaps a 2:1 ratio for a third channel can be essential for the patient who recruits at a different rate for different frequencies. LGOB test results will help the fitter set the crossover frequencies for determining different compression and gain characteristics. It may be useful to have different crossover frequencies for different memory banks so the patient can immediately notice acoustic differences among memories.

Figures 9.17–9.19 illustrate different LGOB results. Note in Figure 9.17 that the loudness growth pattern suggests no need for compression circuitry. Figures 9.18 and 9.19, representing the right and left ears, respectively, of a single patient, suggest significantly different loudness growth patterns. Each example required (a) a different compression kneepoint, and (b) a different compression

ratio. Several systems allow the dispenser to alter the compression kneepoint, though only a few allow for alteration of compression ratio (a critical factor, in this author's opinion). Note how useful this feature would be for the loudness growth pattern shown in Figure 9.18. Also note that there is an unexpected finding of greater recruitment at 500 Hz than at 1000 Hz. For those hearing aid systems that do not permit the dispenser to select the compression ratio, the acoustic output for various input levels (below and above the compression knee) should be examined to ensure maximum audibility and listener comfort for the entire frequency and intensity range.

In addition to the obvious advantage of preselecting a different amount of gain for various frequency ranges, hearing aids having multichannel compression also can

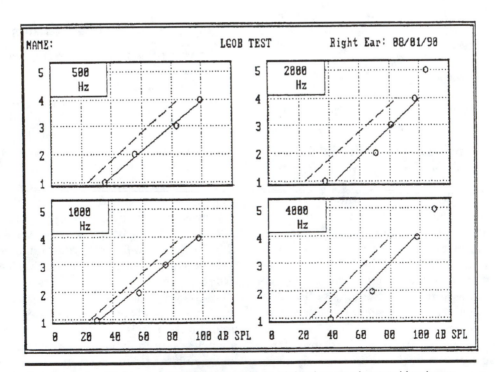

FIGURE 9.17.   Right ear LGOB demonstrating minimal or no abnormal loudness growth.

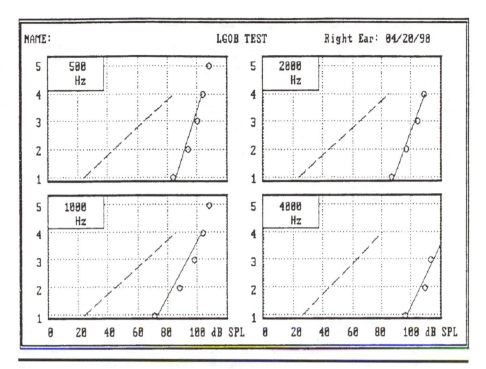

FIGURE 9.18. Right ear LGOB demonstrating abnormally rapid loudness growth for all frequencies. Note that loudness growth is more rapid at 500 Hz than at 1000 Hz.

adaptively adjust the amount of gain in specific frequency regions as a function of the input signal. For example, low-frequency gain can decrease simultaneously with an increase in high-frequency gain. This electro-acoustic feature often helps audibility, though not necessarily discrimination, in noise, since the spectral distribution of environmental noises is broadband. Moore (1990), however, notes that the acoustically impaired ear has about ten critical bands that process information (the normal ear has 35). He theorizes that unless the hearing aid has more than ten bands, it will do little to reduce the masking effects of background noise. He asserts that adaptive filtering may be as effective in noise reduction as multiband AGC. Despite Moore's theoretical construct, there continue to be a large number of multiband hearing aids users

who report enhanced listening comfort in noise. Such improvement is often not achieved with single-channel instruments.

Despite patient reports of the superiority of these multiband compression systems, improvement is not always demonstrable in the laboratory, office, or clinic. Barfod (1976) and Lippman, Braida, and Durlach (1981) contend that multiband compression is not superior to linear amplification when proper frequency shaping has been achieved. However, Villchur (1978) takes issue with this line of reasoning, contending that realistic evaluation of multiband compression amplification must take into account the following factors: (a) Speech test materials do not reflect the true dynamic range of speech in real life; (b) speech test materials have more restricted dynamic range than does real-life speech, so

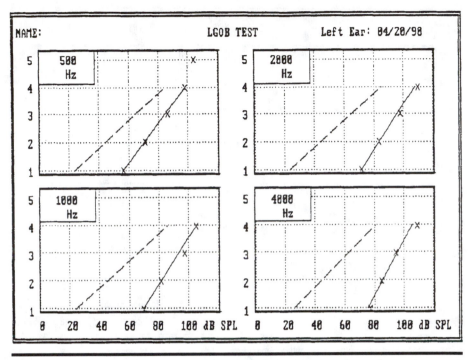

FIGURE 9.19. Left ear LGOB for the patient depicted in Figure 9.18.

there are limited intersyllabic and word-to-word amplitude changes; (c) when compared to linear hearing aid systems, the linear reference must utilize frequency shaping that is realistic and remains within the sound comfort level of the patient; and (d) multiband compression should be restricted to only those patients who demonstrate reduced dynamic range. These statements should be considered when comparing these aids to other amplification systems in the clinical setting. In addition, it should be noted that a period of training and adjustment is often necessary for persons using multiband compression.

The available compression kneepoints vary over a wide range, depending on the system. Some offer kneepoints as low as 45 dB. This low kneepoint seems to minimize pumping and breathing effects often heard in conventional AGC aids by keeping the aid in compression most of the time. It also allows for full dynamic range compression. With single-channel AGC systems, the user's own voice can trigger compression when typical knees of 60–70 dB are used, thus producing an unwanted overall decrease in gain. Considering the nature of most conversation situations, the compression knee may have to be set at a higher-than-desirable level in order to avoid annoying "pumping and fluttering." It is also important to keep in mind that insertion gain measures, typically performed with a 60–70 dB input, force the aid into compression. This produces less insertion gain than functional gain. Therefore, functional gain measures should also be included in the evaluation procedures.

Last, but certainly not least, are considerations relating to attack and release times. Compression can produce waveform distortion, particularly for transient sounds. Therefore, the dispenser needs to obtain a clear picture about the patient's listening environments. The importance of temporal cues is often overlooked because of the preoccupation, with amplifying spectral cues. Crucial formant transition information can be lost or altered during attack and release phases. The patient's ability to detect these rapid frequency changes is crucial. Some vowels (dipthongs) are perceived by formant transitions and by location of the first two spectral peaks. Consonants are very transient and have rapid spectral fluctuations occurring in the range of 10–30 msec. They are acoustically detected by using time and tilt cues—that is, tilt of the amplitude/frequency spectrum at signal onset and how long the tilt remains constant. Listeners differentiate voiced from voiceless initial consonants based on voice onset time following the sound burst (voiced = 5 msec, voiceless = 40 to 60 msec). Perception of speech involves the ability to detect brief, silent intervals of ongoing acoustic stimuli. One method of measuring temporal resolution is by a gap detection task.

Sensorineural-impaired listeners weigh the spectral and temporal cues differently than normal listeners. For normal listeners, spectral cues determine identification of consonants. For hearing-impaired listeners, spectral cues have less influence, while time and tilt cues assume greater importance. This is because frequency selectivity is generally more impaired than temporal resolution for the impaired listener (Drechsler and Plomp, 1980). For severe to profound losses, temporal cues may be the main information-bearing factor utilized by the listener. Drechsler and Plomp presented data suggesting that elevated temporal resolution in impaired listeners does not adversely affect speech

intelligibility. However, if the hearing aid further degrades temporal cues, perceptual problems could occur. This is precisely what could occur if the release time is too fast or too slow for the particular ambient background. That is, reverberant, ambient, and background noise could fill or smear the important silent intervals.

Several years ago, the concept of adaptive compression was introduced to minimize periods of inaudibility that occur as a result of listening in an acoustic environment characterized by loud transient sounds (Smriga, 1986). In this design, release time varies as a function of the duration of incoming noise. For example, a short burst of noise (such as a spoon dropping on a hard surface) produces a shorter release time than an ongoing noise (such as constant background chatter or machine noise). If the release time is too short, the signal-to-noise ratio is decreased. If the release time is too long following transient noises, the aid remains in compression during a period of time in which the listener wants to listen to speech. Such compression activity may render speech components inaudible while the gain recovers to its desired level. While, at the time of this writing, none of the programmable systems has an adaptable release time option, several incorporate different release times for the low- versus high-frequency inputs, and at least one system allows the dispenser to select among three release times for different bands.

Another advantage of multiband instruments is that attack times are longer for lower-frequency inputs. High-frequency sounds fluctuate within a time frame of 40 msec, and vowels may last for 500 msec. It is best to activate low-frequency filtering for long-duration sounds and not for fluctuating sounds of less than 40 or 50 msec. If different time constraints are not used for low- versus high-frequency inputs, normal conversational speech could activate an unnecessary adaptive filtered response.

SUMMARY

This chapter began with the comment that the real advantage of digitally programmable hearing aids is their flexibility. In order to make use of this flexibility, manufacturers of these devices and those who fit them must be imaginative and willing to experiment with new clinical procedures. Advanced test batteries need to be developed, including tests such as the LGOB, temporal gap detection, forward and backward masking, upward spread of masking, MLDs, and brief tone or speech acoustometry (Smith, 1990). These tests need to be presented at different sensation levels. They will need to be evaluated as a test battery. There probably will be conflicting results. For example, LGOB results may suggest the need for compression, but temporal resolution tests may suggest that alterations in the temporal envelope produced by compression may re-sult in unacceptable signal distortion for the individual listener. Real-ear measures are essential, but the use of speech audiometry using continuous discourse and adaptive signal-to-noise measures should not be ignored. This is true even though there is no clinical evidence suggesting that enhanced speech intelligibility is the ultimate goal of the hearing aid fitting process (Pavlovic, 1989). Perhaps listener-preference tasks (sound quality and comfort) represent a higher order of sensitivity.

The future of programmable hearing aids is extremely encouraging. For now, the dispenser must recognize that this technology is still in its infancy, and one must be patient but maintain a determination to push for constant improvement. Support of further research and development of these systems is an obligation that hearing health care professionals should accept and embrace.

REFERENCES

Barfod, J. (1976). Multi-channel compression hearing aids. The Acoustics Laboratory, Report 11. Copenhagen: Technical University of Denmark.

Boothroyd, A., Springer, N., Smith, L., and Schulman, J. (1988). Amplitude compression and profound hearing loss. *Journal of Speech and Hearing Research* 31:362–376.

Bornstein, S., and Randolph, K. (1983). Research on smooth, wideband frequency responses; Current status and unresolved issues. *Hearing Instruments* 12:12–16.

Cox, R. (1983). Using ULCL measures to find frequency-gain and SSPL-90. *Hearing Instruments* 34(7):17–21.

Cox, R., and Risberg, D. (1986). Comparison of in-the-ear and over-the-ear hearing aid fittings. *Journal of Speech and Hearing Research* 51:362–369.

Curran, J. (1991). In: D. Radcliffe, Discord into meaning: Fitting solution for high frequency loss. *The Hearing Journal* 44(3):9–14.

Downs, D. (1991). Viewpoint: Clinical audiologists have lost sight of their clients. *The Hearing Journal* 44(2):18–23.

Dreschler, W., and Plomp, R. (1980). Relationship between psychophysical data and speech perception for hearing impaired subjects. *Journal of the Acoustical Society of America* 68:1608–1615.

Erickson, F., and Van Tasell, D. (1991). Maximum real-ear gain of in-the-ear hearing aids. *Journal of Speech and Hearing Research* 34:351–359.

French, N., and Steinberg, J. (1947). Factors governing the intelligibility of speech sounds. *Journal of the Acoustical Society of America* 19:90–119.

Gartrell, E., and Church, G.T. (1990). Effect of microphone location in ITE vs. BTE hearing aids. *Journal of the American Academy of Audiology* 1(3):151–153.

Hawkins, D., Cooper, W., and Thompson, D. (1990). Comparisons among SPLs in real ears, 2 cm^3 and 6 cm^3 couplers. *Journal of the American Academy of Audiology* 1:154–161.

Hawkins, D., Morrison, T., Halligan, P., and Cooper, W. (1989). The use of probe tube microphone measurements in hearing aid selection for children. *Ear and Hearing* 10(5):281–287.

Hawkins, D., Walden, B., Montgomery, A., and Prosek, R. (1987). Description and validation of an LDL procedure designed to select SSPL 90. *Ear and Hearing* 8:162–169.

Hecox, K. (1988). Evaluation of hearing aid performance. *Seminars in Hearing* 9(3):239–251.

Humes, L., and Roberts, L. (1990). Speech recognition difficulties of the hearing impaired elderly: The contributions of audibility. *Journal of Speech and Hearing Research* 33:726–735.

Killion, M. (1984). Recent earmolds for OTE and ITE hearing aids. *The Hearing Journal* 37:15–22.

Killion, M., Wilbur, L., and Gudmundsen, G. (1988). Zwislocki was right . . . a potential solution to the "hollow voice" problem with deeply seated earmolds. *Hearing Instruments* 1:14–18.

Libby, E., and Sweetow, R. (1987). Fitting the environment: Some evolutionary approaches. *Hearing Instruments* 38(8):8–12.

Lippman, R., Braida, L., and Durlach, N. (1981). Study of multichannel amplitude compression and linear amplification for persons with sensorineural hearing loss. *Journal of the Acoustical Society of America* 69:524–531.

Loven, F. (1991). A real ear speech spectrum based approach to ITE preselection/fitting. *Hearing Instruments* 42(3):6–13.

Lybarger, S. (1982). Acoustic feedback control. In: G. Studebaker and F. Bess (eds.), *The Vanderbilt Report* (pp. 87–90). Upper Darby, PA: Monographs in Contemporary Audiology.

Lybarger, S., and Teder, H. (1986). 2 cc coupler curves to insertion gain curves: Calculated and experimental results. *Hearing Instruments* 37:36–38.

Madell, J., Pfeffer, E., Ross, M., and Chellappa, M. (1991). Hearing aid returns at a community hearing and speech agency. *The Hearing Journal* 44(4):18–23.

Mahon, W. (1989). U.S. Hearing aid sales summary. *The Hearing Journal* 42(12):9–14.

Martin, E., and Pickett, J. (1970). Sensorineural hearing loss and upward spread of masking. *Journal of Speech and Hearing Research* 13:426–437.

Moore, B. (1990). How much do we gain by gain control in hearing aids? *Acta Otolaryngologica* 469(Suppl.):250–256.

Mueller, H., and Jons, C. (1989). Some clinical guidelines for the fitting of certain custom hearing aids. Presented at Annual ASHA Convention, St. Louis, MO.

Newman, A., and Levitt, H. (1990). Selection procedures for digital hearing aids. *Seminars in Hearing* 11(1):79–89.

Pascoe, D. (1985). Hearing aid evaluation. In: J. Katz (ed.), *Handbook of Clinical Audiology*, 3rd ed. (pp. 936–948). Baltimore: Williams & Wilkins.

Pavlovic, C. (1989). Speech spectrum considerations and speech intelligibility predictions in hearing aid evaluations. *Journal of Speech and Hearing Disorders* 54:3–8.

Preves, D. (1990). Approaches to noise reduction in analog, digital, and hybrid hearing aids. *Seminars in Hearing* 11(1):39–67.

Punch, J., and Beck, L. (1986). Relative effects of low frequency amplification on syllable recognition and speech quality. *Ear and Hearing* 7:57–62.

Revitt, L. (1991). New tests for signal processing in multichannel hearing instruments. *The Hearing Journal* 44(5):20–23.

Rosen, S., and Fourcin, A. (1986). Frequency selectivity and the perception of speech. In: B. Moore (ed.), *Frequency Selectivity in Hearing* (pp. 373–487). London: Academic Press.

Schwartz, D. (1991). Hints and kinks for K-hooks and $\frac{1}{32}$" tubing. *The Hearing Journal* 44(5):31.

Seewald, R. (1988). The desired SL approach for children: Selection and verification. *Hearing Instruments* 39(7):18–22.

Seewald, R., and Spiro, M. (1985). Selection amplification characteristics for young hearing impaired children. *Ear and Hearing* 6:48–53.

Silman, S., Gelfand, S., and Silverman, C. (1984). Effects of monaural versus binaural hearing aids. *Journal of the Acoustical Society of America* 76:1357–1362.

Silverman, C., and Silman, S. (1990). Apparent auditory deprivation from monaural amplification and recovery with binaural amplification: Two case studies. *Journal of the American Academy of Audiology* 1(4):175–180.

Skinner, M. (1979). Speech intelligibility in noise induced hearing loss: Effects of high frequency compensation. *Journal of the Acoustical Society of America* 67:306–317.

Skinner, M., Pascoe, D., Miller, J., and Popelka, G.

(1982). Measurements to determine the optimal placement of speech energy within the listeners' auditory area. In G. Studebaker and F. Bess (eds.), *The Vanderbilt Report* (pp. 161–169). Upper Darby, PA: Monographs in Contemporary Audiology.

Smith, D. (1990). Acoustometry. *The Hearing Journal* 41(11):40–44.

Smriga, D. (1986). Modern compression technology: Developments and applications, part 2. *The Hearing Journal* 39(7):13–16.

Staab, W. (1988). Significance of mid-frequencies in hearing aid selection. *The Hearing Journal* 41(6):23–34.

Sung, G., and Sung, R. (1984). Utilizing extended low frequency amplification with precipitous high frequency sensorineural hearing loss. *Hearing Instruments* 12: 6–7.

Surr, R., Montgomery, A., and Mueller, H. (1985). Effects of amplification on tinnitus among hearing aid users. *Ear and Hearing* 6:71–75.

Sweetow, R. (1977). Temporal and spread of masking effects from extended low frequency amplification. *Journal of Auditory Research* 17: 161–170.

Sweetow, R., Cato, P., and Levy, M. (1991). The tinnitus masking efficiency of high frequency hearing aids. *The Hearing Journal* 44(4):24–34.

Sweetow, R., and Mueller, H. (1991). The interfacing of programmable hearing aids and probe microphone measures. *Audecibel* 40(3)11–13.

Tyler, R., and Kuk, F. (1989). Some effects of "noise suppression" hearing aids on consonant recognition in speech-babble and low frequency noise. *Ear and Hearing* 10(4):243–249.

Van Tasell, D., Larsen, S., and Fabry, D. (1989). Effects of an adaptive filter hearing aid on speech recognition in noise by hearing impaired subjects. *Ear and Hearing* 9:15–21.

Villchur, E. (1978). A critical survey of research on amplitude compression. *Scandanavian Audiology* (Suppl. 6):305–314.

CHAPTER 10

CLINICAL COMPARISON OF DIGITALLY PROGRAMMABLE HEARING AIDS

Michael Valente, Margaret W. Skinner, L. Maureen Valente, Lisa Gulledge Potts, Gary L. Jenison, and James Coticchia

Over the past several years, hearing aid dispensers have witnessed many significant technological advances in hearing aid design and circuits. First, components and the physical size of hearing aids continue to miniaturize. Second, compared to transducers having relatively narrow bandwidths (200–6000 Hz) and peaked frequency responses, some recent transducers provide wider (200–16,000 Hz) and smoother frequency responses that contribute to improved speech intelligibility and sound quality. One circuit (K-AMP) (Killion, 1990) has a rising smooth frequency response, with peak gain occurring at around 2800 Hz, and extends the frequency response to 16,000 Hz. Finally, circuit designs incorporating a variety of signal processing schemes have been introduced that reduce, but do not eliminate, the deleterious effects of ambient noise upon speech intelligibility.

Perhaps the most significant advance may be the recent introduction of digitally programmable analog hearing aids. This new technology allows the dispenser to change immediately the performance of the hearing aid in a number of ways. Examples of the ways in which the hearing aid response may be altered include the ability to change the (a) overall gain, (b) output, (c) low-frequency response and slope, (d) high-frequency response and slope, (e) kneepoint for activating an AGC circuit, and (f) frequency bandwidth of two or more channels

for incorporating changes in gain and/or output within each channel. As the parameters of the hearing aid are programmed by the dispenser or the user, the patient can immediately evaluate whether the changes have a significant effect upon either speech intelligibility (Cox and McDaniel, 1989) or sound quality (Gabrielsson, Schenkman, and Hagerman, 1988; Gabrielsson and Sjoren, 1979a; Gabrielsson and Sjoren, 1979b; Hagerman and Gabrielsson, 1985).

When the final parameters are selected, the design is stored in memory within the hearing aid or remote control for immediate retrieval by the patient. If adjustments to the stored design are necessary (e.g., changes in hearing or changes in perception of desired sound quality), the hearing aid can be connected to the programmer and the circuit reconfigured and stored once again in the memory of the hearing aid or remote control. For some systems (ReSound ED2, ED3, and BT2, Starkey Trilogy, and Widex Quattro), the stored design is changed in the remote control instead of the hearing aid.

Interestingly, some programmable hearing aids can store more than one response for immediate retrieval by the patient. For example, the ReSound ED2, ED3, and BT2 can store two responses, the Widex Quattro and Siemens Triton 3004i and 3004b can store four responses, and the Starkey Trilogy I and II can store three responses. With these hearing aids, one response may be programmed to maximize speech intelligibility and sound quality for listening to a male speaker in quiet. A second response may be chosen for listening to a female speaker under the same condition. Still another response can be de-signed for listening to a male or female speaker in noise or perhaps for enhanced enjoyment of listening to music. Although it is estimated that programmable hearing aids currently account for 2–6% of the number of hearing aids dispensed, these aids will prob-

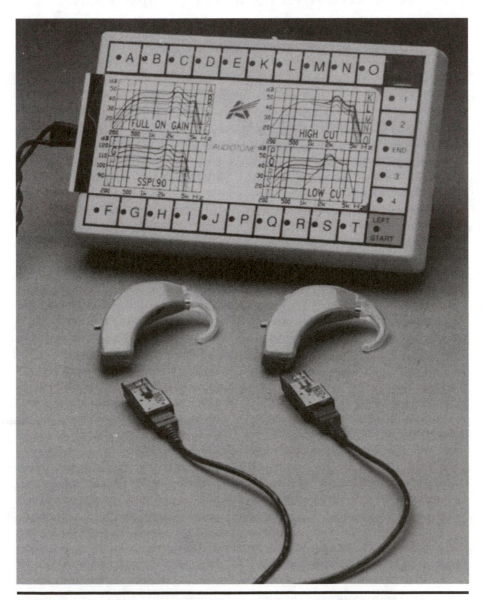

FIGURE 10.1. Audiotone System 2000 programmer and A-2000 BTEs. Reprinted with permission from Audiotone, Inc., 7731 Country Club Drive, Golden Valley, MN.

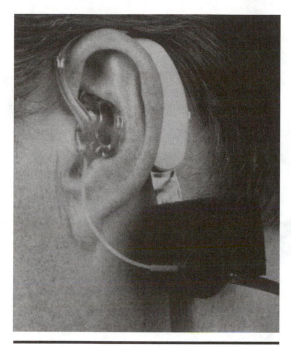

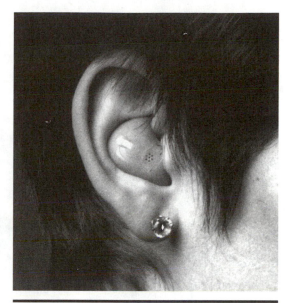

FIGURE 10.3. Ensoniq SSi coupled to the ear. Reprinted with permission from ENSONIQ Corp, 155 Great Valley Parkway, Malvern, PA.

FIGURE 10.2. Ensoniq Sound Selector SSb and probe tube coupled to the ear. Reprinted with permission from ENSONIQ Corp, 155 Great Valley Parkway, Malvern, PA.

ably account for a significantly greater larger percentage in the future (Cranmer, 1990; Powers and Fry, 1991).

Over the past few years, the authors have gained considerable experience using several programmable hearing aids that have been described in great detail in the previous chapters. Our experience includes the following programmable hearing aids:

1. Audiotone A-2000 (Figure 10.1) BTE hearing aid using the System 2000 programmer (Staab, 1988), which is also available in an ITE design (XT-2000).

2. Ensoniq EES SSb BTE (Figure 10.2) and SSi ITE (Figure 10.3) using the Ensoniq Sound Selector fitting system interface and chest pack with an IBM-compatible personal computer (Figure 10.4) (Gauthier, 1989).

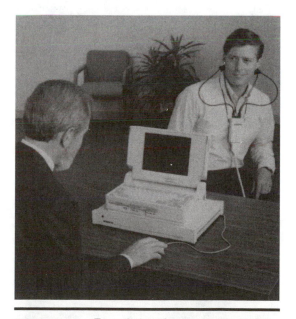

FIGURE 10.4. Ensoniq interface and chest pack used to program Ensoniq hearing aids. Reprinted with permission from ENSONIQ Corp, 155 Great Valley Parkway, Malvern, PA.

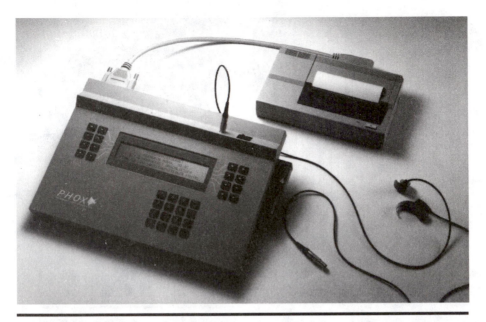

FIGURE 10.5. Bernafon PHOX PX8 programmer, printer, P4, and P2OS. Reprinted with permission from the manufacturer.

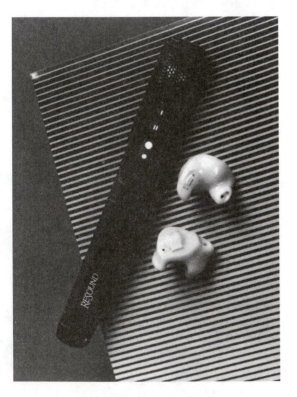

3. Bernafon PHOX P1 and P4 BTE and P20S and P30 ITE using the PX8 programmer (Figure 10.5) (Fiest and Wallace, 1989; Herbst, 1989a and 1989b; Herbst and Larsen, 1991).

4. ReSound ED2 and ED3 ITE and BT2 BTE with remote (Figure 10.6) using the ReSound digital programmer, personal selector, and compact disc player (Figure 10.7) (Johnson, Pluvinage, and Benson, 1989; Moore, Laurence and Wright, 1985; Pluvinage, 1989; Pulvinage and Benson, 1988; Waldhauer and Villchur, 1988). ReSound recently introduced the P³ programmer for programming the ED3 and BT2 hearing aids.

5. Siemens Triton 3004b BTE with the PMC programmer (Figure 10.8) (Branderbit, 1991). Siemens recently introduced the Triton 3004i

FIGURE 10.6. ReSound remote control and ED2. Reprinted with permission from ReSound Corporation, 220 Saginaw Drive, Redwood City, CA.

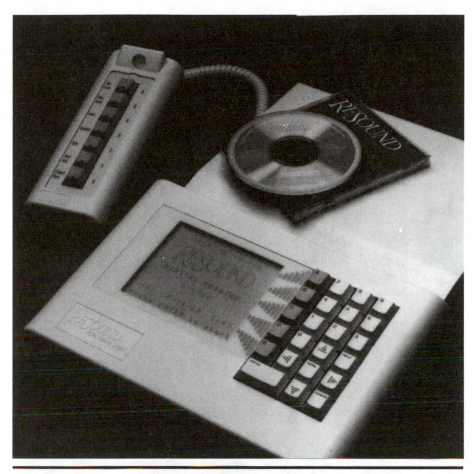

FIGURE 10.7. ReSound DHS programmer, compact disc, and personal selector used to program the ED2. Reprinted with permission from ReSound Corporation, 220 Saginaw Drive, Redwood City, CA.

ITE hearing aid with the capacity to store four responses into memory. Also, Siemens recently introduced the single-channel programmable Infinti ITE/ITC, which can be programmed by the PMC system or a separate programmer.

6. Starkey Trilogy I ITE/ITC and Trilogy II ITE.

7. Widex Quattro Q8, Q9, Q16, and Q32 BTE and the QX ITE/ITC with personal remote (Figure 10.9) (Goldstein, Shields, and Sandlin, 1991; Sandlin and Andersen, 1989).

This experience has provided the authors with a strong foundation to offer suggestions that may be helpful to the dispenser considering entering the arena of programmable hearing aids.

ISSUES AND QUESTIONS THE DISPENSER SHOULD CONSIDER BEFORE DISPENSING PROGRAMMABLE HEARING AIDS

Dispensing programmable hearing aids is something all dispensers will eventually face in the years ahead. Before deciding

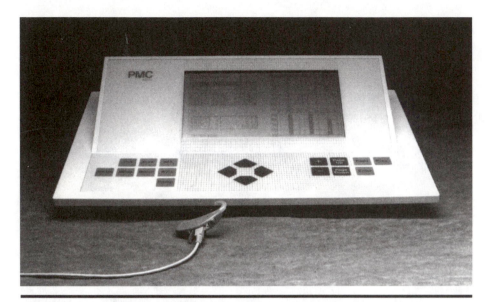

FIGURE 10.8. Siemens Triton® 3004b connected to the PMC programmer.
Reprinted with permission from Siemens Hearing Instruments, Inc., 10 Constitution
Avenue, Piscataway, NJ.

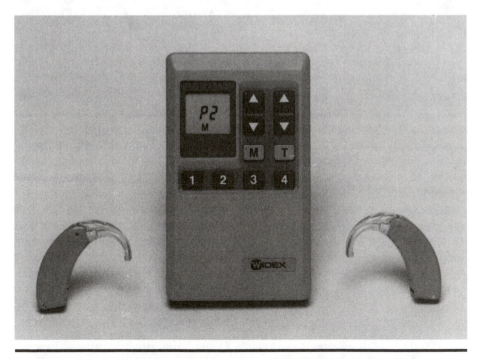

FIGURE 10.9. Widex Quattro remote control and Q8. Reprinted with permission
from Widex ApS, Ny Vertergaardsvej 25, DK-3500 Vaerloese, Denmark.

which system(s) to consider purchasing, it may be beneficial to "network" with colleagues having experience with the system(s) being considered. In addition, it may be helpful to consider the following issues before purchasing and dispensing programmable hearing aids.

Manufacturer Issues

Is the dispenser ready to engage in a long-term relationship with a manufacturer? Once the decision is made to purchase programmable systems, a long-term relationship with the manufacturer is created due to the need to provide continuous, ongoing follow-up service, repairs, or updates. In the past, if the service or product was less than acceptable or a policy or procedure was implemented that was felt to be particularly frustrating or unfair, the dispenser could easily seek the services of another manufacturer. With programmable hearing aids, a permanent umbilical cord is effectively created between the dispenser and the manufacturer in order for the dispenser to provide continued service for his patient. For this reason, the dispenser should carefully investigate the performance of the manufacturer in the critical areas of the quality of the product, pricing, timeliness of repairs, product development, and manufacturer support *before* committing to such a long-term relationship.

What are the manufacturers' plans for updates in software, hardware, and hearing aid product development?

How receptive is the manufacturer to suggestions for changes in the software, hardware, or design of the hearing aid(s)?

What are the plans and procedures for ongoing staff continuing education? Ensoniq, for example, provides an excellent two-and-one-half-day workshop at their headquarters in Pennsylvania. ReSound invites users to attend workshops at their facility near San Francisco. In addition, most manufactures arrange for local and regional workshops.

When problems arise when programming the hearing aid, how accessible is the manufacturer for solving problems? In our experience, it was almost impossible to contact any professional within the plant of one manufacturer when problems arose during the fitting process. On the other hand, another manufacturer flew a software specialist from the plant to spend the day with us to resolve a long-standing problem that could not be resolved over the phone. Thus, it is reasonable to anticipate a wide variation in the capacity of manufacturers to be available for consultation to resolve fitting issues. It would be very beneficial for the dispenser to isolate key individuals within a manufacturing company who would be available for consultation in the event problems arise (and they will).

What is the manufacturer's policy concerning credits? One manufacturer recently began a policy of charging a $35 restocking fee on all hearing aids returned for credit, while most other manufacturers have no such policy. This policy needs to be explained to the patient so that he is informed prior to ordering the hearing aid.

What plans does the manufacturer have for marketing their product? Most manufacturers have rather active marketing services and are willing to work in developing ideas for marketing this technology.

Product Issues

Would it be better to wait until the "bugs" have been eliminated so that the dispenser will be sure to deliver the best product to his patients? This technology will clearly undergo numerous revisions and modifications. All technology, including the technology incorporated in nonprogrammable hearing aids, constantly undergoes refinement and improvement. Therefore, it is not advisable to hesitate in obtaining experience with programmable technology because of fears related to changes occurring to this technology over time.

Should the dispenser wait until more ITE and ITC programmable hearing aids are available before committing to this technology? Most programmable hearing aids are currently available in a BTE design. However, ReSound (ED2 and ED3), PHOX (P20S and P30), Ensoniq (SSi), Starkey (Trilogy I and II), Siemens (Triton 3004i), and Widex (QX) currently provide ITE and/or ITC programmable hearing aids. Current market demands require the ability to dispense ITE and ITC hearing aids. Quite frankly, any current system with the ability to program BTE hearing aids can easily be upgraded (via software and hardware changes) to program ITE and ITC hearing aids when product becomes available. For example, the Ensoniq SSi became available after a year of dispensing the SSb aid. When the SSi became available, it was a simple process of upgrading the software and adding a new connecting cable. The change to dispensing the SSi hearing aid occurred in a few minutes. If a decision was made to wait until the SSi became available, we would have missed the opportunity of dispensing the SSb aid for over a year. ReSound recently introduced the P^3 programmer, which is used to program the new ED3 ITE and BT2 BTE hearing aids.

Does this technology provide significantly greater benefit and flexibility than many current nonprogrammable hearing aids with easy access to potentiometers to adjust the output, overall gain, compression kneepoint, slope, or low- and high-frequency response? If current nonprogrammable hearing aids have easy access to potentiometers providing essentially the same changes as the programmer, then programmable hearing aids probably offer little additional advantage over conventional linear hearing aids. However, one should consider the greater ease of changing circuit designs by pressing a keypad on a programmer than rotating potentiometers (often with limited access) on BTEs, ITEs, or ITCs. That is, under the worst scenario, programmable hearing aids still offer significant advantages for incorporating changes in circuit designs.

When hearing aids are sent for repair, what is the average turnaround time for the repair? Generally, greater repair time is required for many programmable aids. As with nonprogrammable hearing aids, some manufacturers of programmable hearing aids are quicker in returning repaired aids than others.

Do programmable hearing aids require greater repairs than nonprogrammable aids? The need for repairs, for the most part, is not significantly different than nonprogrammable hearing aids.

Is the cost for repairing a programmable hearing aid greater than the cost for repairing a nonprogrammable hearing aid? Generally the cost of repairs is not significantly greater for programmable hearing aids.

What is the warranty for the hearing aid? The warranty is the same as for nonprogrammable hearing aids and generally extends for one year. ReSound, however, provides a three-year warranty. Finally, most manufacturers cover repair, but not loss.

How many bands are optimum and how many bands are too much? Some programmable hearing aids allow for adjustments to the entire frequency band (PHOX, Quattro, Audiotone, Trilogy I). Two programmable aids (ReSound and Trilogy II) have two frequency bands available for adjustments (low- and high-frequency bands divided by one crossover frequency). Still another (Triton 3004b and 3004i) has three frequency bands available to allow for adjusting the gain and

AGC kneepoint in each of the three bands (low-, mid-, and high-frequency bands divided by two crossover frequencies). Yet another (SSb and SSi) has 13 frequency bands available for adjusting gain in reportedly 1 dB increments. Research in this area is ongoing, and the answers will not be available for several years. When the results of the studies are complete and answers provided, do not expect universal agreement on the conclusions from either dispensers or manufacturers.

How many memories are sufficient? Some programmable hearing aids have one memory available for programming (Audiotone A-2000, PHOX, Ensoniq), while others have two (ReSound), three (Trilogy), or four (Widex Quattro and Triton 3004b and 3004i) memories available. Do patients report advantages to having more than one memory? Our few patients having experience using both single-memory and multimemory programmable hearing aids seem to prefer the multimemory hearing aid, depending on the other characteristics of the hearing aid. Those patients who stated a preference for the multimemory hearing aid seem to base their preference on the advantage of changing the response of the hearing aid as their listening environment changed.

What has been the patient response to the remote? Our experience has been quite mixed. Some patients are quite enthusiastic about using a remote to control the volume and/or change the memory of the hearing aid. On the other hand, several patients expressed their desire not to be bothered with carrying around another piece of equipment. One patient was absolutely thrilled with the quality of the amplified sound from her programmable hearing aid, but returned her hearing aid because she simply could not adjust to the remote. One major concern with the ReSound ED2 hearing aid was that if the patient forgets or loses the remote, he can no

longer operate the hearing aid. The hearing aid cannot even be turned on. For this reason, it is suggested that persons purchasing the ReSound ED2 hearing aid consider purchasing a spare remote. In addition, it would be appropriate for the dispenser to purchase one or two additional remotes to provide on loan for their patients in the event the remote is lost or forwarded for repair. The problem with the need for the remote to operate the hearing aid was recently answered by ReSound when they introduced the ED3 ITE and BT2 BTE hearing aids. These hearing aids default to program 1 when the battery door is opened and closed. The remote is still required if the patient wishes to change from one memory to another or increase or decrease the overall volume.

Do previous users report superior performance with programmable hearing aids over nonprogrammable hearing aids? The vast majority of patients having previous hearing aid experience have expressed a very positive response to most programmable hearing aids.

What are the typical problems reported by users of these hearing aids? Are these problems unique to programmable hearing aids? Our experience has revealed that most users report continued problems of unequal performance of the hearing in quiet versus competition. However, most patients report significantly better performance for understanding speech in competition with most programmable hearing aids in comparison to their previous linear hearing aids. This may be related more to the manner in which the programmable hearing aids were fitted in comparison to their nonprogrammable hearing aids and may not be related to superior technology. Continued research in this area will be necessary to asses the benefits of programmable technology on improved communication. Another potential problem was whether any programmable hearing aid lost the program stored in memory. To this date, we know of no such occurrence.

How difficult is it to program the hearing aids using the various systems? The Audiotone system can be learned in a few minutes. The PHOX, PMC, Quattro, and desktop version of the Trilogy systems are more complex, but can be learned in a reasonably short time. The ReSound, Ensoniq, and PC versions of the Trilogy systems are more complex and usually require the greatest amount of time to learn. Most systems contain fairly well-written manuals that can be supplemented by training seminars and telephoning the manufacturer when problems arise.

Cost Issues

Has the patient population within the dispenser's immediate geographical region expressed an interest in such technology?

Is the number of patients who have expressed an interest large enough to warrant investing in the equipment and continuing education necessary to dispense this type of technology?

Can the dispensing practice absorb the additional direct expenses required to purchase the programmer and programmable hearing aids? In addition, many manufacturers provide, and in some cases require, ongoing continuing education for the staff.

Does the practice allow for the required time that will obviously be needed for ongoing continuing education?

Should the dispenser wait for further decreases in the cost of the equipment and hearing aids necessary to dispense this product? All new technology is expensive when first introduced. This is followed, in some cases, by a slow decrease in cost. In fact, costs for several programmable hearing aids (Triton 3000, Bernafon PHOX, and the Ensoniq BTE) and programmers (Bernafon PHOX) have already been reduced in the past year. On the

other hand, the costs for other programmable hearing aids and equipment have risen in the past year.

What are the costs, if any, for updates in the software and/or hardware? Ensoniq, Starkey, and PHOX, for example, provide free and easy updates. ReSound and PMC provide free updates in the first year.

How often does the manufacturer plan updates? Updates are provided sporadically throughout the year to incorporate suggestions from dispensers, as well as product improvements. In the past year, PHOX, Siemens, Starkey, and ReSound have had major software updates. Ensoniq had a major software revision (version 1.3) as well as hardware (probe microphone and battery pills) updates.

How easy is it to update the software and hardware? For the PHOX, PMC, and desktop versions of the Starkey Trilogy systems it is a simple matter of pulling out the old software module from either the side or back of the programmer and inserting the new software. The Ensoniq and PC versions of the Starkey Trilogy provide software updates that arrive as a floppy disk (3.5" or 5¼") with very easy directions for installation. The ReSound update required the entire unit to be shipped to the manufacturer. However, the cost for entire process was covered by ReSound and the unit was back in our office within two days.

How do I determine what to charge my patients for these aids due to the additional direct and indirect costs necessary to dispense programmable hearing aids? These hearing aids will cost more to dispense because of the increased direct costs required to purchase the hearing aids and equipment. Also, more patient time may be required to fit most of these hearing aids in comparison to non-programmable hearing aids. In addition, patients will require additional time for reprogramming. Finally, considerable time will be required for staff continuing education. Clearly a dispenser cannot use the same formula to calculate an appropriate charge for these hearing aids as was done for non-programmable hearing aids.

How should the dispenser counsel the patient about the increased cost for these hearing aids? Suggestions pertaining to this last question will be addressed in a subsequent section of this chapter.

COMPARISON OF ELECTROACOUSTIC CHARACTERISTICS, FEATURES, AND ADJUSTABLE PARAMETERS AMONG PROGRAMMABLE HEARING AIDS

Comparing Electroacoustic Characteristics

In Tables 10.1 and 10.2, the electroacoustic characteristics of the various programmable aids are compared. Generally, the following observations can be made. First, many programmable hearing aids have equivalent input noise levels (Ln) that are generally higher than nonprogrammable hearing aids. This can present problems when fitting a patient having reasonably good hearing below 1000 Hz. It is important that the patient be counseled about this prior to dispensing the hearing aid. Second, battery drain, except for the PHOX and Starkey Trilogy hearing aids, is typically higher for most programmable hearing aids compared to nonprogrammable hearing aids. Again, this fact needs to be discussed with the patient. This is especially true for patients who have previous experience with hearing aids and are accustomed to greater battery life. Third, as a general guideline, the available range of gain and output of the Widex Quattro Q8 and Q9, Audiotone A-2000, ReSound ED2 and ED3, Ensoniq SSb and SSi, PHOX P4, P20S, and P30, and Siemens Triton 3004b and 3004i are appropriate for successfully fitting patients with mild to moderately severe hearing loss. The Quattro

Q16 and Q32, ReSound BT2, and PHOX P1 can be successfully fitted to more severe hearing losses.

Comparing Features Among the Programmable Aids

In Tables 10.3 and 10.4, the general features, adjustable parameters, and selected options are compared. The following sections describe some selected features.

Selecting target gain as a function of frequency.   The software within some programmers allows the dispenser to enter a patient's audiometric data, and the programmable settings required to achieve the selected prescribed gain (as a function of frequency) are determined by the software as long as the volume control is set to approximately ¾ rotation. This feature typically allows the dispenser to select from NAL-R (Byrne and Dillon, 1986), POGO (McCandless and Lyregaard, 1983), Berger (Berger, Hagberg, and Rane, 1977), and the Libby ⅓ or ⅔ rule (Libby, 1986). Some systems (PMC, Ensoniq, and PHOX) allow dispensers to create their own calculated target. The ReSound system selects the desired gain in the low- and high-frequency bands for soft (50 dB) and loud (80 dB) input intensities for both programs I and II by using one of three dispenser-selected algorithms. One algorithm is based on the audiometric thresholds, and a second algorithm is based on the patient response to the Loudness Growth in Octave Bands test (LGOB), which was described in an earlier chapter. A third algorithm is based on the use of both the audiometric data and the LGOB.

It must be stated in the strongest terms that the dispenser needs to be very careful when using this feature for automatic selection of hearing aid parameters because the actual measured gain will almost never approach the prescribed targeted gain. Thus, it is im-

TABLE 10.1. Comparing the electroacoustic characteristics of the Widex, Audiotone, and ReSound programmable hearing aids.

	Widex					Audiotone		ReSound		
	Q8	Q9	Q16	Q32	QX	BTE	ITE	ED2	ED3	BT2
Avg full on gain	48	50	55	70	40	43–70	31–51	52	52	56
Peak gain	55	57	60	N/A	N/A	52–76	36–56	55	57	59
Ref test gain	N/A	N/A	N/A	N/A	N/A	43–53	31–42	N/A	N/A	N/A
Avg SSPL	108–118	110–119	117–127	122–132	103–112	110–130	100–119	114	115	120
Peak SSPL	111–121	111–121	122–132	129–138	108–114	117–139	104–123	118	118	122
Battery drain (mA)	2.0–2.5	2.0–2.5	2.1–2.6	6–10	1.9–2.2	2.0–6.0	1.1	2.3	2.3	2.3
Telecoil	97	94	103	124	87	115	115	N/A	N/A	N/A
Frequency range (kHz)	.17–6.5	.4–6.2	.2–6.0	.9–5.0	.13–6.0	.2–6.4	.2–7.1	.2–6.2	.2–6.0	.2–6.0
Attack (msec)	9	9	9	7	5	6	6	1	1	1
Release (msec)	120	120	120	150	100	185	185	50–100	50–100	50–100
Ln (dB)	N/A	N/A	N/A	N/A	N/A	<30	<30	28	28	28

N/A = Not available

TABLE 10.2. Comparing the electroacoustic characteristics of the Ensoniq, PHOX, Siemens, and Starkey programmable hearing aids.

	Ensoniq		PHOX				Siemens		Starkey	
							Triton		Trilogy	
	SSb	SSi	P4	P1	P2OS	P30	3004b	3004i	I	II
Avg full on gain	54	41	63	59	50	50	53–58	30–45	13–38	13–46
Peak gain	62	46	70	65	56	56	58–63	35–50	20–45	20–50
Ref test gain	54	41	49	46	35	35	52	N/A	13–29	13–29
Avg SSPL	116	118	126	123	112	112	126–129	105–115	103–106	91–106
Peak SSPL	120	118	133	130	120	120	119–133	108–118	110	95–110
Battery drain (mA)	6.5	3.2	1.5	1.6	1.3	1.3	3.1	1.1–2.2	.70	1.1
Telecoil	108	N/A	117	108	90	90	112	N/A	N/A	N/A
Frequency range (kHz)	.2–7.2	.2–7.2	.18–6.4	.18–6.2	.2–6.1	.2–6.1	.11–6.9	.2–7.0	.2–6.7	.2–6.7
Attack (msec)	3	3	4	3	4	4	10–60	10–50	N/A	N/A
Release (msec)	50	50	50	50	40	40	100–700	70–700	N/A	N/A
Ln	31	31	27	25	25	30	30	30	<30	<30

N/A = Not available

TABLE 10.3.   Comparisons of selected features of the Widex, Audiotone, and ReSound programmable hearing aids.

	Widex					Audiotone		ReSound		
	Q8	Q9	Q16	Q32	QX	BTE	ITE	ED2	ED3	BT2
General Features										
Select target	N	N	N	N	N	N	N	Y	Y	Y
Paired comparison	N	N	N	N	N	N	N	N	N	N
REUR response	Y	Y	N	N	Y	N	N	Y	Y	Y
Binaural eval.	Y	Y	Y	Y	Y	Y	Y	Y	Y	Y
Circuit design	L	L	L	L	L	NL	NL	NL	NL	NL
Remote required	Y	Y	Y	Y	Y	N	N	Y	Y	Y
Number of channels	1	1	1	1	1	1	1	2	2	2
Number of memories	4	4	4	4	4	1	1	2	2	2
Directional mic.	N	Y	N	N	N	N	N	N	N	N
Read response	N	N	N	N	N	Y	Y	Y	Y	Y
Type compression	O	O	O	O	O	I	I	—— MBFDR ——		
Adjustable Parameters Available										
Output	Y	Y	Y	Y	Y	Y	Y	N	N	N
Overall gain	N	N	N	N	N	Y	Y	Y	Y	Y
LF gain	Y	Y	Y	Y	Y	Y	Y	Y	Y	Y
HF gain	Y	Y	Y	Y	Y	Y	Y	Y	Y	Y
LF slope	Y	Y	Y	Y	Y	N	N	N	N	N
HF slope	N	N	N	N	N	N	N	N	N	N
Crossover freq.	N	N	N	N	N	N	N	Y	Y	Y
Compression	Y	Y	Y	Y	Y	Y	Y	Y	Y	Y
Selected Options										
CROS/BICROS	Y	Y	Y	Y	N	Y	N	N	N	N
Direct audio input	Y	Y	Y	Y	N	Y	Y	N	N	N
Vol. control avail.	Y	Y	Y	Y	Y	Y	Y	N	N	N

REUR = Real-ear unaided response
Y = Yes
N = No
L = Linear circuit
NL = Non-linear circuit
O = Output compression
I = Input compression
MBFDR = Multiband full dynamic range compression

TABLE 10.4. Comparisons of selected features of the Ensoniq, PHOX, Siemens, and Starkey programmable hearing aids.

| | Ensoniq | | PHOX | | | | Siemens | | Starkey | |
| | | | | | | | Triton | | Trilogy | |
	SSb	SSi	P4	P1	P2OS	P30	3004b	3004i	I	II
					General Features					
Select target	Y	Y	Y	Y	Y	Y	Y	Y	N	N
Paired comparison	Y	Y	Y	Y	Y	Y	Y	Y	N	N
REUR response	Y	Y	N	N	Y	Y	N	Y	Y	Y
Binaural eval.	Y	Y	Y	Y	Y	Y	Y	Y	Y	Y
Circuit design	NL	NL	L	L	L	L	NL	NL	L	NL
Remote required	N	N	N	N	N	N	N	N	Y	Y
Number of channels	1	1	1	1	1	1	3	3	1	2
Number of memories	1	1	2*	2*	2*	2*	4	4	3	3
Directional mic.	Y	N	N	N	N	N	N	N	N	N
Read response	Y	Y	Y	Y	Y	Y	Y	Y	Y	Y
Type compression	FDRC	FDRC	I	I	I	I	I****	I****	O	I
					Adjustable Parameters Available					
Output	N	N	Y	Y	Y	Y	Y	Y	N	Y
Overall gain	Y**	Y**	Y	Y	Y	Y	Y***	Y***	Y	Y
LF gain	Y	Y	Y	Y	Y	L	Y	Y	Y	Y
HF gain	Y	Y	Y	Y	Y	Y	Y	Y	N	Y
LF slope	Y	Y	Y	Y	Y	Y	N	N	Y	Y
HF slope	Y	Y	Y	Y	Y	Y	N	N	N	Y
Crossover freq.	N	N	N	N	N	Y	Y(2)	Y(2)	N	Y
Compression	Y	Y	Y	Y	Y	Y	Y	Y	N	Y
					Selected Options					
CROS/BICROS	N	N	Y	Y	N	Y	N	N	N	N
Direct audio input	N	N	Y	N	Y	Y	Y	N	N	N
Vol. control avail.	Y	N	Y	Y	Y	Y	Y	Y	Y	Y

REUR = Real-ear unaided response
Y = Yes
N = No
L = Linear circuit
NL = Non-linear circuit
O = Output compression
I = Input compression
FDRC = Full dynamic range compression
* = With activation of speech enhancement response
** = 1 dB increments in 13 bands
*** = Three independent bands
**** = Set kneepoint in three independent bands

perative that the dispenser have at his disposal a method for verifying that measured gain (real-ear insertion gain using probe tube measures; functional gain or targeted aided thresholds) approaches the prescribed target. The reasons for making this statement will be illustrated in greater detail in a subsequent section of this chapter.

Paired comparisons of parameter settings. Some programmers can hold in memory two or more programmed sets of parameters for the listener to evaluate, in rapid succession, to select the preferred fit. For example, Ensoniq allows the dispenser to store and recall four sets of frequency/gain characteristics for comparison, while the PHOX allows six responses to be stored and recalled. With the PMC system, 15 responses can be stored for each ear to be recalled.

REUR-type output response. Several programmable hearing aids (Quattro Q8, Q9, and QX, ReSound, Ensoniq, PHOX P20S and P30, Triton 3004i, and Trilogy I and II) have 2 cc coupler frequency responses that mimic the average real-ear unaided response (REUR). This frequency response is characterized by a smooth, gradually rising response that peaks at approximately 2800 Hz and gradually provides less output/gain at frequencies above the peaked response. This response is in contrast to the frequency responses of other hearing aids that have resonances and antiresonances throughout the frequency bandwidth. Interestingly, Trilogy I has the ability for the audiologist to program the peak gain of the hearing aid so that it more closely approximates the peak resonant frequency of the patient.

The authors have observed that the REUR-type frequency response can result in improved sound quality and may be preferred by many hearing-impaired listeners; this observation is based on an unpublished study that was undertaken at our facility in 1990. For this study, ten hearing-impaired listeners with gradually sloping sensorineural hearing loss were provided two pairs of ITE or ITC hearing aids having the same matrix (peak output/peak gain/slope). One pair included the standard peaked frequency response, while the second pair included a REUR-type frequency response. Listeners were asked to keep daily diaries of their listening experiences with the two pairs of hearing aids. After thirty days, the listeners submitted their diaries and were asked if they preferred one frequency response over the other. Nine of the ten listeners clearly preferred the hearing aids having the REUR frequency response.

Ability to program binaural amplification. Most systems allow the dispenser to program binaural amplification in an efficient manner.

Linear versus nonlinear designs. Many programmable hearing aids have linear circuits (PHOX, Quattro, and Trilogy I). That is, the same amount of overall gain is provided regardless of the intensity of the incoming signal up to the point of saturation. On the other hand, Ensoniq, ReSound, Audiotone, Triton, and Trilogy II aids provide greater overall gain for softer input signals (e.g., 50 dB SPL) and progressively less gain as the level of the intensity of the incoming signal is increased. For the ReSound system, the kneepoint at which the compression circuit is activated is 45 dB SPL, while the kneepoint for the Ensoniq system is approximately 55 dB SPL. This type of circuit design is becoming known as full dynamic range compression (FDRC). The authors have observed that this circuit design tends to result in greater user acceptance for most hearing-impaired listeners with reduced dynamic range between threshold and UCL. It is crucial for the dispenser to be aware of the circuit design (linear versus nonlinear) because it will have a significant impact upon how the resulting fit will be verified when using probe tube, functional gain, or targeted aided threshold measures. The importance of this latter statement will be illustrated in greater detail in a subsequent section of this chapter.

Remote control. Some programmable hearing aids require the use of a remote to control the volume or change from one memory to another (Trilogy, Quattro, or ReSound). Again, the ReSound ED2 hearing aids will not operate without the remote. This may present a problem and must be carefully explained to the patient. On the other hand, the Quattro and Trilogy aids do not require the remote for the basic operation of the hearing aid.

One versus several channels. Some programmable hearing aids (ReSound, Trilogy II, and Triton 3004b and 3004i) allow the dispenser to configure the frequency/gain response in more than one frequency region (i.e., channel or band) essentially independently of adjacent frequency regions. For example, the ReSound hearing aid is divided into low-frequency (LF) and high-frequency (HF) bands separated by the crossover frequency (Cf). For example, a selected crossover frequency of 1300 Hz creates a low-frequency band below 1300 Hz and a high-frequency band above 1300 Hz, where the overall gain and compression ratio in one band can be programmed essentially independently of the other band. The Trilogy II has a low and a high band available for programming with the crossover frequency fixed at approximately 2800 Hz. The Siemens Triton 3004b and 3004i allow the dispenser to adjust two crossover frequencies (F1 and F2) that divide the overall frequency response into three channels. One channel is a low-frequency region below F1. The second channel is the mid-frequency region between F1 and F2. The third channel is the high-frequency region above F2. With this system, the dispenser can adjust both the gain and AGC-I kneepoint within each of the three channels almost independently of the adjacent channel.

One versus several frequency/gain memories. Some programmable hearing aids have one frequency/gain memory available for programming, while other programmable hearing aids have two (ReSound), three (Starkey Trilogy), or four (Widex Quattro and Triton 3004b and 3004i) memories available for programming. The ability to program multimemories makes it possible to program each memory for a different listening situation. For example, one memory may be programmed for maximum speech intelligibility and sound quality for listening in quiet surroundings, while an entirely different memory may be more useful for listening in noisy conditions, to music, or to someone with different vocal characteristics (e.g., male versus female versus child).

Directional microphone. Some programmable hearing aids (Ensoniq SSb and Quattro Q9) are available with a directional microphone. Reportedly, a directional microphone allows for greater release from the masking effects of ambient noise than is available with omnidirectional microphones (Beck, 1983; Hawkins, 1986).

Directly reading the response(s) stored in memory. It is advantageous for the dispenser to easily determine what is stored in the memory of the hearing aid or remote when it is reconnected to the programmer for reprogramming. Several programmable aids (PHOX, Triton 3004b and 3004i, ReSound, Trilogy, and Audiotone) have this capability, while with others (Ensoniq and Quattro), this cannot be done as efficiently.

Different methods of compression. Some programmable hearing aids provide output compression (Widex Quattro), while most others provide input compression. In addition to the method of compression, the dispenser may be able to program the kneepoint at which the compression circuit is activated (PHOX and Triton 3004b and 3004i). Other programmable aids provide FDRC that provides compression ratios ranging between 1:1 (linear circuit providing 1 dB output for every decibel increase at the input) to 3:1 (nonlinear circuit providing 0.3 dB output for every decibel increase at the input). The multiband FDRC circuit for the ReSound ED2, ED3, and BT2 can be programmed to provide between 1:1 and 3:1 compression in the LF and HF bands for FIT I and II. The FDRC circuit for Ensoniq is frequency dependent and follows the spectrum of speech (i.e., greater low-frequency intensity than high-frequency intensity is necessary to activate the compression circuit). The FDRC circuit in the Ensoniq provides a consistent 2:1 compression ratio for the entire frequency range. However, it provides linear amplification below the kneepoint and 8:1 compression at intensities greater than 95 dB SPL.

Comparing Adjustable Parameters

Programmable systems vary significantly in the parameters that can be adjusted (see Tables 10.3 and 10.4). Several of the more common parameters available include:

1. The ability to adjust the output.
2. The ability to adjust the overall gain over a wide frequency region of the frequency response or within very narrow frequency regions.
3. The ability to adjust the shape of the low- and/or high-frequency gain.
4. The ability to adjust low- and/or high-frequency slope.
5. The ability to adjust crossover frequency(s).

AVAILABILITY OF SELECTED OPTIONS

Programmable systems are available using a variety of special options. Some of these options may include:

1. *CROS and/or BICROS arrangement.*
2. *Direct audio input.*
3. *Volume control.*   Most programmable hearing aids have a volume control present either on the case of the hearing aid or on the remote control. One other programmable hearing aid (Ensoniq ITE) does not use a volume control. However, Ensoniq recently announced that a volume control will be available as an option in the near future. The Widex QX can be ordered with a volume control on the faceplate in addition to the volume control available on the remote control.

COST COMPARISONS AMONG PROGRAMMABLE HEARING AIDS AND PROGRAMMERS

Figure 10.10 highlights differences in 1992 monaural single-unit costs for selected programmable hearing aids. These costs range from as little as $298 for the Audiotone XT-2000 to as much as $1000 for the ReSound ED3 with remote control. The reader is reminded that it is common for manufacturers to reduce single-unit cost or have promotions that reduce the cost for a limited time.

Figure 10.11 highlights the differences in 1992 costs for purchase of the equipment necessary to program the various hearing aids. These costs range from no cost for the Widex Quattro to $13,500 for the 3M Masterfit system, which also includes a complete computer system. Figure 10.11 illustrates that most programmers cost around $3,000–$5000.

The Ensoniq Sound Selector is quite different in that it requires the purchase of an interface and chest pack for $3495. However, the use of an IBM-compatible computer with an 80286 microprocessor, 640K RAM, 20–40 mg hard drive, Microsoft Windows mouse, one floppy drive (3.5 or 5¼"), and an 80287 math coprocessor is required. The additional cost of the computer, monitor, printer, and peripherals could increase the total cost for the

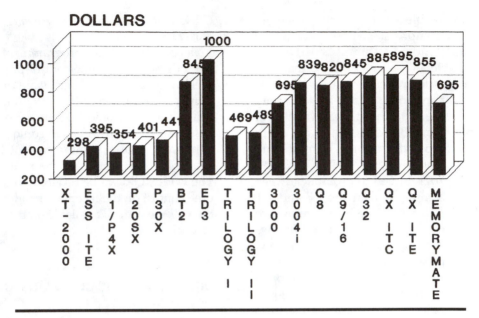

FIGURE 10.10. Comparing 1992 monaural single-unit cost for programmable hearing aids.

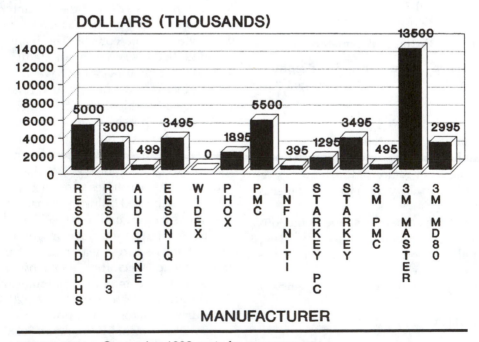

FIGURE 10.11. Comparing 1992 costs for programmers.

Ensoniq system to approximately $5000. The Starkey Trilogy system (I and II) can be programmed via a PC computer. The dispenser can purchase the necessary software and hardware from Starkey for $1295 for connection to his PC.

The PMC programmer is unique in that this unit accepts program modules for up to five manufacturers at a time. Each manufacturer module plugs into the back of the unit to be called up from the main menu. Currently, eight manufacturers (Siemens, 3M, Philips, Rexton, Argosy, Danavox, Qualitone, and Phonak) have agreed to use the PMC system, but only four have the software and hearing aids available at this time (Siemens, Philips, Danavox, and 3M). Several manufacturers have lease/purchase agreements to decrease the initial cost required for the purchase of the programmer so that it is financially feasible for dispensers to fit their programmable hearing aids. It is suggested the dispenser communicate with the manufacturers' representatives to determine if lease arrangements can be made.

EFFECTIVE PATIENT COUNSELING

Dispensing programmable hearing aids can be a double-edged sword. On one hand, this technology provides amplification that is different and, in many ways, superior to the technology of many nonprogrammable hearing aids. On the other hand, the dispenser needs to clearly articulate the potential advantages and disadvantages of programmable hearing aids to the patient and family.

One of the most challenging experiences has been developing methods with which to effectively counsel patients so that the amplification system is selected that is most appropriate for their hearing loss, communication, and personal needs (e.g., financial resources, third-party payment, telephone use, preferred size, etc.). Effective patient counseling has become increasingly complex due to the large number of different amplification systems now available. A counseling tool needed to be developed so informed decisions could be made of which hearing aid(s) was most appropriate. This counseling tool was developed with the understanding that each facility is unique in the types of hearing aids available and policies pertaining to their dispensing. Thus, the following counseling tool was developed to meet our needs and may need to be modified to meet the needs of other facilities. Undoubtedly, it will be modified to make it more effective in the future.

First, Figures 10.12 and 10.13 illustrate that hearing aids are available in three designs (ITC, ITE, and BTE), and all are available using programmable and nonprogrammable technology. If the patient expresses an interest, Figures 10.14 to 10.16 are used to outline the programmable and nonprogrammable options for each of the designs at our facility. Clearly, the numbers of hearing aids and the names of manufacturers appearing on these figures will vary from facility to facility.

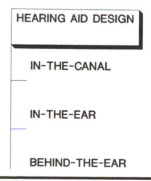

FIGURE 10.12. Organizational chart to counsel patients on three hearing aid designs.

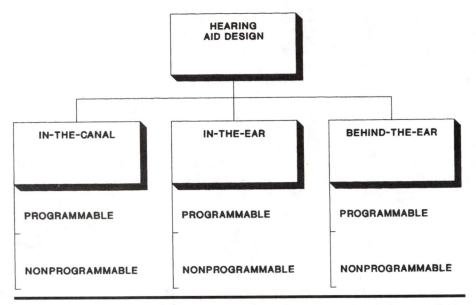

FIGURE 10.13. Organizational chart to counsel patients about the designs available using nonprogrammable and programmable technology.

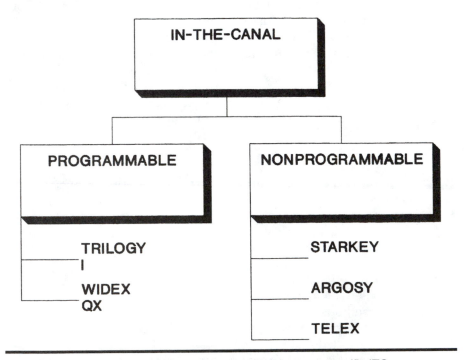

FIGURE 10.14. Organizational chart to counsel patients on specific ITC nonprogrammable and programmable hearing aids available at our facility.

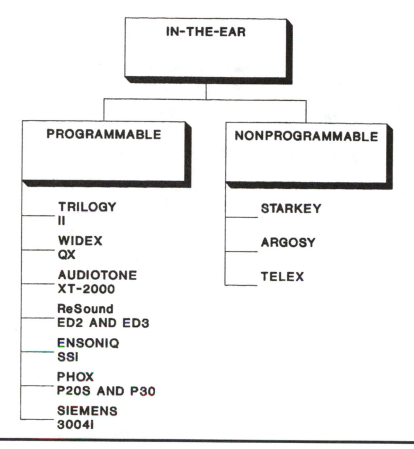

FIGURE 10.15.   Organizational chart to counsel patients on specific ITE nonprogrammable and programmable hearing aids available at our facility.

Six major generic differences between nonprogrammable and programmable hearing aids available are outlined in Figures 10.17 to 10.19. This list of differences often leads to a valuable discussion of the major questions the patient may have concerning advantages or disadvantages of programmable hearing aids. At this point the patient, with the audiologist, typically decides whether to pursue programmable technology. If the decision is made to pursue programmable technology, Figures 10.20 to 10.24 are helpful in expressing our current thoughts of the major advantages and disadvantages of some of the systems. This information serves as a basis for specific questions and discussion, concluding with a decision to purchase a particular programmable system. Please notice that some features may appear as an advantage and a disadvantage (e.g., absence of a volume control and use of a remote). Our experience indicates that many features can be viewed quite differently by individual patients.

BEHIND-THE-EAR
PROGRAMMABLE
NONPROGRAMMABLE
WIDEX
Q8, Q9, Q16, Q32
AUDIOTONE
A-2000
ReSound
BT2
ENSONIQ
SSb
PHOX
P1 AND P4
SIEMENS
3000
BERNAFON
TELEX
OTICON
PHONAK

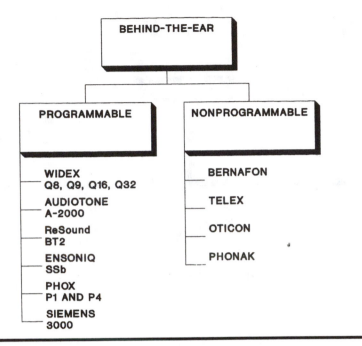

FIGURE 10.16. Organizational chart to counsel patients on specific BTE nonprogrammable and programmable hearing aids available at our facility.

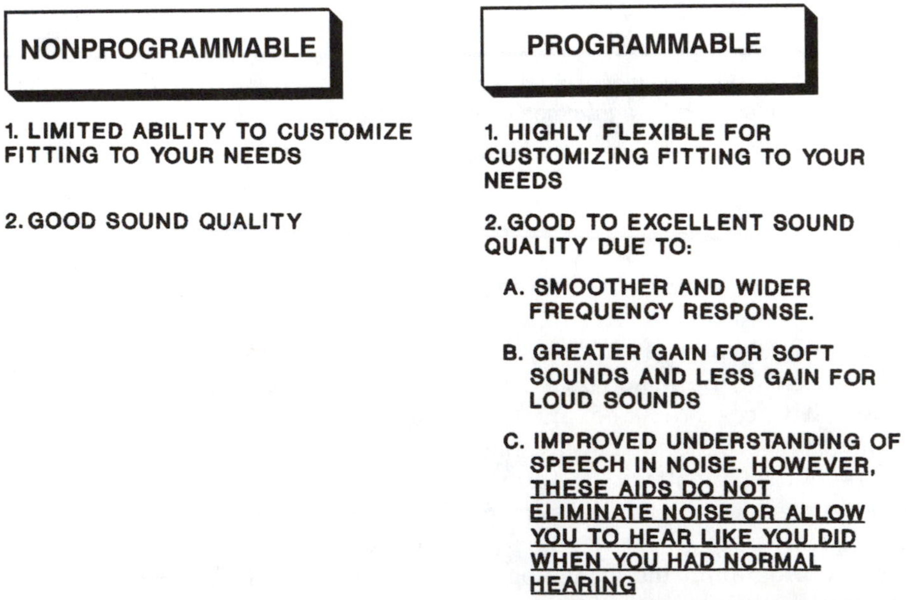

NONPROGRAMMABLE
1. LIMITED ABILITY TO CUSTOMIZE FITTING TO YOUR NEEDS
2. GOOD SOUND QUALITY
PROGRAMMABLE
1. HIGHLY FLEXIBLE FOR CUSTOMIZING FITTING TO YOUR NEEDS
2. GOOD TO EXCELLENT SOUND QUALITY DUE TO:
A. SMOOTHER AND WIDER FREQUENCY RESPONSE.
B. GREATER GAIN FOR SOFT SOUNDS AND LESS GAIN FOR LOUD SOUNDS
C. IMPROVED UNDERSTANDING OF SPEECH IN NOISE. HOWEVER, THESE AIDS DO NOT ELIMINATE NOISE OR ALLOW YOU TO HEAR LIKE YOU DID WHEN YOU HAD NORMAL HEARING

FIGURE 10.17. Page 1 of the counseling guide outlining differences between nonprogrammable and programmable hearing aids.

NONPROGRAMMABLE

3. NEED TO REPLACE OR RETURN THE HEARING AID FOR A NEW CIRCUIT IF PERCEPTION OF SOUND OR CHANGES IN HEARING OCCUR. THIS CAN BE:

   A. INCONVENIENT
   B. EXPENSIVE

4. INITIAL EXPENSE IS LESS THAN PROGRAMMABLE HEARING AIDS.

PROGRAMMABLE

3. CAN REPROGRAM THE HEARING AID OVER AND OVER AGAIN IF SOUND QUALITY OR HEARING SHOULD CHANGE OVER TIME. THIS IS:

   A. CONVENIENT
   B. LESS EXPENSIVE

4. INITIAL EXPENSE IS MORE THAN NON-PROGRAMMABLE HEARING AIDS BECAUSE:

   A. COST OF EQUIPMENT TO PROGRAM THE SPECIFIC HEARING AID.
   B. GREATER TIME REQUIRED TO FIT THESE HEARING AIDS
   C. GREATER COST OF HEARING AIDS
   D. INCREASED EDUCATION TO PROPERLY FIT THESE HEARING AIDS

FIGURE 10.18.   Page 2 of the counseling guide outlining additional differences between nonprogrammable and programmable hearing aids.

NONPROGRAMMABLE

5. GENERALLY LONGER BATTERY LIFE.

6. LITTLE CIRCUIT NOISE

PROGRAMMABLE

5. GENERALLY SHORTER BATTERY LIFE.

6. GENERALLY GREATER CIRCUIT NOISE

FIGURE 10.19.   Page 3 of the counseling guide outlining additional differences between nonprogrammable and programmable hearing aids.

FITTING STRATEGIES FOR PROGRAMMABLE HEARING AIDS

In the previous chapter, Robert Sweetow provided suggestions regarding six fitting strategies for many of the programmable hearing aids reviewed in this chapter. However, his chapter does not include fitting strategies for the Audiotone, Ensoniq, Trilogy, and PHOX programmable hearing aids. Therefore, this next section will present several fitting strategies that may be useful for these and other programmable hearing aids. These strategies include:

ENSONIQ

ADVANTAGES	DISADVANTAGES
AVAILABLE IN ITE AND BTE DESIGN	NO TELECOIL IS AVAILABLE FOR THE ITE
WIDE FREQUENCY RESPONSE	WEAK TELECOIL FOR THE BTE
SMOOTH FREQUENCY RESPONSE	PROGRAMMED FOR ONE FREQUENCY RESPONSE
CAN SHAPE THE FREQUENCY RESPONSE BY ADJUSTMENTS IN 13 BANDS	NOISY IF YOU HAVE HEARING WITHIN NORMAL LIMITS IN THE LOWER FREQUENCIES
PROVIDES GREATER GAIN FOR SOFT SOUNDS AND LESS GAIN FOR LOUD SOUNDS	SHORT BATTERY LIFE FOR THE ITE
LONG BATTERY LIFE FOR THE BTE DESIGN	NO VOLUME CONTROL ON THE ITE DESIGN. WILL BE AVAILABLE AS AN OPTION IN THE NEAR FUTURE
NO VOLUME CONTROL ON THE ITE DESIGN	

FIGURE 10.20.   Counseling tool outlining the advantages and disadvantages of Ensoniq hearing aids.

PHOX

ADVANTAGES	DISADVANTAGES
TWO RESPONSES AVAILABLE WHEN ORDERED WITH THE NOISE REDUCTION SWITCH	PEAKED FREQUENCY RESPONSE WHICH MAY RESULT IN SOME REDUCTION IN SOUND QUALITY
EXCELLENT TELECOIL SWITCH	SAME GAIN FOR SOFT OR LOUD SOUNDS
AVAILABLE IN BTE AND ITE DESIGNS	CIRCUIT NOISE MAY BE NOTICEABLE FOR THOSE WITH NORMAL LOW-FREQUENCY HEARING
VERY FLEXIBLE FIT	HIGH-FREQUENCY RESPONSE IS NOT AS WIDE AS SOME OTHER PROGRAMMABLE HEARING AIDS

FIGURE 10.21.   Counseling tool outlining advantages and disadvantages of PHOX hearing aids.

ReSound

ADVANTAGES	DISADVANTAGES
HEARING AID CAN BE PROGRAMMED WITH TWO RESPONSES	MOST EXPENSIVE PROGRAMMABLE AID
WIDE FREQUENCY RESPONSE	NEED REMOTE CONTROL TO OPERATE ED2, BUT NOT ED3 AND BT2
USE OF REMOTE: A. TO ADJUST VOLUME B. TO SWITCH MEMORIES	LARGE BATTERY DRAIN
PROVIDES GREATER GAIN FOR SOFT SOUNDS AND LESS GAIN FOR LOUD SOUNDS	CIRCUIT MAY SOUND NOISY IF YOU HAVE NORMAL LOW-FREQUENCY HEARING
ITE AND BTE DESIGN	

FIGURE 10.22.   Counseling tool outlining advantages and disadvantages of ReSound hearing aids.

Triton 3000

ADVANTAGES	DISADVANTAGES
WIDE FREQUENCY RESPONSE	PEAKED FREQUENCY RESPONSE WHICH MAY RESULT IN SOME REDUCTION IN SOUND QUALITY
FLEXIBILITY OF PROGRAMMING THREE FREQUENCY BANDS	SAME GAIN PROVIDED REGARDLESS IF THE SIGNAL IS SOFT OR LOUD
GOOD TELECOIL	MAY SOUND NOISY IF YOU HAVE NORMAL LOW-FREQUENCY HEARING

FIGURE 10.23.   Counseling tool outlining advantages and disadvantages of Triton 3000 hearing aids.

1. Using the programmer software to determine the programmable adjustments necessary to achieve the frequency/gain requirements for a selected prescriptive procedure.

2. Using several verification measures (e.g., probe tube, functional gain, or aided thresholds) to guide the dispenser in providing the appropriate programmable adjustments so that the measured real-ear insertion response (REIR), functional gain, or aided thresholds match the prescribed response for one of several popular prescriptive procedures.

3. Using probe tube measures to verify that the real-ear aided response (REAR) lies within the user's dynamic range.

4. Programming the hearing aid so the cou-

Widex

ADVANTAGES	DISADVANTAGES
HEARING AID CAN BE PROGRAMMED WITH FOUR DIFFERENT FREQUENCY RESPONSES	RELATIVELY EXPENSIVE
WIDE FREQUENCY RESPONSE	USE OF REMOTE CONTROL
SMOOTH FREQUENCY RESPONSE FOR THE Q8, Q9 AND QX	SAME GAIN PROVIDED FOR LOUD OR SOFT SOUNDS
USE OF REMOTE TO: A. ADJUST THE VOLUME B. SWITCH BETWEEN MEMORIES	PEAKED FREQUENCY RESPONSE (Q16) WHICH MAY RESULT IN SOME REDUCTION OF SOUND QUALITY
GOOD TELECOIL	
DIRECTIONAL MICROPHONE (Q9)	

FIGURE 10.24.   Counseling tool outlining advantages and disadvantages of Widex Quattro hearing aids.

pler response is reasonable for the magnitude and configuration of hearing loss.

5. Training the patient to program his/her own frequency/gain response.

6. Using a paired comparison procedure that is available in the Ensoniq, PHOX, and PMC systems. With this feature, the patient can immediately retrieve and compare any two stored responses to select the response (4 with Ensoniq, 6 with PHOX, and 15 with PMC) that is judged by the patient to provide the best speech intelligibility and sound quality.

Software-Selected Real-Ear Insertion Response (REIR)

PHOX.   The Ensoniq, PHOX, and Siemens PMC fitting systems contain software that allows the dispenser to select a prescriptive procedure (NAL-R, ENSONIQ, POGO, or ⅓ for Ensoniq; NAL-R, POGO, Berger, or ⅓–⅔ for PHOX; and NAL-R, POGO, Berger, ⅓, or ½ for Siemens PMC) or create his own fitting formula. Then, the dispenser enters the au-

diometric thresholds and the software calculates and selects the necessary programmable settings (i.e., gain, low- and high-frequency cutoff, low- and high-frequency slope, etc.) to provide an approximation of the prescribed REIR. Then the dispenser stores the software-selected settings into the memory of the hearing aid and often assumes that the software-selected fitting provides the frequency/gain response to achieve the prescribed REIR.

Figure 10.25 illustrates the initial measured REIR (thinner lower curve) for a PHOX fitting using speech-weighted composite noise presented at an overall level of 70 dB SPL. The frequency gain characteristics for this measured REIR were obtained after the "autoselect" segment of the software calculated and selected the parameters necessary to achieve the prescribed NAL-R REIR. It is clear that the measured REIR is significantly lower than the prescribed NAL-R REIR (thicker upper curve). At this point, the dispenser used the programmer to adjust the response to obtain the final fit as shown in

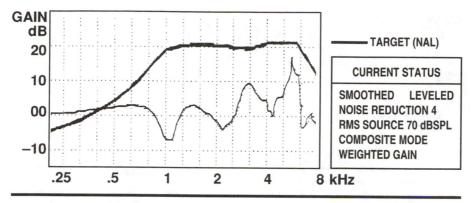

FIGURE 10.25.   Initial measured REIR (light curve) using the "autoselect" feature of the PHOX PX8.

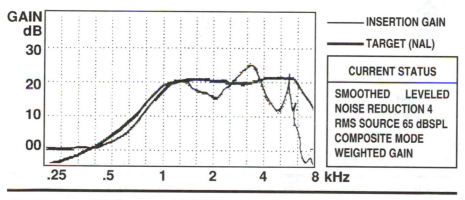

FIGURE 10.26.   Final measured REIR (light curve) versus prescribed NAL-R REIR (dark curve) after adjustments to the "autoselect" fit.

Figure 10.26. The measured REIR is now closer to the prescribed NAL-R REIR; however, some resonances and antiresonances still remain.

Figure 10.27 illustrates another example of parameters selected using the PHOX autoselect option. Here, the initial measured REIR (thinner lower curve) was reasonably close to prescribed NAL-R REIR (thicker upper curve). However, with several adjustments the measured REIR (thinner curve) matched

the prescribed NAL-R REIR (thicker curve) more closely (Figure 10.28).

Ensoniq.   The software of the Ensoniq system matches the hearing aid parameters to the prescriptive target in a manner quite different from the PHOX. With the Ensoniq, the dispenser can either enter audiometric thresholds, obtained using insert receivers, onto the displayed worksheet on the monitor or the dispenser can obtain and enter thresholds via

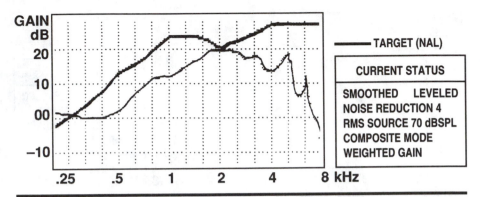

FIGURE 10.27.   Initial measured REIR (light curve) versus prescribed NAL-R REIR (dark curve) for another patient using the "autoselect" feature of the PHOX PX8.

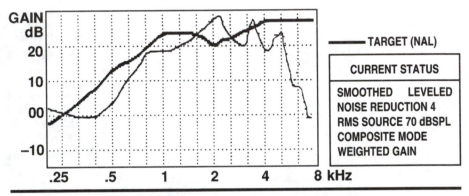

FIGURE 10.28.   Final measured REIR (light curve) versus prescribed NAL-R REIR (dark curve) for the same patient after adjustments to the "autoselect" fit.

the hearing aid while using the software available with the Ensoniq system. After the audiometric data is entered, a required calibration procedure is initiated to measure the performance of the instrument in the individual ear to correct for individual variations of the transmission line characteristics of the hearing aid and ear canal. After the calibration procedure is completed, the dispenser clicks the mouse in the "calculate" box to select one of four possible prescriptive targets (ENSONIQ, NAL-R, POGO, or Libby ⅓). At this point, the selected target is calculated and displayed on the monitor. Finally, the dispenser clicks the mouse in the "fit" box and the software calculates the hearing aid settings necessary to achieve the prescribed target. In a short time, the fitted and calculated responses are displayed on the monitor. In most cases, the calculated and fitted responses are superimposed, leading the dispenser to the assumption that the measured REIR would be very close to the prescribed REIR.

Figure 10.29 illustrates the initial mea-

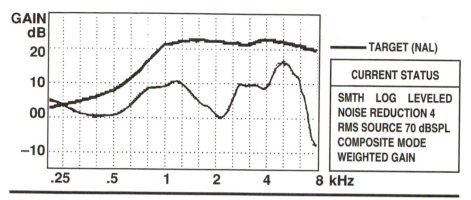

FIGURE 10.29. Initial measured REIR (light curve) versus prescribed NAL-R REIR (dark curve) using the Ensoniq software to calculate the fit.

sured REIR (lower thinner curve) for the SSb fitting displayed with the prescribed NAL-R REIR response (thicker curve) using speech-weighted composite noise. Although this hearing aid incorporates full dynamic range compression with a kneepoint at 55 dB SPL, an input of 70 dB SPL was chosen because NAL-R is based on the frequency/gain response required to amplify average conversational speech (overall level of 70 dB SPL) to the patient's most comfortable level (MCL) (Byrne and Dillon, 1986, p. 260). As can be seen, the measured REIR does not match the prescribed NAL-R REIR, although the En-

soniq monitor earlier had indicated that the calculated and fitted responses were virtually superimposed. Figure 10.30 illustrates the final measured REIR upon completing several adjustments. Now, measured REIR is closer to prescribed NAL-R REIR.

Figure 10.31 shows another example of the initial measured REIR (re: the NAL-R REIR) fitted with an Ensoniq SSb hearing aid. Again, the initial measured REIR is substantially different from the prescribed NAL-R REIR at all frequencies. Figure 10.32 illustrates the final measured REIR after completing the adjustment process. Again, measured

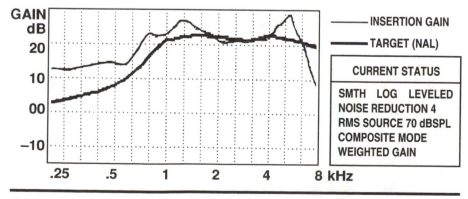

FIGURE 10.30. Final measured REIR (light curve) versus prescribed NAL-R REIR (dark curve) for the Ensoniq SSb after adjustments to the calculated fit.

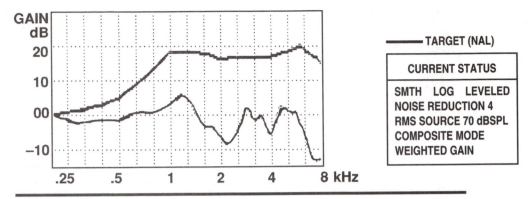

FIGURE 10.31. Initial measured REIR (light curve) for another patient using the Ensoniq software to calculate the fit.

REIR is now closer to the prescribed NAL-R REIR at most frequencies.

Interestingly, the same findings of large differences between the measured and prescribed REIR were not as large when fitting the Ensoniq SSi hearing aid. For most SSi fittings, very small differences were seen between the initial measure of the REIR relative to the prescribed REIR. In early 1992, Ensoniq introduced their updated version 1.3 software. Interestingly, significantly smaller differences are now seen between the initial measure of the REIR when compared to the prescribed REIR for both the SSb *and* SSi hearing aids.

Several reasons may account for the significant differences seen between measured and prescribed gain when fitting and verifying the output of the Ensoniq hearing aid us-

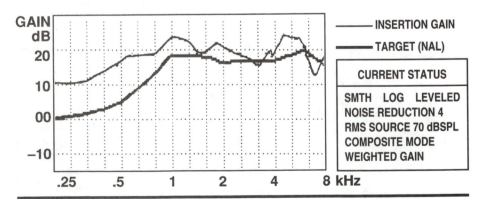

FIGURE 10.32. Final measured REIR (light curve) versus prescribed NAL-R REIR (dark curve) for the same patient after adjustments to the fit calculated by the Ensoniq software.

ing the version 1.0 software. First, the prescribed REIR (NAL-R, for example) was developed using hearing aids with linear circuitry. With linear hearing aids, measured gain is essentially unchanged regardless of the input intensity level of the signal unless the output is saturated. Hearing aids with full dynamic range compression provide varying degrees of measured gain depending on the overall intensity of the input signal. Since full dynamic range compression aids have only been available since 1990, prescriptive targets for full dynamic range compression hearing aids simply do not exist. Furthermore, it may be inappropriate to use linear targets for fitting and adjusting hearing aids incorporating full dynamic range compression.

A second reason may be related to the type of signal used to measure the real-ear response. In the measures reported above, the signal was speech-weighted composite noise. Although the overall level was 70 dB SPL, the input level to the microphone of the hearing aid decreases as frequency increases in a manner similar to average conversational speech. However, the software contained within the Ensoniq fitting system was developed assuming the hearing aid will be measured using narrow bands of noise that are relatively (+/–5 dB) constant in intensity as a function of frequency (personal communication, Gauthier, 1991). As will be described in a later section, there are significant differences in hearing aid output (i.e., REAR measures) when using an input signal that is relatively constant in intensity (ie., pure tones, narrow bands of noise, or warble tones) compared to a signal that decreases in intensity as frequency increases (i.e., speech-weighted composite noise).

A third reason may be related to the fact that the microphone of the hearing aid is inactive during the Ensoniq fitting process. However, when using external verification procedures (e.g., probe tube measures) the

microphone is active. A fourth reason is that the equalization method incorporated in the Ensoniq fitting system is based on the substitution method for a diffuse field that is stored in the software memory. On the other hand, the Frye 6500 (with which these comparison were made) uses a real-time modified equivalent substitution with differential comparison. The major difference between these two methods of equalization is that the substitution method includes the effects of head and body baffle as well as head shadow, whereas the real-time modified equivalent substitution with differential comparison method excludes these effects.

Finally, the software within the Ensoniq fitting includes a real-ear unaided response (REUR) that is based on average data. The REIR measures with the Frye 6500 were based on the individual REUR. A recent study by Valente, Valente, and Goebel (1991) clearly illustrates the wide intersubject variability of the REUR. Therefore, differences in the measured REIR should appear if one system is using average REUR data while another system uses the actual individual data.

A Word of Caution: As mentioned earlier, it is important that the dispenser realize that prescriptive formulas were established using hearing aids with a single frequency response and linear circuitry. However, several programmable hearing aids contain full dynamic range compression circuity (e.g., ReSound and Ensoniq) in which the frequency gain characteristics change as a function of the incoming sound level and spectrum. Dispensers must be cautious if they use prescriptive targets developed with linear aids to verify the performance of hearing aids having full dynamic range compression.

For example, the PHOX is a programmable hearing aid containing linear circuitry with a single-frequency response. Therefore (if the output is programmed at maximum), measured REIR will remain essentially the same regardless if the input signal was 50 dB to approximately 85 dB SPL as long as the output level is below saturation. For this hearing aid, the use of prescriptive targets is appropriate for verification.

In contrast, the Ensoniq hearing aid contains full dynamic range compression with a kneepoint of 55 dB SPL. With this aid, the measured REIR will decrease as the input signal increases; conversely, the REIR will increase as the input level decreases.

For example, Figure 10.33 shows two REIR responses measured on the same Ensoniq hearing aid. The upper curve was measured using a 60 dB SPL, speech-weighted composite noise, while the lower curve was measured using 70 dB SPL. The prescribed NAL-R REIR is shown as the thicker curve. If the dispenser was not aware of this interaction it would be tempting to conclude the aid was providing greater than prescribed gain (re: the NAL-R target) when using 60 dB. However, if the dispenser had used 70 dB SPL he probably would conclude this was an appropriate fit, although it was exactly the same fit. Also notice that the shapes of the two frequency responses are slightly different; the low-frequency slope is

steeper (below ~1200 Hz) for the 70 dB input than for the 60 dB input.

Figure 10.34 illustrates another example. Again, the thick curve represents the prescribed NAL-R REIR. The lower thin curve was measured using 70 dB SPL speech-weighted composite noise, while the upper thin curve was measured using a 65 dB SPL input. There is greater measured REIR for the 65 dB SPL input and less REIR for the 70 dB SPL input. Again, notice differences in the shapes of the insertion gain responses. There is little difference in the gain below 1000 Hz between the two input levels, whereas with the 65 dB input there is greater high-frequency gain than with the 70 dB input.

This caution is intended to help dispensers select the appropriate settings for their patients. In summary:

1. It is the responsibility of the dispenser to select an appropriate frequency/gain response. In addition, it is his or her responsibility to verify that the prescribed response was attained to the degree it is clinically feasible.

2. It is the responsibility of the dispenser to know how the hearing aid response changes as the level of the input signal changes.

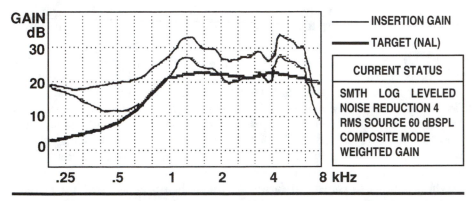

FIGURE 10.33.   Measured REIRs for inputs of 60 dB SPL (upper light curve) and 70 dB SPL (lower light curve) for the Ensoniq SSb.

Using Probe Tube or Functional Gain Procedures to Adjust the Measured Response

Probe Tube Procedures Using REIR. A second strategy involves active dispenser interaction with the programmer to adjust the hearing aid response to match the prescribed real-ear insertion response (REIR) using probe tube procedures. In fact, this strategy was used to obtain the fittings in Figures 10.26, 10.28, 10.30, and 10.32–10.34.

An example of the steps followed with this strategy are described as follows while dispensing an Audiotone A-2000 BTE. First, the prescribed NAL-R REIR for a patient (thicker curve) was calculated by the software of the probe tube system as shown in Figure 10.35 (thicker curve). With the hearing aid in place, the volume control was adjusted to the most comfortable level (MCL) using 70 dB SPL of speech-weighted noise. This overall level was used because Walden, Schuhman, and Sedge (1977) found that using 70 dB SPL for adjusting the volume control wheel was likely to result in the same volume control setting used in daily life. At this point, the dispenser adjusted the programmable parameters until the measured REIR (thinner curve) matched as closely as possible the prescribed NAL-R REIR. Once this was accomplished, the fitting was locked into the memory of the hearing aid for trial in everyday life.

One Final Point. A hearing aid fitting strategy in which success is based solely on measured REIR arriving close to prescribed REIR may be open to question. This strategy does not utilize dispenser interaction with the patient, and it assumes that achieving the prescribed REIR will always yield the most appropriate frequency/gain response. One major weakness with this strategy is that it assumes all patients having the same audiometric configuration require the same frequency/gain response (homogeneous) regardless of individual variations in preferred sound quality or loudness growth (heterogenous). In essence, individual differences and preferences are discounted because this strategy effectively states that the dispenser knows what is best for the patient and that the patient will adapt to it.

Desired Aided Thresholds Using Functional Gain Measures. All dispensers do not have the equipment necessary to perform probe tube measures. However, similar results can be obtained using functional gain to adjust a

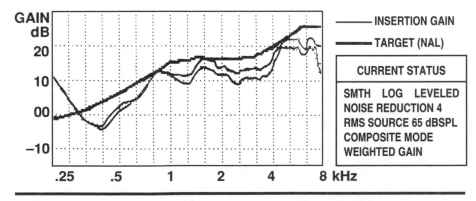

FIGURE 10.34. Measured REIRs for inputs of 65 dB SPL (upper light curve) and 70 dB SPL (lower light curve) for the Ensoniq SSb.

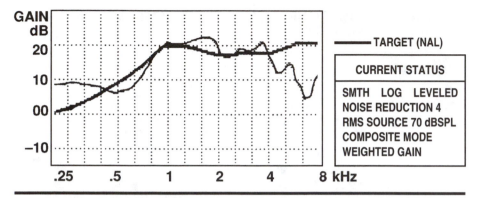

FIGURE 10.35. Measured REIR (light curve) versus prescribed NAL-R REIR (dark curve) for the Audiotone A-2000.

hearing aid with linear circuitry to a pre-scribed aided threshold contour.

Figure 10.36 illustrates prescribed aided thresholds (A--A) using the same NAL-R re-sponse reported in Figure 10.34 for a patient with unaided monaural sound-field thresh-olds (U--U) between 250 and 6000 Hz. The prescribed functional gain (NAL-R) varies between 1 dB at 250 Hz and 21 dB at 1000 and 6000 Hz, as shown near the bottom of Figure 10.36. The prescribed aided threshold target (A--A) is calculated by subtracting functional gain from the unaided threshold. For ex-ample, the unaided monaural threshold for a 1000 Hz warble tone at 0° azimuth is 45 dB HL. Prescribed functional gain is 21 dB. Therefore, the desired aided threshold is 45 minus 21 or 24 dB HL. Thus, the dispenser can adjust the programmable aid until the aided threshold, using a 1000 Hz warble tone at 0° azimuth, approaches 24 dB HL while the opposite ear is muffed and/or plugged. This procedure would be completed for the other test frequencies.

One major disadvantage of functional gain measures was reported by Rines, Stelmacho-wicz, and Gorga (1984). They cautioned that ambient noise and internal noise of hearing aids may interact to mask the aided sound-field threshold. If the threshold is elevated by the presence of this noise, the actual func-tional gain will be underestimated. This situ-ation is most likely to occur for patients with normal or near-normal hearing in frequency regions where significant gain is provided. In these cases, probe tube measures will provide a more accurate measure of real-ear gain. In addition, functional gain measures can only evaluate real-ear gain at discrete frequencies, while probe measures can measure real-ear gain at all frequencies between approxi-mately 200 and 6000 Hz.

Real-Ear Aided Response (REAR) Within the Dynamic Range of the User

A third strategy uses probe tube measures to verify that the REAR provides sufficient gain to amplify the speech spectrum to within the listener's dynamic range. Using this proce-dure, the real-ear output (input level plus gain) of the hearing aid is measured to deter-mine its position within the dynamic range of the listener.

Figure 10.37 illustrates a listener's dynamic range (dB SPL) measured with an insert re-ceiver and probe tube near the tympanic mem-brane (TM) for threshold (O—O), MCL (◇—◇), and LDL (□—□). The dynamic range at each frequency was obtained using pure tones from

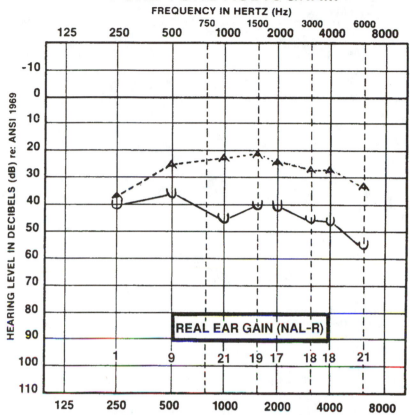

FIGURE 10.36. Prescribed aided thresholds (A--A) calculated from functional gain requirements (reported at the bottom) for the NAL-R procedure using the unaided (U--U) thresholds.

an audiometer, an ER-3A (50 ohm) insert receiver, and a loudness rating scale procedure described by Skinner (1988, pp. 127–128). Using this procedure, threshold was equivalent to a loudness judgment of "very soft," while MCL was equivalent to a loudness judgment of "OK" and LDL was equivalent to a loudness judgment of "loud."

To establish the listener's dynamic range, a probe tube is marked 30 mm from the tip and the mark placed at the tragal notch. In an average adult ear, this should place the probe approximately 4–6 mm from the TM. At this position, measured SPL would be within 2 dB of the SPL at the TM to 6000 Hz (Gilman and Dirks, 1986).

With the probe tube taped in place, the ER-3A insert receiver is placed into the ear canal

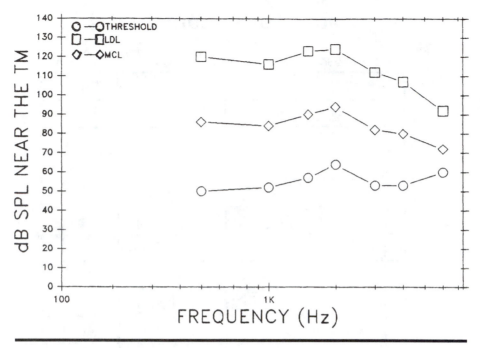

FIGURE 10.37.   Probe tube measures (dB SPL near the TM) of threshold, MCL, and LDL.

using a 7–8 mm immittance probe tip to hold it in place. The insert receiver is connected to a calibrated audiometer (ANSI-1989) and threshold, MCL, and LDL are obtained for continuous discrete tones between 500 and 6000 Hz. The SPLs corresponding to these thresholds were recorded from the real-ear analyzer and plotted at a later time. One note of caution: Due to problems related to the amount of ambient noise in the test suite as well as the noise floor of the probe microphone system, it is not possible to measure threshold SPL if the hearing loss is less than approximately 45–50 dB HL.

Next, the unaided speech spectrum for overall levels of 50, 60, 70 and 80 dB SPL are calculated and superimposed over the measured dynamic range using spreadsheet and scientific graphing software (Figure 10.38). The calculated unaided speech spectrum for soft to loud conversational speech (50, 60, 70

and 80 dB) is based on applying two corrections. First, the 70 dB speech spectrum was based on the data reported by Cox and Moore (1988). This reference speech spectrum (70 dB SPL) was adjusted to reflect the changes in the spectrum of composite speech noise for overall levels of 50, 60, and 80 dB SPL as a result of varying vocal effort as reported by Pearsons, Bennett, and Fidell (1976). In addition, the speech spectrum for 50–80 dB was adjusted to account for the real-ear unaided response (REUR) of the listener. The final result shown in Figure 10.38 is the theoretical unaided speech spectra (50–80 dB) measured near the eardrum of the individual and the relation of each to the individual's dynamic range.

Figure 10.39 illustrates REAR measures (dB SPL near the TM) for input levels of 50–80 dB SPL of speech-weighted composite noise obtained with a linear ITE adjusted to MCL. It is clear that soft conversational speech (repre-

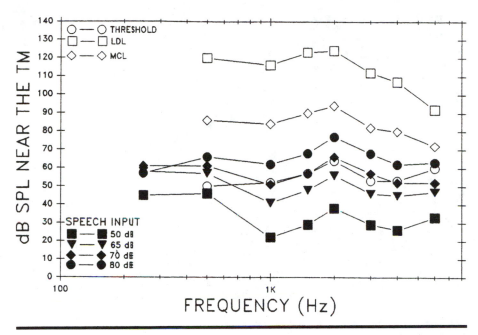

FIGURE 10.38. Calculated REAR for the unaided speech spectrum for input levels of 50–80 dB SPL (see text for description).

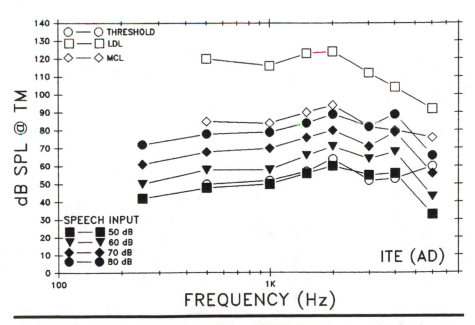

FIGURE 10.39. REAR measures (dB SPL near TM) for speech-weighted noise at input levels of 50–80 dB SPL for a linear ITE hearing aid.

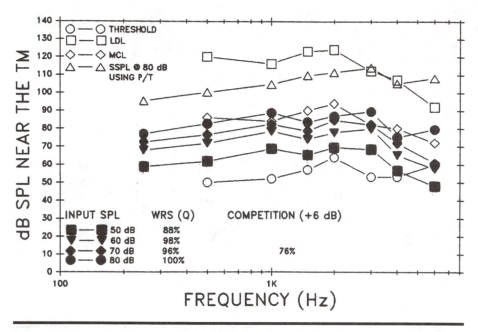

FIGURE 10.40. REAR measures (dB SPL near TM) for speech-weighted noise at input levels of 50–80 dB SPL for an Ensoniq SSb hearing aid that was programmed by the patient.

sented by the 50 dB input) is below or near threshold for all test frequencies. Except for 6000 Hz, the REAR for the 60 dB input is about 10 dB SL (re: threshold). For this patient, word recognition in quiet was 72% (NU-6 monosyllabic words; Auditec recordings) (overall level of 68 dBC) and 58% using a +6 dB S/N ratio (multitalker babble).

Figure 10.40 illustrates a procedure where the frequency response of an Ensoniq SSb was shaped so that the REAR output was above threshold at all frequencies (except 6000 Hz) using a 50 dB speech-weighted signal. Then, REAR was measured at 60, 70, and 80 dB to verify that the REAR approached MCL, but was below LDL. This fit improved the word recognition score in quiet to 100% and in noise to 76% Figure 10.41 illustrates the REAR measures one week later. It is clear that REAR measures are slightly greater compared to the previous week. This difference is

related, in part, to the test/retest reliability of probe tube measures (Valente, Meister, Smith, and Goebel, 1990; Valente, Valente, and Goebel, 1991). However, part of the difference is related to a partially clogged 2200 ohm damper, which was removed and replaced prior to this measure.

In addition, the REAR was measured using an 80 dB SPL, pure tone sweep (△). It is felt this may represent a more valid measure of the output of the hearing aid, relative to the LDL, than using an 80 dB speech-weighted composite noise because the LDL was measured using pure tones.

Two things become clear when examining the relation between the REAR for pure tones and speech-weighted noise in Figure 10.41. First, the measured REAR for the pure tone sweep is below or near LDL at all frequencies except for 4000–6000 Hz. This latter finding is of some concern, and perhaps the frequency

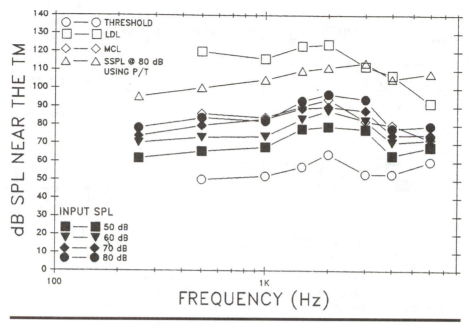

FIGURE 10.41.   REAR measures (dB SPL near the TM) for speech-weighted noise at input levels of 50–80 dB SPL for an Ensoniq hearing aid one week later. Also reported is the REAR for an 80 dB pure tone sweep signal.

response should be reprogrammed to maintain the same shape, but reduce the overall gain (using region adjust) approximately 3 dB. The obtained LDL at 6000 Hz is not the "true" LDL because LDL could not be measured due to the limited output of the insert receiver and audiometer. More importantly, it is clear that significantly different measures of REAR will be obtained depending upon the type of signal (pure tone versus speech-weighted noise) used to make the measure. Calculations using our probe system (Frye 6500) indicated that the measured REAR using a pure tone sweep was 10–30 dB greater than the measured REAR using a speech-weighted composite noise. Also, calculations revealed that these differences increased as frequency increased.

At this point, the authors believe the speech-weighted composite noise may have greater face validity for adjusting the fre-

quency/gain response to fit within the dynamic range of a listener for improved speech intelligibility, and it is more appropriate to use a pure tone sweep to verify that the output does not exceed the LDL of the patient.

The REAR has been used successfully for programming hearing aids. The following is an outline describing this procedure:

1. As described above, measure the output near the TM (in dB SPL) using a probe microphone system and the ER-3A insert receiver with audiometer to produce the pure tones for threshold, MCL, and LDL. This procedure will provide the dynamic range of the listener.

2. With the probe tube in the same position, place the hearing aid in the ear canal and have the patient adjust the volume control to MCL using speech-weighted composite signal at 70 dB SPL or a recorded version of connected discourse spoken by a male or female.

	VERY		RATHER		MIDWAY		RATHER		VERY			
	0	1	2	3	4	5	6	7	8	9	10	
BLURRED												DISTINCT
UNPLEASANT												PLEASANT
UNNATURAL												NATURAL
DULL												SHARP
NOISY												QUIET
CRINKLING												SMOOTH
TINNY												FULL
	0	1	2	3	4	5	6	7	8	9	10	

FIGURE 10.42. Worksheet used to determine quality judgments. Modified after Gabrielsson, Schenkman, and Hagerman, 1988.

3. Present speech-weighted composite noise at 50 dB SPL (representative of soft speech). Program the hearing aid response so that the measured REAR (output in dB SPL near the eardrum) is approximately 3–6 dB above the measured threshold of the patient at most test frequencies. This may not be possible in the higher frequencies for patients having sharply sloping or precipitous audiometric configurations.

4. Present speech-weighted composite noise at 80 dB SPL and a pure tone sweep at 80 dB SPL to verify that the measured REAR does not exceed the measured LDL.

5. If these measures verify that soft speech-weighted composite noise (i.e., 50 dB) is audible and loud speech (80 dB) does not exceed the LDL, then it should not be necessary to determine the REAR for inputs of 60 and 70 dB.

6. As frequency shaping is being adjusted with the programmable hearing aid, it is suggested that sound quality judgments (Figure 10.42) and speech intelligibility ratings (SIR)

(Cox and McDaniel, 1989) be obtained to assist in determining the frequency/gain response to be stored in the hearing aid. The worksheet illustrated in Figure 10.42 is used during the process of shaping the frequency response so that the REAR for a 50 dB signal is above threshold and quality judgments are as close to the 10 rating for most of the categories. Unfortunately, a recent report by Surr and Fabry (1991) suggests that the SIR may not be beneficial in revealing differences among frequency responses if the volume control of the hearing aid is adjusted to MCL for each change in the parameters. It is important for the individual to wear the hearing aid(s) in everyday life and then return to the dispenser to describe observations about the amplified sound. If indicated, further adjustments in the hearing aid parameters should be made to improve the usefulness of the amplified sound.

Unfortunately, current probe tube systems do not allow for measuring and reporting results in this manner. These data were calculated using a spreadsheet software program and then integrated with scientific graphing software to plot the results after the patient left. We believe that this information, presented in real time with a probe tube system, could serve as a valuable counseling and fitting tool.

Coupler Response

As mentioned earlier, not all dispensers have the equipment required to perform probe tube measures. However, the dispenser could program the hearing aid so that the coupler response matches a prescribed coupler response appropriate for the hearing loss, type of hearing aid (ITC, ITE, BTE), prescriptive procedure (Berger, NAL-R, POGO, ⅓, etc.), and volume control setting.

In fact, one hearing aid analyzer (Frye) contains software that allows the dispenser to achieve this goal. Using the analyzer, the dispenser:

1. Enters the audiometric thresholds
2. Selects the desired prescriptive procedure (NAL-R, POGO, Berger, ⅓, ⅔, etc.)
3. Selects the type of hearing aid (ITE, ITC, BTE)
4. Selects the reserve gain to approximate the volume control the user would select. For example, the NAL-R and Libby procedures assume the volume control is 15 dB below maximum rotation, while POGO and Berger procedures assume the volume control is 10 dB below maximum rotation.
5. Selects the average real-ear unaided response (REUR). Recent reports by Valente, Valente and Goebel (1991), Valente, Valente, and Vass (1990), Valente, Valente, and Vass (1991), and Valente and Valente (1989) illustrate how individual variations of the REUR can prevent the prescribed REIR from being achieved in the frequency region around the ear canal resonance of

the patient. Measuring and incorporating the individual REUR into the calculations would enable the dispenser to more closely achieve the prescribed REIR.

After entering this information, the monitor displays the 2 cc full-on coupler response required to achieve the prescribed real-ear gain for the average ear at 15 dB below full-on gain. Figure 10.43 illustrates an example using such a procedure. The upper curve is the prescribed NAL-R for a mild to moderate hearing loss gradually sloping in configuration. The lower curve is the calculated full-on 2 cc coupler gain required for a BTE fitting assuming that the hearing aid user would set the volume control 15 dB below maximum rotation in everyday life. Figures 10.44 and 10.45 show the same full-on 2 cc coupler data for ITE and ITC hearing aids, respectively. Note the need for less coupler gain for an ITC (3–9 dB between 2 and 6 kHz) relative to a BTE fitting for the same hearing loss and prescribed gain. The difference between coupler response for an ITE fitting (re: BTE) is 2–5 dB less required coupler gain in the same frequency region.

At this point, the dispenser can connect the programmable hearing aid to the appropriate coupler (HA-1 or HA-2); turn the volume control to maximum rotation; and program the hearing aid so the measured coupler response matches, as closely as possible, the coupler response displayed previously on the monitor. For dispensers not having access to hearing aid analyzers with this capability, research was recently published (Valente, Valente, and Vass, 1990, 1991; Skinner, 1988) allowing the dispenser to make the necessary calculations to achieve the same goals. Finally, if the dispenser has an audiometer and a calibrated sound field, the real-ear gain (or only aided thresholds for those with severe to profound hearing loss) provided by the hearing aid can be obtained.

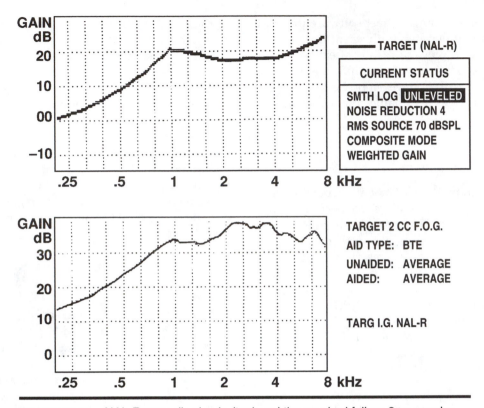

FIGURE 10.43.   NAL-R prescribed gain (top) and the required full-on 2 cc coupler gain for a BTE hearing aid (bottom).

Patient-Selected Frequency/Gain Shaping

As mentioned earlier, there are two concerns when hearing aids are programmed based solely on measured REIR matching prescribed REIR and no further adjustments of the parameters are made. These concerns are: (a) prescriptive procedures calculate the gain required to amplify conversational speech to MCL for the average listener, and (b) the lack of allowance for intersubject differences in loudness growth and preferred sound quality.

A fitting strategy that can be used with all the programmable hearing aids is training the user to use the programmer to adjust the frequency/gain response judged to be most satisfactory. With this procedure, the volume control is adjusted to MCL while listening to recorded female connected discourse at 70 dB SPL. A female talker is usually selected because most patients report greater difficulty understanding female than male speakers. Next, 55 dB SPL of multitalker babble (+15 dB signal-to-babble ratio) is added through the same loudspeaker (0° azimuth) while the patient adjusts the frequency/gain response to obtain the best sound quality and intelligibility. Once this has been accomplished, the response is stored into the hearing aid.

For hearing aids having multiple memories (e.g., ReSound, Starkey Trilogy I and II, Siemens 3004b and 3004i, or Quattro), one response may be programmed while listening to male connected discourse in quiet (overall level

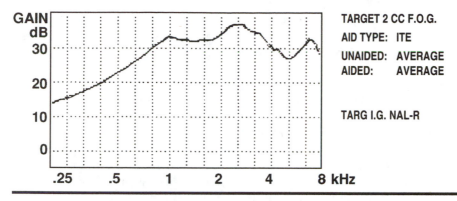

FIGURE 10.44.   Required full-on 2 cc coupler gain for an ITE hearing aid for the same NAL-R prescribed gain illustrated in Figure 10.43.

of 70 dB SPL). A second response may be programmed while listening to female connected discourse in quiet (overall level of 70 dB SPL). Another response may be programmed while listening to male or female discourse presented in a background of multitalker babble (+6 to +10 dB signal-to-babble ratio). For several patients, one response was programmed for listening to music.

The intrinsic attractiveness of this strategy is that the patient assumes responsibility for the selected programmed response. Using other strategies, the success or failure of the selected response lies entirely on the shoulders of the dispenser. In addition, the patient-selected response allows for interpatient differences in judgments of sound quality and intelligibility as well as loudness growth. Finally, this strategy can provide significant insights for dispensers who select, in advance, what they feel is most appropriate for the patient. We have found that responses patients have selected have provided a basis for reassessing our criteria for preselecting frequency/gain characteristics.

Paired Comparisons

One final strategy is the use of paired comparisons. As mentioned earlier, the Ensoniq,

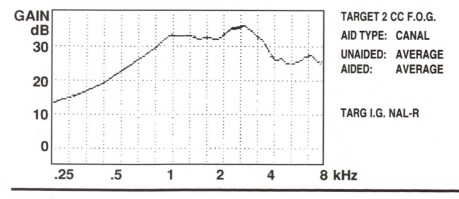

FIGURE 10.45.   Required full-on 2 cc coupler gain for an ITC hearing aid for the same NAL-R prescribed gain illustrated in Figure 10.43.

PHOX, and PMC allow four or more programmed responses to be stored in temporary memory for immediate retrieval as part of a paired-comparison fitting process.

Any of the fitting strategies described above can be used to generate frequency/gain responses and to place the programmed responses into one of the available memories. For example, using the first fitting strategy, the dispenser can have an NAL-R fit programmed and placed into memory 1 and a POGO fit programmed and placed into memory 2. This process can be repeated for the other prescriptive procedures and the responses stored in the other available memories. Then the dispenser can retrieve any two stored responses for a paired comparison.

Using this procedure, any two responses held in memory are alternately compared using, for example, sound quality and/or intelligibility ratings scales, until one response is ultimately eliminated by the listener. The "winning response" is then successively compared with the other stored responses. This process is continued until an ultimate winner is selected by the listener from among the stored responses and then programmed into the memory of the hearing aid. The process of comparing the winner with each of the remaining responses to select the final winner has been referred to as a single elimination (SE) tournament by Montgomery, Schwartz, and Punch (1982) and Studebaker, Bisset, Van Ort, and Hoffnung (1982). As new prescriptive procedures for selecting frequency/gain characteristics of a hearing aid evolve, they can be included in the alternatives that are compared.

ADVANTAGES AND DISADVANTAGES AMONG THE DIFFERENT SYSTEMS

Over the past few years the authors have had the opportunity to use these programmable hearing aids for clinical and research purposes. This experience has allowed us to document our current thoughts concerning the advantages and disadvantages of some of the systems (see Figures 10.20–10.24).

Audiotone A-2000

Advantages

1. It is very easy to program. With this system, the dispenser can immediately program his first hearing aid. The manual is short and well written. Furthermore, several patients have already been trained to program their own hearing aid circuits while listening to recorded signals (male or female connected discourse) in quiet (70 dB SPL) or competition (e.g., +10 to +15 dB signal-to-babble ratio) at one meter at 0° azimuth.

2. The programmer and hearing aid are relatively inexpensive.

3. The dispenser can connect the hearing aid to the programmer via the programming cable, and the parameters of the stored response are instantaneously visible via red light-emitting diode (LED) lights on the programmer.

4. It is very easy to program binaural hearing aids. The dispenser simply presses the red button to program the right hearing aid. He then presses the blue button to program the left hearing aid.

Disadvantages

1. The number of parameters available for programming is very limited. There are five settings for each of the following parameters: output, gain, and adjusting the low- and high-frequency cutoffs. In most respects, the flexibility of this system is not significantly greater than using potentiometers present on most BTE and some ITE hearing aids.

2. Occasionally our programmer locked up, and it was necessary to hit the programmer to continue.

3. There is no provision for a hard copy.

4. There are many resonances and anti-resonances in the coupler-measured frequency response.

5. A directional microphone is not available.

Ensoniq

Advantages

1. The coupler frequency response is smooth and gradually rises to a peak at approximately 2800 Hz. As pointed out earlier, this REUR type of response appears to be preferred by patients for enhanced sound quality.

2. A full dynamic range compression circuit is present with a kneepoint at 55 dB SPL. As pointed out earlier, this circuit is considered advantageous because it provides greater gain for soft sounds and progressively less gain for louder sounds. This circuit design results in reduced distortion for loud input sounds and increased sound quality. In addition, the reduction of gain for loud sounds lessens the possibility of amplified sound exceeding the patient's threshold of discomfort.

3. It is very easy to fit binaurally.

4. The unit can be used as an audiometer for determining threshold (and MCL and LDL) at the standard audiometric frequencies or at the center frequency of the thirteen bands used with this system. The advantage is that the individual's auditory area is "mapped" in the same environment as that for the hearing aid fit.

5. The cost of the SSb and SSi is close to that for conventional linear hearing aids.

6. Manufacturer support has been excellent. Several staff members are always available to help when fitting, software, or hardware problems arise.

7. The fitting system is the most flexible of the programmable aids that are currently available.

8. The user can compare sound perceptions with four sets of frequency/gain parameters before selecting the preferred fit to be stored in the hearing aid memory. This paired-comparison procedure has proven to be very successful in selecting the final fit for several patients.

9. There is a printout of patient data, probe microphone calibration, and noise floor, as well as the audiometric and fitting data.

10. Software updates are free. The instructions for installing new software are well written so that the update is very easily implemented.

11. The SSb has a directional microphone.

12. All fitting data can be saved to a hard or floppy disk for easy retrieval when changes are required to the hearing aid.

Disadvantages

1. The programmer is relatively expensive when the costs for the computer, monitor, and printer are combined with the costs for the interface and chest pack.

2. The telecoil gain is low on the SSb and not available on the SSi.

3. The O-T-M switch is poorly designed. The switch is not aligned with the "O," "T," and "M" on the case, which causes confusion. In addition, the battery falls out of the SSb very easily when it is opened at night or to replace the battery.

4. The circuit noise is noticeable to patients having normal hearing below 1000 Hz.

5. The dispenser needs to determine (with real-ear insertion or functional gain) whether the measured frequency/gain response reasonably approaches the prescribed frequency/gain response and then change the parameters to achieve this goal. As mentioned earlier, the frequently used methods for prescribed real-ear gain were developed with linear amplification systems, and the Ensoniq is a full dynamic range compression system. Therefore, it may be important to further modify the frequency/gain characteristics to meet the needs of the individual patient.

6. Although our experience is limited, we are concerned that the elimination of the volume control on the SSi will not give the patient sufficient control over the sound intensity in everyday life. Recently, Ensoniq announced that a volume control will be available as an option in the near future.

7. On several occasions, patients reported the SSb aid to be inoperative. Close inspection revealed the fused mesh damper (2200 ohms) was clogged. This problem has been resolved by ordering dri-tubing with earmolds or inserting a 680 or 1000 ohm damper before performing the calibration procedures recommended by Ensoniq.

Bernafon PHOX

Advantages

1. It is available in an ITE (P20S and P30) that has been successfully fitted on many patients. Either #13 or #312 batteries may be used in the battery drawer. We recommend the #13 battery because of longer battery life.

2. The programmer is very easy to operate. Several users have programmed their own hearing aids as they listened to a variety of recorded signals (male or female talker at 70 dB SPL) in quiet or noise (+10 to +15 dB signal-to-babble ratio) at one meter and at 0° azimuth. In addition, the programmer operates on AC or DC power (four D cell batteries).

3. The hearing aids are relatively inexpensive.

4. The noise-reduction circuit (optional "X" switch) has been helpful to our patients. By setting the switch to the "X" position the user

has two responses. In the microphone position, the response has more low-frequency gain and is useful for listening in reasonably quiet environments. In the "X" position, the response has a reduction of low-frequency gain to improve performance in noisy situations. It is important to know that the hearing aid cannot be programmed while the user has the switch in the "X" position; it must be in the microphone (M) position.

5. All PHOX aids have excellent telecoil switches. Many patients with past difficulties using telecoil switches remark how well they perform on the telephone with the PHOX.

6. The updates, although infrequent, are easy to install. The updated software module arrives in the mail and the dispenser simply pulls out the old module and snaps in the new module.

7. The new BTE (P1) has been significantly reduced in size and is attractive as an option for many patients. Recently, the software was updated to provide approximately 6 dB greater overall gain for the smaller P1 aid. Surprisingly, the same software did not incorporate any new changes for the older P4 BTE.

8. The dispenser (see Tables 9.3 and 9.4) has many parameters available for changing the frequency/gain response and, consequently, a great deal of flexibility during the fitting process.

9. The dispenser can store and recall six user-selected frequency/gain responses to use with a paired-comparison strategy to select the final fit. The ability to store and recall each of the six responses is easy and efficient.

10. The unit is delivered with eight setup frequency/gain responses programmed by Bernafon, and the dispenser can program an additional four. Thus, at any time the dispenser can easily call up twelve frequency/gain responses for the fitting process.

Disadvantages

1. Hard copy is of limited value. For example, a section of the hard copy plots the calculated insertion gain, which is an inaccurate estimate of the actual insertion gain.

2. The coupler response for the P1 and P4 aids is peaked as reflected by numerous resonances and antiresonances.

3. Repairs take longer than desired.

4. Gain and output can only be programmed in 6 dB increments or decrements. This step size is too large; a suggestion for 3 dB increments has been forwarded to the manufacturer for their consideration.

5. As with other programmable systems having target select functions, the "autoselect" function does not provide the prescribed real-ear gain as calculated by the software.

6. The hearing aid (especially the P20S) is rather noisy and can be annoying for patients having hearing within normal limits at or below 1000 Hz.

7. The cable for programming the ITE is poorly designed. The contact points easily bend. This prevents contact with the ITE hearing aid. We have had many cables replaced over the past three years.

8. The hearing aid provides linear amplification when output is set at maximum.

9. The BTE and ITE do not have a directional microphone.

10. Numerous real-ear measures revealed insufficient insertion gain above 3000 Hz for many patients.

ReSound

Advantages

1. It has a smooth and gradually rising frequency response that extends to 6200 Hz and peaks at approximately 2800 Hz. As pointed out earlier, this REUR-type response appears to be preferred by patients for enhanced sound quality.

2. It has full dynamic range compression with a kneepoint at 45 dB SPL. This system is different from the FDRC circuit present in the Ensoniq hearing aid in that the compression ratio can be adjusted from 1:1 (linear) to as great as 3:1 (nonlinear) depending on the differences in selected gain in each band (low and high frequency) for soft (50 dB) and loud (80 dB) inputs.

3. After considerable practice, integrated with careful reading of the recently revised manual, the hearing aid is reasonably easy to program. Recently, we were able to train a more sophisticated listener to program his own hearing aid. The dispenser is encouraged to use the compact disc recordings for adjusting the hearing aid response and to follow the recently published protocols for fitting FIT I and FIT II.

4. Two responses are available to the patient through the use of a remote control. FIT I is usually programmed for maximum benefit for understanding speech in reasonably quiet environments. FIT II may be programmed for improved understanding of speech in competition. Recent fitting notes from ReSound report that FIT I, if programmed using their guidelines, can be used successfully in quiet and competition. On the other hand, consideration should be given to program FIT II for enhanced listening to music or for improved communication on the telephone.

5. The remote may be considered either an advantage or disadvantage. Most patients enjoy the remote because of the ease in which it operates in changing FIT I to FIT II or volume. However, if the remote is lost or not functioning for the ED2, the patient cannot turn on nor adjust the gain of his/her hearing aid. Although one experienced hearing aid user thoroughly enjoyed the benefits provided by the ReSound hearing aid, she could not adjust to the small controls on the remote. During the counseling process described earlier, several patients rejected the ReSound hearing aid simply because of having to use the remote. On the other hand, several patients selected ReSound because they believed the remote would be an advantage. This scenario illustrates the importance of the counseling process in selecting the most appropriate hearing aid for the patient.

6. It is available in an ITE (ED2 and ED3) and BTE (BT2).

7. The support from ReSound has been excellent. Improvements are constantly being made to the programmer, hearing aid, and software. They are very open to suggestions and, in fact, encourage suggestions from dispensers to improve the entire ReSound system. In addition, representatives often schedule continuing education so that dispensers can become more skilled in using their system.

8. The 2 dB incremental change in gain is appropriate for fine-tuning the final fitting.

9. The hard copy is excellent. However, the DHS must be connected with an IBM-compatible computer (using ReSound software) and a printer to obtain a hard copy. The P^3 programmer currently does not have supporting software to provide a hard copy.

10. It is easy to fit binaurally. In fact, the software calculates a correction for a binaural fit after each ear has been fitted monaurally.

11. The sound quality of the ED2, ED3, and BT2 is excellent.

12. Data retrieval is easy and efficient for incorporating changes in the hearing aid design.

Disadvantages

1. As mentioned earlier, the ED2 will not operate if the remote is lost, misplaced, or in need of repair. It would be beneficial to coun-

sel the patient to purchase a backup remote. In addition, it would be beneficial if the dispenser purchased several remotes to loan to patients while the remote was being replaced or repaired. The loaner remote would need to be programmed to match the programs stored in the patient remote.

2. It is the most expensive programmable hearing aid. This high cost may prevent a number of patients from purchasing the ReSound hearing aid.

3. The battery drain is fairly high (~2.5 mA).

4. A telecoil is not available. However, the use of telephone foam pads may allow for telephone communication without introducing feedback. In addition, ReSound recently forwarded information on how FIT II can be programmed for telephone use (e.g., significant gain reduction in the high-frequency band).

5. The equivalent input noise level is fairly high (~28 dB). This noise may be annoying to patients having hearing within normal limits at or below 1000 Hz.

6. A directional microphone is not available.

Triton 3004

Advantages

1. The ability to program gain and the kneepoint of the AGC-I in three separate bands makes the aid very flexible for achieving the desired fit. Probe tube measures have verified the ability to program one band with minimal change occurring in adjacent bands.

2. It is very easy to fit binaurally via a keypad on the PMC programmer.

3. It has a wide bandwidth (110–6900 Hz).

4. Software updates are easy to install. The dispenser pulls out the old software module and inserts the new module into the same slot at the rear of the PMC.

5. There has been excellent support from the manufacturer.

6. The dispenser has immediate access to nine manufacturer-selected sets of hearing aid characteristics permanently stored in memory A. In addition, the dispenser can store nine dispenser-generated hearing aid characteristics in memory B. These characteristics reside permanently in memory B until the dispenser changes the design.

7. The dispenser can store up to 15 patient-selected frequency responses for each ear in memory C. Any two of the 15 stored responses can be retrieved for paired comparisons during the fitting procedure to select the final response to be transferred to the hearing aid. The responses in memory C are eliminated when the PMC programmer is turned off.

8. New software was introduced recently that allows the dispenser to enter hearing thresholds and UCLs. The dispenser uses a few keystrokes and the software calculates the fit (i. e., Cf1, Cf2, gain, and kneepoint of the AGC-I for each of the three bands) necessary to achieve the dispenser-selected prescribed target (e.g., NAL-R, POGO, Libby ⅓–⅔; Berger or POGO-II). As mentioned earlier, the dispenser needs to verify if the measured response matches the prescribed response when using this feature.

9. The ability to "read" the stored response is efficient. The hearing aid is connected to the PMC and the READ button is pressed. Immediately, the stored response is illustrated on the visual display.

10. The PMC programmer is easy enough to use that several patients have been easily trained to program their own hearing aid characteristics.

11. Four memories are available without the need for a remote.

Disadvantages

1. The coupler response reveals numerous resonances and antiresonances

2. A directional microphone is not available.

3. Battery drain (~3.1 mA) is fairly high, which will lead to reduced battery life. The patient needs to be informed of this.

4. The hearing aid has a fairly high equivalent input noise level (~28 dB), which can be annoying to patients having hearing within normal limits at or below 1000 Hz.

Widex Quattro

Advantages

1. A directional microphone is available on the Q9.

2. The frequency response of the Q8 and Q9 extends to 6500 Hz (6300 Hz for the Q16) and has a peak that mimics the average REUR response. As mentioned earlier, this type of response appears to be preferred by patients for enhanced sound quality.

3. The remote allows for easy programming of a binaural fit.

4. After minimal practice, it is easy to program any of the Quattro hearing aids. Many patients have been easily trained to program their own frequency/gain responses.

5. There is no cost to the dispenser for purchasing a programmer because the remote is the programmer.

6. Four responses can be stored for each ear.

7. All Quattro aids have an excellent telecoil. For maximum benefit, it is suggested that one response be dedicated to the T switch and all parameters set to the frequency response with the maximum gain as a function of frequency.

8. Manufacturer support has been excellent.

Disadvantages.

1. The hearing aid provides linear amplification.

2. The hearing aid and remote are rather expensive.

3. No hard copy is provided unless the dispenser choses to download to an IBM-compatible PC (software available from Widex).

4. Some patients dislike the need for a remote control.

DISPENSER RESISTANCE TO PROGRAMMABLE HEARING AIDS

As mentioned earlier, programmable hearing aids account for 2–6% of the hearing aids dispensed in the United States. Several reasons may account for why dispensers have not readily accepted this technology. These may include:

1. *Cost of programmers.* As reported in Figure 10.11, programmer costs vary between approximately $500 and $5500. This may prevent some dispensers from considering programmable hearing aids.

2. *Cost of hearing aids.* As reported in Figure 10.10, monaural single-unit costs for programmable hearing aids range between $298 and $1000. This has prevented some dispensers from considering these hearing aids for two reasons: first, the additional expense to operate their practice, and second, the belief that these aids are "too expensive for my patients."

3. *Avoidance of new technology.* New procedures or technologies seem to create a lag of several years before they enter the mainstream of patient care (Schnier, 1988). Some professionals may be reluctant to learn new techniques because they feel they are quite proficient and comfortable with their current procedures.

4. *Need to select fitting parameters.* As mentioned earlier, approximately 80% of dispensed aids are either ITE or ITC. Several years ago one of the authors informally polled several manufacturers to determine

what percent of the dispensers requested the manufacturer to select the matrix. Results indicated that 70–90% requested the manufacturer to select the matrix. If this is true, it would be easy to see how some may hesitate to be involved in a method of dispensing where they need to determine how to adjust the hearing aid.

5. *Future of the market.* Dispensers may be concerned about investing in equipment that only recently has been made available. Many may have past experiences with new procedures touted as the "way of the future" that required investment in equipment. Unfortunately, the new procedures were not as successful as planned, and the equipment is now used as an end table.

6. *Manufacturer solvency.* The hearing aid industry has undergone significant changes in the past few years. Several companies are no longer in business or have been purchased by larger companies. A legitimate concern exists about purchasing equipment and hearing aids only to learn the manufacturer is no longer able to provide ongoing service.

7. *Questionable advantages.* As indicated earlier, some dispensers may feel programmable hearing aids offer only minimal advantages over nonprogrammable hearing aids. Dispensers may feel that these minimal advantages do not justify the investment.

8. *Decreasing costs.* A common belief exists that technology is expensive when first introduced and costs decrease as time increases. This belief is partially true because several companies have already reduced charges for programmers and hearing aids.

CONSUMER RESISTANCE TO PROGRAMMABLE HEARING AIDS

Several factors may account for consumer hesitancy in purchasing programmable hearing aids in greater numbers. These may include:

1. *Expense.*   Programmable hearing aids are generally more expensive than nonprogrammable hearing aids. Many consumers feel costs will have to decrease before they consider pursuing this technology.

2. *Use of remote.*   While most patients like the remote control, other patients have decided not to purchase these hearing aids because they would prefer not to carry around another piece of equipment.

3. *Performance in noise.*   The most common complaint of hearing aid users is decreased ability to understand speech in noise when wearing the hearing aid. Many users have tried, and failed, with recent approaches at signal processing for improving speech intelligibility in noise. These failures have led many hearing aid users, and their friends, to take a very cautious attitude toward new technology that claims to resolve some of these complaints. Some are convinced that the quality of the amplified signal provided by programmable hearing aids is not significantly better than their present nonprogrammable aids.

4. *Availability of a telecoil.*   Some programmable aids exclude a telecoil (ReSound,

Ensoniq SSi) or contain a weak telecoil (Ensoniq SSb). For this reason, a number of patients have rejected these programmable aids.

5. *Noisy circuits.*   Several programmable aids have internal noise levels that are distracting or annoying to patients with normal hearing at or below 1000 Hz.

CONCLUSION

These are truly exciting times for individuals who have chosen a profession aimed at improving the communication skills of persons with diminished hearing. Recent technological advances in all aspects of hearing health care have provided real hope for patients with diminished hearing to experience significant benefits in understanding speech under difficult listening conditions.

One example is the availability of programmable hearing aids. Programmable hearing aids are providing exciting benefits and opportunities for the dispenser and those patients who seek their expertise. In the years ahead, this technology will improve, and this improvement will further enhance the lifestyle of persons with hearing loss.

REFERENCES

American National Standards Institute (1989). Specification of audiometers (ANSI-S3.6-1989). New York: *American National Standards Institute.*

Beck, L. (1983). Assessment of directional hearing aid characteristics. *Audiological Acoustics* 22:178–191.

Berger, K., Hagberg, N., and Rane, R. (1977). *Prescription of Hearing Aids.* Kent: Herald Publishing House.

Branderbit, P. (1991). A standardized programming system and three-channel compression hearing instrument technology. *Hearing Instruments* 42:24, 29–30.

Byrne, D., and Dillon, H. (1986). The National Acoustic Laboratories' (NAL) new procedure for selecting the gain and frequency response of a hearing aid. *Ear and Hearing* 7:257–265.

Cox, R., and McDaniel, D. (1989). Development of the speech intelligibility rating (SIR) test for hearing aid comparisons. *Journal of Speech and Hearing Research* 32:347–352.

Cox, R., and Moore, J. (1988). Composite speech spectrum for hearing aid gain prescriptions. *Journal of Speech and Hearing Research* 31:102–107.

Cranmer, K. (1990). Hearing instrument market analysis. *Hearing Instruments* 41:6, 8, 10.

Feist, C., and Wallace, B. (1989). Implementing digitally programmable technology. *Hearing Instruments* 40:16–19, 58.

Gabrielsson, A., Schenkman, B., and Hagerman, B. (1988). The effects of different frequency responses on sound quality judgments and speech intelligibility. *Journal of Speech and Hearing Research* 31:166–177.

Gabrielsson, A., and Sjoren, H. (1979a). Perceived sound quality of sound-producing systems. *Journal of the Acoustical Society of America* 65:1019–1033.

Gabrielsson, A., and Sjoren, H. (1979b). Perceived sound quality of hearing aids. *Scandanavian Audiology* 8:159–169.

Gauthier, E. (1989). Bringing high fidelity out of the lab and into the office. *Hearing Journal* 42:40–43.

Gilman, S., and Dirks, D. (1986). Acoustics of ear-canal measurement of eardrum SPL in simulators. *Journal of the Acoustical Society of America* 80:783–93.

Goldstein, D., Shields, A., and Sandlin, R. (1991). A multiple memory, digitally-controlled hearing instrument. *Hearing Instruments* 42:18, 20–21.

Hagerman, B., and Gabrielsson, A. (1985). Questionnaires on desirable properties of hearing aids. *Scandanavian Audiology* 14:109–111.

Hawkins, D. (1986). Selection of hearing aid characteristics. In: W.R. Hodgson (ed.), *Hearing Aid Assessment and Use in Audiologic Habilitation*, 3rd ed. (pp. 128–151). Baltimore: Williams & Wilkins.

Herbst, G. (1989a). The digitally programmable hearing instrument. Part 1: Digital technology applied to hearing instruments. *Hearing Instruments* 40:38, 40.

Herbst, G. (1989b). The digitally programmable instrument. Part 2: The PHOX. *Hearing Instruments* 40:36, 38, 40.

Herbst, G., and Larsen, A. (1991). The PHOX: A two-year review and outlook for the future. *Hearing Instruments* 42:16–17.

Johnson, J., Pluvinage, V., and Benson, D. (1989). Digitally programmable full dynamic range compression technology. *Hearing Instruments* 40:26–29, 30.

Killion, M. (1990). A high fidelity hearing aid. *Hearing Instruments* 41:38–39.

Libby, E.R., (1986). The ⅓–⅔ insertion gain hearing aid selection guide. *Hearing Instruments* 37:27–28.

McCandless, G., and Lyregaard, P. (1983). Prescription of gain/output (POGO) for hearing aids. *Hearing Instruments* 34:16–21.

Montgomery, A., Schwartz, D., and Punch, J. (1982). Tournament strategies in hearing aid selection. *Journal of Speech and Hearing Disorders* 47:363–372.

Moore, B., Laurence, R., and Wright, D. (1985). Improvements in speech intelligibility in quiet and noise produced by two-channel compression hearing aids. *British Journal of Audiology* 19:175–187.

Pearsons, K., Bennett, R., and Fidell, S. (1976). Speech levels in various environments. Report #312. Canoga Park, CA: Bolt, Beranek and Newman.

Pluvinage, V. (1989). Clinical measurement of loudness growth. *Hearing Instruments* 39:28–29, 32.

Pluvinage, V., and Benson, D. (1988). New dimensions in diagnostics and fitting. *Hearing Instruments* 39:28, 30, 39.

Powers, T., and Fry, D. (1991). An environmentally sound hearing system. *Hearing Instruments* 42:34, 36, 39.

Rines, D., Stelmachowicz, P., and Gorga, M. (1984). An alternate method for determining functional gain of hearing aids. *Journal of Speech and Hearing Research* 27:627–633.

Sandlin, R., and Andersen, H. (1989). Development of a remote-controlled, programmable hearing system. *Hearing Instruments* 40:33–34, 60.

Schnier, W. (1988). Capitalizing on the digital opportunity. *Audecibel* Winter, 10–13.

Skinner, M.W. (1988). *Hearing Aid Evaluation*. Englewood Cliffs, NJ: Prentice-Hall.

Staab, W. (1988). Development of a programmable behind-the- ear hearing instrument. *Hearing Instruments* 39:22, 24, 26, 39.

Studebaker, G., Bisset, J., Van Ort, D., and Hoffnung, S. (1982). Paired comparison judgments of relative intelligibility in noise. *Journal of the Acoustical Society of America* 72:80–92.

Surr, R., and Fabry, D. (1991). Comparison of three hearing aid fittings using the speech intelligibility rating (SIR) test. *Ear and Hearing* 12:32–38.

Valente, M., Meister, M., Smith, P., and Goebel, J.

(1990). Intratester test-retest reliability of insertion gain measures. *Ear and Hearing* 11:181–184.

Valente, M., and Valente, M. (1989). Selection of gain for ITE/ITC hearing aids. *Journal of Hearing Instrumentation and Technology* 1:23–29.

Valente, M., Valente, M., and Goebel, J. (1991). Reliability and intersubject variability of the real ear unaided response (REUR). *Ear and Hearing* 12:216–220.

Valente, M., Valente, M., and Vass, W. (1990). Selecting the appropriate matrix for ITE/ITC

hearing aids. *Hearing Instruments* 41:20, 22–24.

Valente, M., Valente, M., and Vass, W. (1991). Use of real ear measures to select the gain and output of hearing aids. *Seminars in Hearing* 11:53–61.

Walden, B., Schuhman, G., and Sedge, R. (1977). The reliability and validity of the comfort level method of setting hearing aid gain. *Journal of Speech and Hearing Disorders* 42:455–461.

Waldhauer, F., and Villchur, E. (1988). Full dynamic range multiband compression in a hearing aid. *Hearing Journal* 42:29–32.

CHAPTER 11

DISPENSER ACCEPTANCE OF DIGITALLY CONTROLLED (PROGRAMMABLE) ANALOG HEARING AID SYSTEMS

Wayne J. Staab

Hearing aids using digital control of analog circuitry have been available commercially since 1988 (Staab, 1990). In spite of this, and the manufacturers' published advantages, hearing aid dispensers have only lukewarmly endorsed their utilization. This chapter discusses dispenser attitudes toward these systems to evaluate why overwhelming usage has not occurred—why resistance to their use by the consuming public and dispensers has resulted in a more limited application than expected. Hearing aids that employ digital control by use of a programmer (digitally controlled programmable analog hearing aids) to access analog function within the hearing aid circuitry will be referred to as "digitally programmable" hearing aids in this chapter for ease of writing. Discussion related to true digital hearing aids is not addressed generally because these systems are not a part of this market at this time. Still, the discussions are as appropriate to them as they are to digitally controlled programmable hearing aids, perhaps even more so. Much of the information contained in this chapter comes from the author's almost nine years of involvement with digital/digitally programmable hearing aids and from hundreds of conversations with dispensers relative to this topic. The author believes that digitally programmable hearing aids are the wave of the future, and as such,

this chapter should not be construed as a justification against their use.

CONSIDERED ADVANTAGES OF DIGITALLY PROGRAMMABLE HEARING AIDS

A rather extensive listing of considered advantages of digitally programmable hearing aids includes (Staab, 1990):

1. *True in situ circuit selection.* These systems allow for the selection of various performance characteristics (such as gain, saturation output, low-frequency adjustment, etc.) while the person is actually wearing the aid, listening with the earmold coupling and with the hearing aid he/she will actually be wearing.

2. *Multiple hearing aid configurations.* Hundreds or thousands of electroacoustic configurations are possible in the same hearing aid. Basically, and for the first time, these systems are "true" master hearing aids.

3. *Individualized fitting*

4. *Independent trimmer function adjustment*

5. *More precise adjustment of desired electroacoustical performance settings*

6. *Programmability and reprogrammability*

7. *Automatic electroacoustic selection.* Some digitally programmable hearing aid systems allow for automatic electroacoustic selection from audiometric data. The selection may be based on formulas, and so forth.

8. *Difficult-to-fit cases.*   These systems are considered desirable for medically fluctuating losses, for children (and other unusual cases) where uncertainty exists about the loss, and even for use during new-user adjustment periods.

9. *Immediate hearing aid comparisons.*   The ease with which electroacoustics can be modified and recalled without having to constantly change hearing aids and earmolds allows for simplified paired-comparison judgments.

10. *Inventory control.*   Being able to program a wide range of circuit changes in a single hearing aid allows for fewer hearing aids in stock. This is primarily true for BTE hearing aids.

11. *Minimization of remakes and credits.*   The opportunity to reprogram a hearing aid without being required to return the instrument to the manufacturer for modification minimizes remakes and credits, especially for custom-molded hearing aids.

12. *Future performance change adaptability.*   The programming devices themselves can be reprogrammed to accommodate future modifications.

13. *Practical alternative to true digital hearing aids.*   Digitally programmable hearing aids provide a practical alternative to true digital hearing aids because they address the two primary obstacles to true digital hearing aids—size and power. Digitally programmable hearing aids function on 1.4 V and have current drains similar to hearing aids in standard use.

14. *Dispenser and client confidence builder.*   The adjustability and fitting technology of the digitally programmable system can build dispenser confidence in fitting the product and, as a result, can build the patients' confidence in the dispenser.

SPECULATIONS CONTRIBUTING TO LIMITED DIGITALLY PROGRAMMABLE HEARING AID USE AND ACCEPTANCE

The advantages of the digitally programmable hearing aid appear to be numerous. Therefore, what are the conditions impeding digitally programmable hearing aids from significantly penetrating the total hearing aid sales unit volume? Since the dispenser, rather than the consumer, is the real purchaser, manufacturers must first convince the dispenser that digitally programmable hearing aid systems are viable and that they offer marketing and fitting advantages. Evidently, this has not been accomplished. Following are some speculations as to why this has not occurred.

Manufacturer/Marketing

An Appropriate Product?   Manufacturers themselves provided the greatest obstacle to the initial lack of sales. Most manufacturers made the first units available in low- to moderate-gain behind-the-ear (BTE) units, in spite of the fact that 80% of the market was purchasing custom-molded products. Most individuals who could wear these initial hearing aid offerings were the primary candidates for custom-molded in-the-ear (ITE) and in-the-canal (ITC) aids. As a result, dispensers were less than excited about selling BTE aids to populations they had been fitting satisfactorily with custom-molded products. Even if this were the only marketing error, the result would be limited sales. Unfortunately, the error was compounded by setting a higher wholesale price to compensate for extensive developmental and promotional costs, additional equipment requirements for selection and programming, extended test time, and procedural protocol. The lack of immediate evidence of improved performance over what already existed and the approach of trying to force the sale of a product neither the user nor the dispenser wanted (a BTE hearing aid), and at a substantially higher retail price, required more sales effort than most dispensers were willing to put forth.

Additionally, within existing industry BTE sales, a very high percentage were to individuals who could not wear the moderate-gain BTE aids introduced (primarily because of insufficient gain/output). This scenario was the industry rule, not the exception. Attempts at justifications stating that the additional space of the BTE was required to contain the electronics did not justify the error. If indeed this were the case, why weren't the first units large, powerful BTE aids that could have been more appropriately used by the BTE market? (It has been the author's experience that approximately 80% of the BTE hearing aids sold in the U.S. are power BTE instruments). Attempts to justify the moderate power of the hearing aids introduced by suggesting that better user satisfaction was available from BTE aids than from ITE aids, as suggested by some manufacturers, have not been supported in the literature. The truth, most likely, is that manufacturers actually did want to build ITE units, but unable to because of component size, attempted to fabricate the smallest BTE units they could in anticipation of eventual downsizing to ITE aids and did not give any real thought as to what the greatest and most acceptable BTE market consisted of.

The Distribution Trap.   The author's observation is that hearing aid dispensers and their hearing aid fitting/selection patterns tend to fall within a normal distribution curve (the bell curve). This observation suggests that 20% of the dispensers fall at the extremes of the distribution (10% at each end), and the majority (80%) fall within the main portion of the distribution curve. It is generally the 10% of the dispensers at one end of the distribution that respond most readily to new tech-

nology. Manufacturers have historically devoted their developmental and promotional time and dollars to forcing the interests of this 10% (rightly or wrongly) upon the remaining 90% of the dispenser network. History suggests that the majority of dispensers tend to be relatively conservative. As such, they tend to be slow followers and must be totally convinced that the new technology is essential to their livelihood for them to embrace it.

Unrealistic Market Penetration Expectations. When digitally programmable hearing aids were introduced, dispensers were informed by the manufacturers that the instruments would be better than analog hearing aids, that the advantages would be sufficient to overcome the cosmetic disadvantages, that this technology would eventually dominate hearing aid sales, that specialized fitting equipment would be required to dispense these aids, and that they would be more expensive than analog hearing instruments (Zelski, 1990). With this mixed-bag introduction, it shouldn't be surprising that market penetration has been less than expected. Also, the higher price tag of digitally programmable hearing aids may have inflated market penetration expectations with the manufacturer's calculation of greater overall revenues and erroneous combination of those revenues with average nondigitally programmable unit sales—resulting in artificially high market penetration expectations.

Some dispensers intentionally limit the digitally programmable market. For example, Price (commenting in Mahon, 1989) stated that rather than market broadly, because of the higher cost, she was hand-selecting those patients from her files for whom she thought the aid was appropriate and promoting directly to them. In an eight-month period, Navarro et al. (1990) fitted 4.3% of their patients with digitally programmable hearing aids and suggested that the low percentage might partly be due to the fact that most of the audiologists in their group were very price oriented and tended to discuss the price of the units in less than enthusiastic terms. Benevides (1991) reported that in a series of seminars in which a number of manufacturers of digitally programmable systems participated, nearly all participating manufacturers echoed the comment that this new technology was not for everyone. Their statements, setting the market potential for no more than 3–5% (and most of these were BTE products) of the total hearing aid market, seem to be sending mixed signals to the dispensers—here is a new and advanced technology, but let's limit its use. Additionally, published articles appear to focus more on the ability of the various systems to address the difficult-to-fit client rather than the routine cases, which these systems must address if an increase in overall market penetration is to occur.

Digitally programmable hearing aids have been referred to by some as "electronic screwdrivers." Whether accurate or not, does this suggest that their use requires skilled personnel? If this is a limitation of the technology, does it limit the number of dispensers who can use it successfully, and hence, the client population penetrated?

Additionally, as reported by a dispenser (Mahon, 1989), it is not logical to think that purchasers of premium-priced digitally programmable hearing aids will ever constitute more than, say, 25% of the overall market. In other words, there will always be a larger market for Chevrolets than there is for Cadillacs. As the author sees it, eventually, digitally programmable technology will be the rule and not the exception and will become the Chevrolet. However, expect the market penetration to be linked to the availability of digitally programmable technology to cosmetically acceptable ITE and ITC hearing aids.

New Product Introduction Factors.   Pivotal factors in the introductory stage of the product life cycle for digitally programmable hearing aids relate closely to (1) the higher cost of the hearing aids and system (value for the money), (2) cosmetic compromises, (3) convenience (ease of use by both the dispenser and client), and (4) performance—the client must hear better, then a market will exist. If these issues are not resolved appropriately, the market for this product will be limited. A realistic expectation should be of gradual resolution of these issues over time and, hence, a slow but steady market growth.

Dispenser Expectations and Needs.   For the most part, manufacturers have developed the technology for these systems and have forced it on the dispenser by stating that the advantages would be good for both them and their clients. Literally nothing has been surveyed and reported relative to anticipated needs of the dispenser (and, indirectly, the consumer) with the exception of the following investigation by Staab and Nunley (1986), which provides some interesting insights.

In a mail survey, 5023 questionnaires were sent to hearing aid professionals to determine their expectations and needs from a digital hearing aid introduction. The return rate to the single mailing was 14.6%. Surveys returned were almost equally divided between dispensing audiologists and hearing aid specialists/dispensers. These 732 usable responses to 19 questions were entered into a computer data base and analyzed. (Although the survey was related to true digital hearing aids rather than to digitally programmable hearing aids, the fact that only 7.5% of the 732 returns indicated they were even remotely familiar with hearing aid programming technology would suggest that the results would have been the same if the questions had been asked about digitally

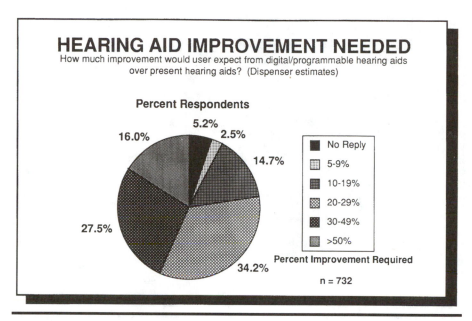

FIGURE 11.1. Reprinted with permission from Staab and Nunley (Tempe, AZ: Forward Concepts, 1986).

programmable hearing aids.) The percent-improvement-required ranges were provided in the questionnaire. The responses to questions in Figures 11.1 and 11.2 were without cost taken into consideration. (Percent responses may not equal 100% due to rounding.)

When dispensers were asked how much improvement over present hearing aids would be needed (by the user) to be considered an advantage, the breakdown in Figure 11.1 was provided. Approximately 45% of the dispensers felt that at least a 30% improvement over present hearing aids would be required by the user.

How much increase in hearing aid benefit would be provided if the hearing aid also provided noise canceling? Over half of these dispensing professionals indicated that they perceive that such a hearing aid would provide greater than a 30% increase in hearing benefit, while a third indicated that the increase in hearing benefit would be greater

than 50% (Figure 11.2). (Noise canceling was not defined.)

When asked what wholesale price , of four suggested price ranges, the dispenser would pay for a hearing aid that provided noise cancellation, programmability, and feedback suppression, the mean response was $455 for BTE aids and $460 for ITE aids. It should be pointed out that of all price ranges, the mode reflects the lowest price range for both BTE and ITE aids (Figure 11.3). From the responses it is expected that whatever the lowest price range had been (even if a lower range offering had been made available in the questionnaire), that range would have received the most responses.

Three additional trends seem evident. First, by reviewing the slope of the lines comparing ITE and BTE aid prices, dispensers are more willing to pay a higher wholesale price for an ITE aid than they are for a BTE aid, regardless of the price. Second, the lowest

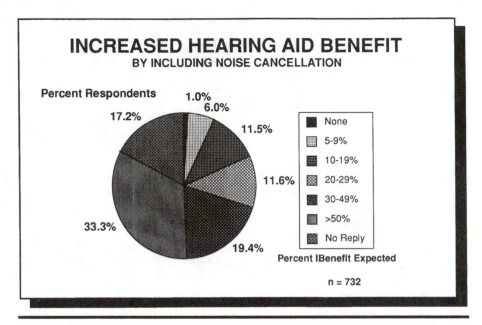

FIGURE 11.2.   Reprinted with permission from Staab and Nunley (Tempe, AZ: Forward Concepts, 1986).

price range is most likely to be paid for a BTE aid. This shows a greater resistance to high prices for BTE aids. Third, a higher percentage of dispensers are willing to pay for noise cancellation as a primary feature than for programmability as a feature, and even fewer for feedback suppression for both BTE and ITE hearing aids.

Although not shown in the graph, when the features of programmability, noise cancellation, and feedback suppression were compared, for BTE hearing aids the desirability for noise cancellation and programmability features were about equal, with feedback suppression ranked lower. For ITE aids noise cancellation was deemed the most important, followed by programmability, with feedback suppression last.

Perceived client retail prices averaged $703 for a BTE aid and $797 for an ITE unit. This was an indication of what the dispenser felt comfortable with. It is interesting to note the greater disparity in retail than in wholesale pricing between the models and also that the retail price did not reflect the traditional three-times markup. Also, dispensers selling in small volumes (100 or fewer units per year) projected that their clients would pay less, while dispensers selling large volumes (500 or more units per year) indicated that their clients would pay more for these hearing aids.

The survey audience was asked to rank the kind of support needed to sell the new technology hearing aids. Surprisingly, advertising, usually the favorite, came in second. Because the concepts and technology were new, dispensers ranked training seminars as their first choice, followed by advertising, then technical literature, as indicated in Figure 11.4.

Dispensers' Concerns with the Systems

Why is it that dispensers are self-restrained in recommending the digitally programmable systems available?

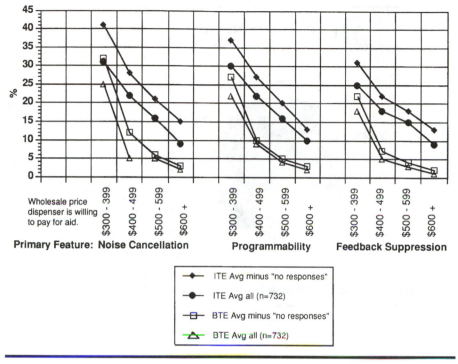

FIGURE 11.3.   Wholesale price dispenser is willing to pay for digital/programmable hearing aid. Reprinted with permission from Staab and Nunley (Tempe, AZ: Forward Concepts, 1986).

Performance. Interestingly, all reports (research and anecdotal) on digitally programmable systems report increased success of their units over nondigitally programmable hearing aids (Johnson et al., 1988; Rapisardi, 1989; Schnier, 1989; Sandlin and Meltsner, 1989; Navarro et al., 1990; Hall and Jacobs, 1991a and 1991b; Endo et al., 1991). Is this because digitally programmable hearing aids are inherently better? The latter statement may be difficult to justify, especially when performance and electronics are essentially similar to nondigitally programmable units. It might be suggested that some performance appears improved because of the possibility of having a smoother response, better (more controlled) adjustments, compression, and because of a "halo" effect fostered by the con-

sumer in which justification for having purchased this new technology occurs.

The hearing aid must do more than provide a different way of doing the same thing. How is this product better? Has the product really been improved? It must represent a fundamental change in the way the hearing aid operates and in the benefit it provides to the user. There is no advantage if these larger and more expensive hearing aids represent little more than a high-tech, more expensive way of performing the same functions that a smaller and less costly sophisticated analog hearing aid can perform.

Much digitally programmable technology is designed to provide fitting flexibility with regard to frequency response, compression, gain, output, and so forth. Many of the same

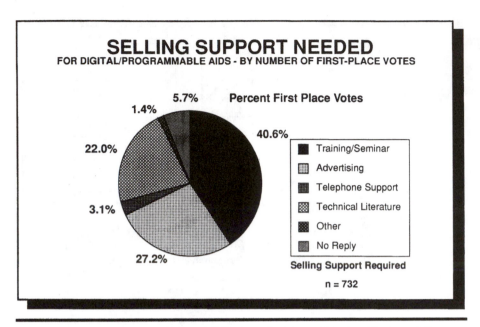

FIGURE 11.4.   Reprinted with permission from Staab and Nunley (Tempe, AZ: Forward Concepts, 1986).

objectives can be achieved with a multiple-performance analog-signal aid that is cosmetically appealing and at a lower cost.

Electroacoustics Selection.   Dispensers currently send hearing evaluation data to the manufacturer and have them select the electroacoustics for the product, especially with most custom-molded hearing aids. Most dispensers feel comfortable with this approach, having used it for the past ten years or so. The procedure places the onus on the manufacturer and removes the burden of making decisions relative to the recommendation from the dispenser. What skills and confidence does this approach leave the dispenser in selecting electroacoustic performance? A reasonable concern of the dispenser is that the fitting of digitally programmable hearing aids may expose a weakness or suggest a certain ignorance of hearing aid selection procedures.

A renewed emphasis on custom-molded

product electroacoustics selection is required to foster the growth in digitally programmable sales. Training (or retraining) will be required. As opposed to BTE aids, this may not be as elementary as it first appears. The reason is that custom-molded products may not have as much variability in performance as BTE units and, hence, leave the custom-molded product with fewer, and perhaps less evident to the client, modification possibilities. If this is indeed the case, what advantage does a digitally programmable system provide? The systems concentrate generally on frequency response to match some curve predicted by a gain formula, with few paying attention to the need for appropriate saturation output limiting in the selection protocol.

What is the goal of a successful digitally programmable hearing aid fitting? Any fitting system will be better when we know where we are going with it. All dispensers are salespersons/marketers, and as such, understand that a procedure and/or guideline to use to recommend the fitting requires that a goal be identified. The difficulty exists in defining the (or even an) ultimate hearing aid fitting. What is unfortunate is that we still do not know what a satisfactory fitting or what the ultimate fitting should be. If this information were known, the design of hearing aid circuitry to meet those needs might be better met. Certainly today, technology is much farther advanced than our knowledge of the requirements of the impaired hearing mechanism.

Ironically, digitally programmable hearing aids for the first time provide a "true" master hearing aid capable of hundreds of thousands of electroacoustical combinations and available in situ. Still, there is no assurance that these hundreds of thousands of combinations of performance changes available have the possibility of satisfactorily meeting the real needs of the hearing impaired. This is evidenced by the renewed necessity of relying on client responses as to when the digitally programmable master hearing aid is functioning acceptably. Have we progressed? Years ago this type of acceptance criterion was criticized because of its lack of objectivity.

It is not necessarily wrong that with advanced technology we have returned to subjective client tasks qualifying how the aid(s) sound, to holding fitting formulas and insertion gain measurements as appropriate goals, and to returning to MCL (most comfortable loudness) measurements. However, we might legitimately ask whether we have advanced any farther than when in our unabashed sincerity we counseled the client, "Mr. Jones, without a hearing aid(s) you understand 76% of the words presented, and with the hearing aid(s) on your ability to understand is now 76%!"

Cosmetic Compromises.   Most hearing aids sold today in the United States are of the ITE and ITC type, which also coincides with what the hearing aid wearer desires. Up to now, the majority of digitally programmable hearing aids have been of the BTE type. The "hearing aid effect" is related to the negative perceptions that others have for those wearing hearing instruments, and hearing aid wearers with larger instruments are rated more negatively (Mulac, Danhauer, and Johnson, 1981; Iler, Danhauer, and Mulac, 1982; Johnson, Danhauer, and Edwards (1982). Too big a size in the eyes of the consumer and dispenser, along with a high retail price for a BTE, makes this a real selling job to all but a few hearing aid users. The size of most contemporary units (BTE and ITE) must be further decreased to satisfy the consumer's desire for a small, inconspicuous instrument that is easy to adjust.

Cost.   The cost of the programmer and programmable hearing aids, plus accessory equipment such as printers, real-ear measurement devices, and so on, covers a wide range—all more costly than what the dispenser currently has invested in his/her current selection process. Programmers range in cost from approximately $500 to $15,000, and the wholesale cost of individual hearing aids from approximately $250 to $1000. The wide disparity in system and hearing aid costs makes it difficult for many dispensers to make rational comparisons. Many believe they must wait for the costs to equalize (suggesting comparable products that allow comparable comparisons) before they can make their decisions. Other dispensers question the practice of being required to invest significant dollars in programming equipment simply for the right to sell a given manufacturer's product, for which the dispenser is asked to pay a premium price. Some dispensers feel that the cost is too high for the use of what they refer to as an electronic screwdriver.

Low unit projections and developmental

investment have been used as arguments by some manufacturers of the devices to justify their elevated pricing schedule to the dispenser. Justifiably, these are legitimate arguments to allow them to withstand selling costs that would otherwise erode profitability. On the other hand, technology that is priced beyond the ability of a significant consumer population to purchase the product will not allow for amortization of the technology. Additionally, how do these costs impact third-party payments?

Cost/Benefit. The higher cost of the technology must be justified both to the dispenser and to the user.

To the Dispenser. The purchase of additional equipment, often expensive and with uncertainty about the consequences of rapid changes in technology, hinders some dispensers from becoming involved. Why invest in equipment that may be obsolete within the year, especially when reports abound about technology along these lines changing rapidly? To assume that hearing aid dispensers are not cost conscious is to grossly miscalculate one of their primary concerns. Dispensers invest in technology to help increase sales. Are unit sales increasing for those dispensers who have purchased this technology? Or, is it as Metz (*The Hearing Journal,* 1991) laments ". . . my gross was up, my units were down. We're selling fewer units and we're selling them for a higher price, and we're all doing worse." Cost/benefit must exist. Merely trading business to fit an existing customer base into digitally programmable hearing aids may not provide the return necessary to maintain a successful office.

To the user. Unquestionable support for these systems providing significantly improved performance to the user does not appear to be present based on sales statistics. The marginal improvement reported by some may not be sufficient to justify the investment in

the technology. Consumers are not likely to pay an elevated price for a hearing aid just because it is digitally controlled. However, if the aid provides significantly better hearing, especially for existing wearers, then it may warrant a higher price, cosmetic disadvantages, and so forth.

In a condemnation of the pricing structure and how it relates to the cost-to-benefit relationship offered by digitally programmable hearing aids, Benevides (1991) states, ". . . too little attention is being given to . . . how these instruments can be made affordable for the average hearing instrument user. Such commercial issues must be addressed if the new technology is to benefit the greatest possible number of hearing-impaired persons." He suggests further that the user of this costly new technology will quickly dismiss its value unless the consumer's high expectations of performance are met or exceeded. For example, if the hearing aid costs an additional $1000 over his previous aid, won't $1000 worth of improvement be expected? If the product has attractive features and valuable benefits that can be clearly demonstrated to the consumer, it will be purchased; and, if it is attractive price-wise to the major portion of the normal distribution curve, it will also reach its anticipated market share.

Wait-and-See Approach. Most dispensers feel they are fitting hearing aids fairly well. Customers generally express satisfaction with the fitting recommended. The dispenser understands the system and product and feels comfortable with it. The lack of generalized customer dissatisfaction inhibits exploration into unknown and unproven approaches. The majority of hearing aid dispensers tend to act conservatively to technology changes, even when performance appears overwhelmingly convincing, as happened with binaural hearing aids, directional hearing aids, ASP (automatic signal processing), and even custom-molded products.

Change is Too Great a Step for Many Dispensers. In going from point A (dispenser's current fitting procedure) to point Z (digitally programmable technology), the jump may be too great. Without strong demand from the customer, the dispenser needs something to fall back on or relate to in the fitting procedure that is not too dissimilar to what he is currently using. Therefore, the steps may have to be smaller, but perhaps more frequent, to generate more intensive dispenser involvement. In being able to fall back on the known, the dispenser will be able to maintain his integrity and maintain customer confidence. He also maintains a bond with what he knows with a gradual introduction to the unknown. It is not easy to leave the comfort of one's fitting approach and knowledge to delve into the unknown.

Some Dispensers See This as Only Another Step Toward the Ultimate Hearing Aid System. Because they believe that the ultimate hearing aid system does not yet exist, they do not want to invest heavily in intermediate steps.

Confusion. Confusion in terminology alone makes it difficult to accept the new technology. Are these hearing aids and systems really "digital" or "digitally programmable?" What is the level of integrity in advertising these products? ... in the use of terms? What is the true status of technology, benefits, test protocol, and so forth?

Dispensers find it difficult to generalize about the nature and market potential of these instruments because technology and its terminology are being applied in different ways. The term "digital" as applied by overzealous and/or abusive marketers contributes to this confusion. Until this terminology/technology bridge is gapped, successes or failures in fitting applications will be painted by the same brush—continuing to result in dispenser confusion.

What is known is that there are rather substantial differences in the equipment involved, the prices of the hearing aids, and the programmability of the hearing aids. The question is often asked as to why minimal and fairly inexpensive equipment is required to program one system and substantial, expensive equipment is required to program another system. Does this reflect on the technology levels involved? Does it mean that the system with less programming equipment and cost is less technologically advanced? Dispensers have heard different stories from manufacturers and do not know who or what to believe.

Are too many hearing aid combinations available in a single instrument? Do all the combinations available make it too confusing to the dispenser and to the user in electroacoustical selection? At what point is a satisfactory decision made? Is the decision best arrived at by the use of formulas, in situ measurements, client comments, a combination of these, or by other factors?

Dispenser Knowledge/Sales Skills. In a roundtable discussion on high-technology hearing aids and the dispenser's ability to keep pace (*The Hearing Journal*, 1991), a general consensus was that technology can be a double-edged sword. And, although advances in equipment and techniques offer dispensers the potential to provide better care to the hearing impaired, these same advances make it difficult for dispensers to remain current in their profession. It is important to realize that these advancements are not limited to digitally programmable hearing aids, but also apply to real-ear measurement systems, office automation, new hearing aid circuitry, data base management, new diagnostic technology, and so on—the combination of which makes it difficult to keep current.

Some of the devices are becoming quite complicated for dispensers to understand and for what they are intended to do. In a turnabout of dispenser involvement in the fitting process, digitally programmable hearing aid technology may again force the dispenser to learn to be the selector of the hearing aid and its performance, no longer relying on the manufacturer. A concern is that attempting to try something new may expose an ignorance of hearing aid selection procedures developed over the past few years that the dispenser may not wish to address. Certainly, this concern may not be justified for a number of reasons, but it could exist.

Dispensers may have to hone their sales skills, particularly to clients who have purchased conventional hearing aids in the past, and at considerably lower prices. This may be especially difficult with clients who have been well satisfied with their old hearing aids and who may be the most difficult to interest in this new technology—and its new prices (Radcliffe, 1991).

The Fear of "Getting Stuck" With a Given Manufacturer's Hearing Aids. Many dispensers purchase hearing aids from a variety of manufacturers. Losing this independence does not sit well with some dispensers. Attempts to develop a universal programming unit for use by a number of manufacturers have not yet met the challenge of an appropriate product with decided advantages.

Purchasing dedicated equipment turns some dispensers away from digitally programmable systems. Many complain that their storage rooms are filled with non-used equipment from previous "new technology" or with equipment that rapidly became obsolete as improvements were introduced. They speculate as to what better use the non-used equipment dollars could have been spent. Would an advertising or promotional investment have been a wiser decision?

Some dispensers disdain the necessity of limiting their digitally programmable purchases from the supplier of their programming device. This group would prefer a fitting system that allows immediate and compatible programming of various brands of hearing aids that meet the users' needs, not the manufacturers' abilities, from the same programmer. This means ITC and ITE hearing aids—not BTE units—as exists with one such current system. Hearing aid dispensers are less likely to purchase equipment that has as its primary focus a product (BTE aids) that constitutes less than 10% of their market, regardless of what possibilities the future holds. The immediate applications determine the purchasing decision making. This is true even when the equipment provides for true data base management or record keeping as an additional feature, as some do. Modifying a record-keeping system is a major endeavor, and most dispensers will move slowly on this, or not at all, if they feel that their equipment needs may soon change. Additionally, some dispensers feel they compromise their purchasing powers and flexibility by purchasing from a single supplier. The alternative is to purchase programming systems from a variety of manufacturers to be used with each of their hearing aid lines.

Must Learn New Fitting System Protocols. Each of the digitally programmable hearing systems has its own fitting protocol, and justifiably so. If not, there would be little or no difference between the systems and, hence, no marketing distinctions. In some cases the procedure calls for a new, more complicated, or proprietary protocol—not always consistent with ease of application by the dispenser.

What most of the systems lack is a good, defensible, reference point as to where to begin the selection process. Also, systematic protocols to evaluate the advantages and disadvantages of digitally programmable cir-

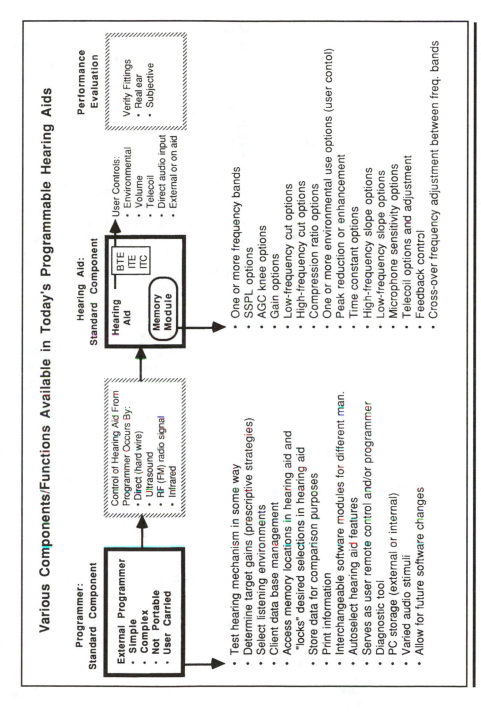

Various Components/Functions Available in Today's Programmable Hearing Aids

Programmer:
Standard Component

External Programmer
- **Simple**
- **Complex**
- **Not Portable**
- **User Carried**

- Test hearing mechanism in some way
- Determine target gains (prescriptive strategies)
- Select listening environments
- Client data base management
- Access memory locations in hearing aid and "locks" desired selections in hearing aid
- Store data for comparison purposes
- Print information
- Interchangeable software modules for different man.
- Autoselect hearing aid features
- Serves as user remote control and/or programmer
- Diagnostic tool
- PC storage (external or internal)
- Varied audio stimuli
- Allow for future software changes

Control of Hearing Aid From
Programmer Occurs By:
- Direct (hard wire)
- Ultrasound
- RF (FM) radio signal
- Infrared

Hearing Aid:
Standard Component

Hearing Aid
BTE
ITE
ITC

Memory Module

User Controls:
- Environmental
- Volume
- Telecoil
- Direct audio input
- External or on aid

Performance Evaluation
- Verify Fittings
- Real ear
- Subjective

- One or more frequency bands
- SSPL options
- AGC knee options
- Gain options
- Low-frequency cut options
- High-frequency cut options
- Compression ratio options
- One or more environmental use options (user contol)
- Peak reduction or enhancement
- Time constant options
- High-frequency slope options
- Low-frequency slope options
- Microphone sensitivity options
- Telecoil options and adjustment
- Feedback control
- Cross-over frequency adjustment between freq. bands

FIGURE 11.5. Reprinted with permission from Staab and Lybarger (Baltimore: Williams & Wilkins, 1994).

269

cuitry are needed. Interestingly, most dispensers believe that client input is a strong consideration in the total evaluative process.

The issue of candidacy is a real educational problem according to Preves (*The Hearing Journal*, 1991). Along with this are the issues of how to evaluate what these devices do. What kinds of assurances exist that the manufacturer's approach is merited?

New Technology Idiosyncrasies. All new technologies have a "burn-in" time period during which reliability of the product is questionable and modifications occur. Dispensers are aware of this and have a tendency to wait for the product to stabilize prior to committing to the market. Many dispensers prefer not to be the first to purchase new technology. They prefer to let others take the first steps and work out the problems and procedures, and only then consider becoming involved.

Premium Product During a Soft Market. From a cost view, the digitally programmable hearing aid is considered a premium product. During soft hearing aid markets many dispensers believe their clientele are not ready candidates for such a product.

Concentration on Features Rather Than on User Performance. Promotional approaches to dispensers by manufacturers emphasize the multitude of features available with the different systems, rather than providing unquestionable evidence of successful advantages. As an example, Figure 11.5 is a partial listing of features provided by manufacturers (Staab and Lybarger, 1994). A comparable list of user advantages is not available.

Extended Hearing Aid Selection Time. Fitting a digitally programmable hearing aid may lengthen the time period involved with each patient (Fortner, in Mahon, 1989; Vekovius and Mendoza, 1989). For example, Fortner (in Mahon, 1989) reported that the

selection and programming process required an additional hour per hearing aid initially, but even with experience, required an additional 30 minutes per instrument. However, in *The Hearing Journal* roundtable (1991), Valente suggested that their actual fitting time for most, not all, units was actually less than with their more conventional-type application.

In that same roundtable discussion, McFarland echoed another aspect of time reported previously by others—the time (and cost) aspect of more frequent involvement with the client by the dispenser who suggests to the client that the hearing aid performance can be changed as frequently as necessary to improve its performance. And while the higher unit cost to the client partially covers this involvement, many dispensers who were excited about the new technology are having second thoughts because of the extended time required to adapt the instruments to the clients. However, with a very limited patient population Navarro et al. (1990) found their users to return less frequently than other patients with conventional instruments.

Is "Different" "Better"? Digitally programmable hearing aids are different. But, does that make them better? The expectation that digital technology will produce a miracle hearing aid tends to be fueled by the term itself, based on consumers' beliefs that digital technology is somehow inherently better and has capabilities not available from other nondigital products. When little or no expected advantage is realized over nondigitally programmable hearing aids, the more-costly, highly-touted product can easily become an object of scorn. If the functions and benefits that the hearing aid are expected to serve are not realized, the higher cost becomes a critical issue.

Decisions. Beyond the fundamentals of programmability and reprogrammability, the dispenser is subjected to distinct differences among the manufacturers that reflect fundamental decisions regarding fitting philosophy and control, equipment purchases, breadth of product line, and other practical approaches to the application of digitally programmable technology. Perhaps even more fundamental and important is how the higher cost to the dispenser, and thus client, relates to one's overall marketing decisions on product introduction, promotion, timing, and price. Will a given market support the product?

QUESTIONS NOT RESOLVED ADEQUATELY ACCORDING TO DISPENSERS

The following list of questions echoed by dispensers is not intended to duplicate the previous discussions, nor is the list assumed to be comprehensive. Still, it reflects dispenser questions and/or concerns.

- How much difference in an ITE or ITC aid can be expected (electroacoustically) from a digitally programmable versus a non-digitally programmable hearing aid? Is the difference sufficient for the consumer to be willing to pay the increased costs?
- Will the system eliminate the fullness-of-ear feeling some clients experience?
- Will the system help the client hear better in noise?
- Will the system help the client hear better on the telephone?
- Will the instrument be small?
- How interested are the majority of consumers in technology—especially the elderly?
- Are digitally programmable hearing aids being pushed by manufacturers to increase their margins, without regard to the needs of the dispenser?
- Are environment-to-environment patient adjustment abilities necessary, and for whom?

- Are digitally programmable hearing aids designed only for customers who can afford the price? If the technology is good, shouldn't it be available to all customers at affordable pricing?
- What is the need for a portable programmer?
- Is the system easy to program and easy to remember—without having to read manuals after periods of infrequent use—for both the dispenser and client?
- Is user remote control necessary?
- Is it more desirable to have the programmable memory stored in the aid or in the programmer?
- At what price should the hearing aids sell? How affordable could/should they be?
- Do real improvements exist over non-digitally programmable hearing aids currently available?
- Does the unit have too many electroacoustic combinations? Not only is it difficult to know where to start, but it is even more difficult to know when to end.
- Which patients need digitally programmable hearing aids? What is the customer profile?
- Should the user have at his/her control multiple hearing aid responses? If so, how many?
- Should the digitally programmable hearing aid system fit the hearing loss or fit the listening environment?
- Should the dispenser invest in a dedicated hearing testing system?
- What percentage of the customer population actually needs a digitally programmable device?
- Should approximations to fitting targets be considered successful fittings, or should subjective impressions carry more weight?
- Will direct audio input become a feature (if not a standard) on digitally programmable hearing aids?

SUMMARY

Dispenser questions continue to await appropriate answers in their decision making relative to digitally programmable hearing aids. Paramount are those answers that relate to the goal(s) of a successful fitting: what the different programmable hearing aids provide—what they really do, pragmatic test protocols, and how they differ from conventional hearing aids, among others. Dispensers should be interested in what the digitally programmable hearing aids provide, rather than being interested in the digital mechanics, which may only confuse the issue. The realization exists that we still do not know what a hearing aid should do and if it is functioning properly to meet that need.

Although the market penetration is not yet what some manufacturers and dispensers have projected, a normal evolution toward hearing aids that use digital control of analog signal processing will take place. As with most new technologies, digitally programmable hearing aids will require time to reach their full potential. In spite of this, and in spite of those factors delaying wholesale dispenser involvement as reported in this chapter, their potential advantages would appear to assure their long-term success for both the client and the dispenser. In reality, the current digitally programmable hearing aids represent the first widespread practical use of digital technology in the discipline of aural rehabilitation. With respect to the involvement by hearing aid dispensers in digitally programmable hearing aids, it appears that the dispenser has decided to make haste slowly.

REFERENCES

Benevides, J.R. (1991). Digitally programmable hearing aids must be made more affordable. *The Hearing Journal* 44:34.

Endo, J., Lake, T.M., McFarland, W.H., and Sandlin, R. (1991). *Hearing Instruments* 42:9–10, 44.

Hall, C.M., and Jacobs, E.L. (1991a). A review of a digitally programmable, full dynamic range hearing device. *Hearing Instruments* 42:16, 18.

Hall, C.M., and Jacobs, E.L. (1991b). Evaluation of a digitally programmable, full dynamic range hearing device. *Hearing Instruments* 42:18–19.

The Hearing Journal (1991). In the high-tech future of hearing aids, can the dispenser keep pace? a roundtable discussion. *The Hearing Journal* 44:2, 9–17.

Iler, K., Danhauer, J., and Mulac, A. (1982). Peer perceptions of geriatrics wearing hearing aids. *Journal of Communication Disorders* 47:433–438.

Johnson, C., Danhauer, J., and Edwards, R. (1982). The "hearing aid effect" on geriatrics—fact or fiction? *Hearing Instruments* 33:24–26.

Johnson, J.S., Dirvy, V.M., Hodgson, W.A., and Johnson, L.J. (1988). Clinical study of a programmable multiple memory hearing instrument. *Hearing Instruments* 40(11):44.

Mahon, W.J. (1989). What does digitally controlled performance mean for fitters and wearers? *The Hearing Journal* 42(5):11–16.

Mulac, A., Danhauer, J., and Johnson, C. (1981). Attitudes toward geriatric hearing aid wearers. Presented at the Annual Convention of the American Speech-Language-Hearing Association, Los Angeles, CA.

Navarro, R., Engels, T., Wilkens, A., Busald, L., Wright, W.J. III, and Hicks, G. (1990). Clinical experience with the PHOX hearing instrument. *The Hearing Journal* 43:22, 24–25.

Radcliffe, D. (1991). Programmable hearing aids: Digital control comes to analog amplification. *The Hearing Journal* 44:9–12.

Rapisardi, D. (1989). Bridging the gap between product R&D and the consumer. *Hearing Instruments* 40:20, 22.

Sandlin, R. E., and Meltsner, R. (1989). Clinical trials with a remote control, programmable hearing instrument. *Hearing Instruments* 40:34–35, 37, 39.

Schnier, W.R. (1989). Practical experiences with a digital/analog hybrid instrument. *Hearing Instruments* 40:31–32.

Staab, W.J. (1990). Digital/programmable hearing aids—an eye towards the future. *British Journal of Audiology* 24:243–256.

Staab, W.J., and Lybarger, S.F. (1994). Characteristics and use of hearing aids. In: J. Katz (ed.), *Handbook of Clinical Audiology*, 4th ed. Baltimore: Williams & Wilkins.

Staab, W.J., and Nunley, J. (1986). *Digital Hearing Aid Survey*. Project No. 132, Forward Concepts, Tempe, AZ.

Vekovius, G.T., and Mendoza, L. (1989). Digital amplification: Clinical perspectives. *Hearing Instruments* 40:23–24, 58.

Zelski, R.F. (1990). The future of dispenser programmable hearing instruments. *Hearing Instruments* 41:32.

CHAPTER 12

CURRENT AND FUTURE APPLICATIONS OF DIGITAL HEARING AID TECHNOLOGY

David A. Preves

Recent technological advances are rapidly bringing the time when hearing aids will routinely have digital computers in them. In the last five years, there has been a proliferation of digitally programmed analog hearing aids in the marketplace. Although rich in new fitting features, since most of these devices do not process the signal in a digital form, the real promise of digital technology in hearing aids has yet to be fulfilled. While several true digital hearing aids have been advocated and have been reported on by various organizations and laboratories (e.g., Nunley et al., 1983; Morely et al., 1988; Harris et al., 1988), few have been actively marketed to date. Certainly, digital signal processing (DSP) will offer significant improvement in the performance of hearing aids in the future (Hecox and Punch, 1988; Miller, 1988; Widin, 1987).

Various ratios of digital to analog electronics are encountered in what some persons now call "digital" hearing aids. The ratios range from hybrid analog/digital hearing aids, in which an analog form of the signal is controlled digitally, to true digital hearing aids, in which digital processing is performed on a digital representation of the signal. In order to have true digital processing, the incoming signal must first be converted from analog to digital format so that a digital computer can

perform the signal processing algorithms (Staab, 1985; Nielsen, 1986; Preves, 1987).

A useful historical milestone chart for incorporation of digital technology in hearing aids has been formulated by Sammeth (1989) and is reproduced in Figure 12.1. The chart shows that the introduction of the first wearable digital hearing aid in body aid form was reported some years ago, but the device was never marketed for general distribution (Nunley et al., 1983). An early (1987) commercial effort for a true digital hearing aid was not successful. The product was subsequently discontinued. This hearing aid consisted of a body-worn processor connected with a cord to a postauricular (BTE) housing containing the microphone and receiver. Four batteries were required, three in the body pack and one in the BTE housing. Although published information is lacking at this date as to how effective this true digital hearing aid was, one study concluded it provided more benefit and was preferred by some hearing aid wearers over their own hearing aids (Roeser and Taylor, 1988). It appears that the demise of this true digital hearing aid may have been due to a combination of factors, including size, operating cost, and, perhaps, selling price with not enough offsetting performance benefit as compared to conventional hearing aids. However, at this

True Digital

1967	Researchers at Bell Laboratories simulate digital amplification with a large laboratory computer.
1975	Graupe and Causey report the development of a nonwearable model of a digital hearing instrument using an 8080 microprocessor.
1980	Moser receives a patent for a digital hearing instrument.
1982	Levitt reports the development of a nonwearable digital hearing instrument based on an array processor.
1983	First report in the literature of an experimental body-worn digital hearing instrument by Nunley et al.
1987	First commercial introduction of a digital hearing instrument with a body-worn processor from Nicolet Instrument Corp.
199?	Expected introduction of a true digital hearing instrument housed entirely in behind-the-ear packaging.

Hybrid Analog-Digital

1977	Graupe and Causey receive a patent for a hybrid adaptive filtering algorithm.
1979	Mangold and Leijon report experimental multichannel compression hearing instrument using hybrid technology.
1986	Commercial release of the Zeta Noise Blocker™ chip for signal processing based on the Graupe-Causey algorithm.
1987	First commercial introduction of a digitally programmable hybrid BTE by Audiotone.
1988–89	Introduction of six additional digitally programmable instruments to the market, including some ITE models and models with multiple memories, digital remote control and advanced fitting systems.

FIGURE 12.1. Some important events in the history of digital technology in hearing instruments. Reprinted with permission from Sammeth, 1989.

writing, a true digital processing post-auricular hearing aid has just been introduced for the purpose of suppressing acoustic feedback oscillation in high-gain fittings (Dyrlund and Bisgaard, 1991).

The hearing aid marketplace in the United States has been dominated by in-the-ear (ITE) and in-the-canal (ITC) hearing aids. Recent HIA statistics reveal that over 75% of hearing aids sold in this country are ITE and ITC types. The challenge of incorporating true digital technology into these devices is much more difficult than it is to package it into BTE hearing aids. Consequently, most design efforts have concentrated on providing partially digital hearing aids. These devices take advantage of the best performance enhancements possible with a combination of analog-based techniques and as much digital technology as will physically fit into head-worn hearing aid packages. As a result, there are several hybrid analog/digital hearing aids currently being marketed in BTE, ITE, and even in ITC housings. These devices generally utilize analog processing acting under digital control. Some of these hybrid analog/digital hearing aids offer significant performance features, as compared to those of purely analog hearing aids, without a dramatic increase in size or operating cost. Included in the hybrid analog/digital category are programmable hearing aids with digital memory, remote-controlled hearing aids, and digitally based signal processing hearing aids such as those incorporating the Zeta Noise Blocker.

The following discussion attempts to review some of the recent trends in newly emerging digital hearing aid technology for addressing the issues of noise reduction, feedback reduction, and speech enhancement. Before addressing the promise of digital technology for these applications, it is appropriate to review some of the limitations of analog electronics and some of the technological problems responsible for the limited use of digital circuitry in commercially available hearing aids.

ANALOG HEARING AIDS USING BIPOLAR AND CMOS CIRCUITRY

Historically, hearing aid circuitry has been implemented with bipolar analog semiconductor technology. This type of circuitry, which is still used in the majority of hearing aids, has low noise and high output drive capability, both ideal for hearing aid amplifiers.

However, to implement signal processing circuitry with bipolar technology, and particularly filters and compressors for multichannel hearing aids, relatively large value capacitors must be used that are frequently too large to be located on the chip. Because of hearing aid size constraints, these large capacitors (1 per filter pole) limit the amount of multichannel filtering and signal processing possible with bipolar technology. Thus, hearing aids with fewer frequency bands, less-sophisticated signal processing, and filters with shallower slopes are associated with bipolar integrated circuitry technology.

Extending Analog Performance Capability with CMOS and Switched Capacitor Filters

Many of the currently available hybrid analog/digital hearing aids utilize sampled analog data, in which switched capacitor filters sample and process the incoming analog signal at discrete points in time. Filters are constructed with capacitors and resistors. A switched capacitor filter is a type of active filter in which very small on-chip capacitors are used. Instead of using actual resistors in the filter, they are simulated by switches that transfer voltages at high speed via small capacitors between two points in the filter. With this approach, the analog signal is not converted to digital form but, instead, is changed from a continuous analog signal in the time domain to a discrete analog sample (Levitt, 1987). Using switched capacitor filters in sampled analog hearing aids may be considered a form of digital processing because the analog waveform is periodically sampled (by the switches under digital control) and values are stored by the capacitors. This sampling scheme is similar to that employed in true digital hearing aids prior to analog-to-digital conversion.

Switched capacitor filters are made with CMOS (complementary metal oxide semiconductor) integrated circuitry implemented on smaller chip sizes and with fewer components external to the chip than comparable filters made with bipolar semiconductor technology. CMOS integrated circuitry is very high density, which generally permits more transistors, resistors, and capacitors to be included per unit chip area than bipolar integrated circuitry.

The capabilities of CMOS circuitry are just beginning to be exploited in hybrid analog/digital type hearing aids. Sophisticated analog signal processors employ switched capacitor filters for greater filter slope. Unfortunately, CMOS semiconductor circuitry tends to be more noisy than bipolar semiconductor circuitry, which has rendered its use questionable for low-noise preamplifiers required in hearing aids. Consequently, hearing aid circuits are beginning to be made with a combination of bipolar and CMOS circuitry on one chip—called BICMOS circuitry. Inherent with BICMOS semiconductor technology are the advantages of low-noise bipolar circuitry for hearing aid preamplifiers, together with higher-order switched capacitor filters with on-chip capacitors to provide the maximum possible signal processing capability for restricted hearing aid sizes.

Frequency Response Shaping with Switched Capacitor Filters

Many current hearing aid fittings utilize real-ear probe microphone measurements to verify electroacoustic performance specified by prescription formulas. With this approach, precise matching of the predicted targets and actual gain/frequency characteristics provided by the hearing aids has been found to be difficult with current analog technology (Pascoe, 1975; Conger, 1987; Bratt et al., 1987; Sammeth et al., 1993). Finer control of gain by frequency for selectively producing peaks or dips in real-ear insertion gain is required to match more exactly an electroa-

coustic prescription. Such a requirement can be better met with switched capacitor filters than with bipolar filters in small hearing aids.

Several multichannel hearing aids have been introduced with switched capacitor filtering that provides good capability for controlling frequency response. These hearing aids essentially incorporate graphic or parametric equalizers similar to those utilized in stereo receivers and automobile radios. For example, the electrical frequency response of the switched capacitor filters in a three-channel hearing aid are shown in Figure 12.2. Because the cutoff frequencies of switched capacitor filters are determined by the frequency of a digital oscillator or clock, it is relatively easy, as shown in Figure 12.3, to shift the response of a bank of switched capacitor filters up or down in frequency simply by changing the clock frequency. The function of the equalizer can be quite complex if phase is controlled as well as frequency response so as to ensure the smoothness where the filters overlap (e.g., Moorer and Berger, 1986).

With multichannel hearing aids, dips or notches in a particular frequency range(s) can be implemented. An example of such a notch filter implemented in the same three-channel

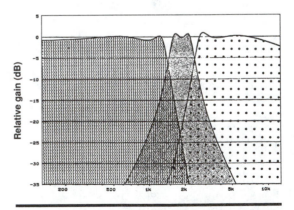

FIGURE 12.2. Electrical frequency response of Argosy Electronics 3-Channel-Clock hearing aid implemented with switched capacitor filters.

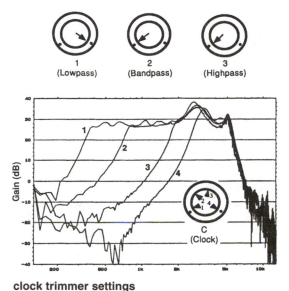

clock trimmer settings
1:500 Hz; 2: 800 Hz; 3: 2600 Hz; 4: 3500 Hz

FIGURE 12.3. Example of simultaneously varying the cutoff frequencies of the three switched capacitor filters in Figure 12.2 by changing their clocking frequency. The acoustic frequency response of the hearing aid in a 2 cc coupler is shifted to higher frequencies as the clocking frequency is increased.

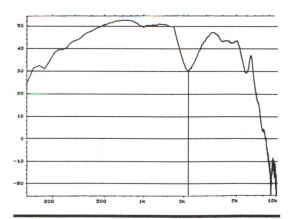

FIGURE 12.4. Example of a notch filter response in a 2 cc coupler implemented by turning the gain down with the middle (bandpass) channel trimmer of the three-channel hearing aid in Figure 12.2.

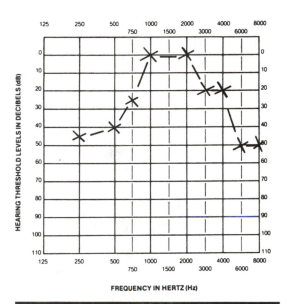

FIGURE 12.5. Audiogram for which the frequency response of Figure 12.4 may be appropriate.

ITE hearing aid used for Figures 12.2 and 12.3 is shown in Figure 12.4. This configuration may be useful in attenuating peaks in the frequency response and for suppressing acoustic feedback oscillation. Additionally, this frequency response may be useful for fitting those persons having an inverted, "cookie-bite" audiometric configuration—normal hearing in the mid-frequencies and elevated hearing threshold levels at higher and lower frequencies, as shown in Figure 12.5.

DIGITAL SIGNAL PROCESSING

It is important to note that many digital algorithms for hearing aid applications were originally analog algorithms. The advantage of true digital processing in hearing aids is that, because it is software based, it may offer more performance features within a given hardware package than analog processing can—that is, with software, several sophisticated algorithms can be performed simultaneously once the digital computer hardware is in place. DSP software, in conjunction with digital computer hardware, replaces such conventional analog components as transistors, resistors, capacitors, and diodes. Functions such as filters, oscillators, limiters, modulators, and demodulators are implemented in software rather than in analog circuitry (Levitt, 1987; Nunley et al., 1983). However, lest we think that analog technology will become totally obsolete, even in hearing aids performing true DSP, there must still be analog input circuitry that conditions the incoming analog acoustic signal properly in preparation for digital processing. Also, unless a digital-switching, class-D output stage is used, there must still be analog output circuitry that converts and smoothes the output of the digital signal processor to accurately reproduce the processed signals in analog form.

While the prospects of improved performance offered by digital technology in hearing aids are exciting, true digital processing should not be regarded as the panacea for all of the problems in currently marketed hearing aids. Because of the analog-acoustic input and output required in hearing aids, the preamplifier and power amplifier (and their attendant headroom problems) that are found in analog hearing aids must also be present in digital hearing aids (Figure 12.6)—that is, the preamplifier and power amplifier (output stage) may have their own distortion problems that can extend to digital hearing aids. It should be understood that the same distortions that are introduced at high levels by the preamplifier, power amplifier, and receiver and, to a lesser extent, by the microphone in analog hearing aids will also be present in digital hearing aids.

Unless carefully implemented, the use of digital technology in hearing aids can also introduce other types of distortions that are unique to the digital process. Among these

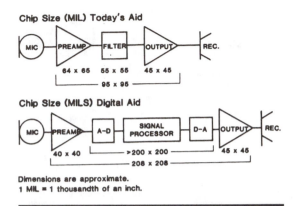

FIGURE 12.6. Comparing component blocks and typical chip sizes of an analog hearing aid to those of a true digital hearing aid. Reprinted with permission from Nielsen, 1986.

distortions are aliasing, quantization error, and imaging. Aliasing occurs when signals in a band centered at the sampling frequency overlap the original baseband signal at a lower frequency. This is caused by too low a sampling rate for the spectral bandwidth of the incoming signal. Quantization error results from too gross an approximation of the analog signal by the analog-to-digital converter. This is caused by too large a digital step size, resulting from too few bits. Imaging produces a jagged rather than a smooth analog output waveform. This is caused by inadequate smoothing of the output signal from the digital-to-analog converter after digital processing.

Real-Time Processing and Digital Electronics Packaging Considerations

One requirement for a DSP hearing aid is performing all of its functions to modify the incoming signal in real time, as opposed to offline as is commonly done in computer simulations of DSP hearing aids. The problem with packaging sophisticated digital signal processing devices into small head-worn hearing aids is that the appropriate digital devices require considerable size and power to function adequately for this real-time application (Levitt, 1987; Staab, 1987). By using specially designed, custom DSP integrated circuit chips, it is possible to have true DSP BTE and even ITE hearing aids. For example, some investigators have proposed a two-chip implementation, based on extensive considerations of battery voltage and power consumption for a two-battery, two-microphone, four-channel, true digital hearing aid. One chip is for a custom digital signal processor and the other chip is for peripheral analog processing functions (Morley et al., 1988). The additional microphone is used as a probe microphone to measure the output of the hearing aid in the hearing aid wearer's ear during the fitting process.

According to Nielsen (1986), for just the added digital portion of the hearing aid circuit, typical chip size would be about 40,000 square mils for the analog-to-digital converter, the digital signal processor, and the digital-to-analog converter, as seen in Figure 12.6 (1 mil is 1/1000 of an inch). Together with the area needed for an analog preamp and output stage and external components, the combination would be too large to fit into most ITE hearing aids and even some BTE hearing aids. Contrast this to the 3025 square mils for a relatively simple analog filter of the type used in many currently marketed ITE hearing aids plus the area for the preamp and output stage (Nielsen, 1986). Obviously, as integrated circuit feature size continues to get smaller and smaller, more and more components can be squeezed in, and the area required for both the digital and analog portions of the circuit will shrink. However, at this time, standard, off-the-shelf DSP chips that are sufficiently high speed to perform the desired signal processing functions in real time are too large and require too much current drain. Instead, true digital hearing aids

will likely incorporate custom DSP chips that have been designed specifically to perform the desired algorithms while meeting the required packaging size and battery current goals (Levitt, 1987; Preves, 1987).

Frequency Response Shaping with Digital Technology

The ability to control peaks and dips finely in the real-ear insertion response is required to match a specified target gain by frequency prescription. Such a requirement can be provided to an even greater degree with digital filtering than with switched capacitor filtering. One result of converting the analog signal to digital form in a hearing aid is the ability to implement frequency responses with a high degree of gain-frequency resolution (Studebaker, Sherbecoe, and Matesich, 1987). As an example, Nielsen et al. (1990) developed an algorithm for controlling with great precision the frequency response and phase of hearing aids via a digital filter. Controlling both the gain and the phase are important for minimizing the possibility of acoustic feedback oscillation. Their system was evaluated for a moderate flat hearing loss and a steeply sloping, high-frequency hearing loss using the real-ear target gain/frequency values of the NAL prescription formula. The degree of matching to the target frequency response and target phase for the steeply sloping hearing loss is shown in Figure 12.7.

In another example, French St. George (1992) reported a 2.4 dB average rms fit error with a four-channel digital hearing aid for 14 subjects over the frequency range of 500 to 2000 Hz. In order to provide precise control of frequency response in the ear canal under microprocessor control, Gilman (1986) has suggested splitting the frequency range up into a bank of $1/3$ octave bandpass filters. In this system, a probe microphone in the ear canal of the hearing aid wearer provides an

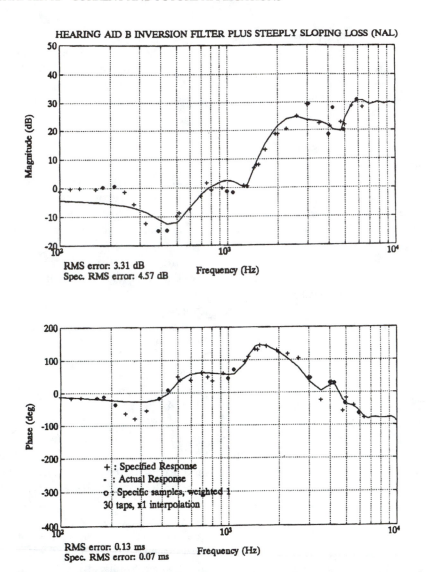

FIGURE 12.7. Ability of digital filtering to closely fit NAL target frequency response. Specified versus actual magnitude (upper) and phase (lower) responses for subjects with steeply sloping hearing loss are shown. Reprinted with permission from Nielsen et al., 1990.

update of the spectrum levels produced by the hearing aid. The microprocessor adjusts the frequency response of the hearing aid according to the difference between the actual spectrum levels produced and the target real-ear response. Achieving such performance with analog circuitry of the type now used in hearing aids would take many transistors, capacitors, and resistors, which would result in a very large hearing aid size.

ANALOG PROCESSING USING DIGITAL TECHNOLOGY (HYBRID ANALOG/DIGITAL HEARING AIDS)

It is important to note that DSP techniques can also be implemented using digitally controlled analog signal processing (Levitt, 1987). A digitally controlled analog hearing aid is practical from a packaging view because of its smaller size and lower power consumption than a true digital hearing aid. This size and power reduction is accomplished via a sampled-data scheme, similar to that used for switched capacitor filters, in which the audio signal is sampled at discrete times and the samples are retained in analog form. Then, digital filtering is implemented by choosing the weights or coefficients, under digital control, for the outputs of a tapped analog delay line (Figure 12.8). The analog output at any moment in time is the sum of the weighted, tapped analog delay line outputs. Values of the analog signal at the discrete sampling times are stored via capacitors, one analog value at each tap. As each succeeding sample is taken, the previously stored sampled values are shifted one tap to the right to make room for the next sample. In a DSP approach, the tapped analog delay line would be replaced by a digital shift register loaded from the output of an analog-to-digital converter.

Digitally Programmable Analog Hearing Aids

This topic is covered by several other chapters in this text. The interested reader is also referred to Staab (1990) for an overview.

Addressing the Headroom Problem with Hybrid Analog/Digital Technology

Hearing aid sound quality is frequently criticized in comparison to that of the high-quality audio components used in high-fidelity sys-

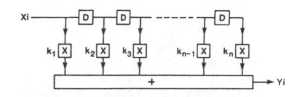

FIGURE 12.8. Tapped analog delay line or digital shift register forming a digital filter. D indicates a delay for each tap. X indicates a multiplier for each of the k tap weights. Reprinted with permission from Levitt, 1987.

tems. This problem is partially caused by inadequate headroom, the difference between the level at which saturation begins and the peak input signal level plus amplifier gain. In order to keep amplified signals from being peak clipped due to saturation, and to limit the associated distortion produced, there must be adequate headroom.

The level at which saturation begins in a hearing aid is determined by the combination of amplifier, receiver, and battery. Inadequate headroom can occur in the hearing aid preamplifier, the signal processing section, or the output stage. A primary cause of inadequate headroom in hearing aids is the result of reducing current drain to improve the life of the low-voltage batteries (1.3 V) used in hearing aids (Preves and Newton, 1989). In contrast, high-quality audio components have the advantages of a large power supply voltage—110 V from the wall power outlet, combined with circuitry that draws enough current to allow large signals to pass without clipping. These factors increase the available headroom into which the dynamic range of amplified audio signals can fit without clipping.

Given that about the same range of incoming acoustic signal levels must be processed by subminiature hearing aids as by high-fidelity audio components, how can one expect the same high-quality performance with a tiny 1.3 V battery? It seems amazing that a hearing aid with such low battery voltage and a tiny hearing aid receiver can even produce sound pressure levels exceeding 120 dB. Even though such high-output sound pressure levels can be produced by subminiature hearing aids, because of headroom limitations, considerable harmonic and intermodulation distortion may be generated as well. The resultant sound quality may be noisy or muddy, especially for hearing aids with linear circuitry, from the distortion created by peak clipping at frequencies other than those in the original input signal (Agnew, 1988). The net effect of the distortion components contributed by inadequate headroom is to decrease the signal-to-noise ratio (SNR) of hearing aid-processed signals.

Headroom has been increased in preamplifier and signal processing stages within analog, hybrid A/D, and DSP hearing aids by using voltage multipliers formed by digital switching circuits. These voltage multiplier circuits essentially double or triple the battery voltage to extend the headroom of the hearing aid amplifier. Additionally, compression or adaptive low-frequency response circuitry in the hearing aid amplifier may also help to increase headroom by preventing saturation.

Another way of extending the headroom achievable in hearing aid fittings without increasing the supply voltage is to utilize a push-pull (class AB) output stage instead of a single-ended (class A) output stage. A push-pull output stage has a theoretical capability of providing up to four times more output signal amplitude into a hearing aid receiver than a single-ended output stage before the onset of clipping (Lenk, 1974).

In the past few years, the class D type of output stage has been incorporated in hearing aids. The class D output stage is not a new idea and has been used for many years in public address systems and other applications. This type of output stage is based on a digital on/off switching or pulse-width modulation of a high-frequency carrier signal

with the audio signal. With a class D output stage, obtainable headroom and gain are comparable to that of a push-pull output stage, but with less current drain required at levels near saturation.

One popular implementation of the class D output stage packages the circuitry inside the hearing aid receiver with little or no additional space required (Knowles, 1988). As shown in Figure 12.9(a), a high-frequency digital square wave "carrier" (e.g., 100 kHz) is applied to the hearing aid receiver. The digital carrier signal is integrated [Figure 12.9(b)] and is combined with the audio signal, shown in the form of a comparatively low-frequency sinusoid [Figure 12.9(c)]. The sum [Figure 12.9(d)] is fed to a comparator whose rectangular output waveform is digital. The higher the audio amplitude, the more the resulting rectangular modulated carrier wave is high; conversely, the lower the audio amplitude, the more the rectangular modulated carrier wave is low [Figure 12.9(e)]. The receiver then filters out this high-frequency rectangular carrier wave to extract the audio acoustically (Carlson, 1988).

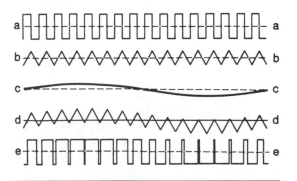

FIGURE 12.9.   Waveforms for a class D output stage. (a) High-frequency carrier. (b) Integrated carrier. (c) Audio signal. (d) Carrier summed with audio signal. (e) Pulse-width modulated output to receiver. Reprinted with permission from Knowles, 1988.

ENHANCING SPEECH AND IMPROVING SIGNAL-TO-NOISE RATIO WITH DIGITAL TECHNOLOGY

Utilization of digital technology for enhancing speech intelligibility for hearing aid wearers includes two areas: improvement in signal-to-noise ratio (SNR) and enhancement of the speech signal itself. Hearing aid wearers miss or confuse unvoiced consonants more than any other type of speech phoneme, especially in noise. Consequently, it is assumed that more consonant emphasis relative to vowel amplification is desirable in a hearing aid fitting. To date, there have been relatively few investigations to substantiate this hypothesis. Improving consonant-to-vowel intensity ratio (CVR) simply by making consonants audible may be more important for good speech perception than enhancing the CVR itself (Freyman and Nerbonne, 1989). In the past, most published efforts to increase CVR have been implemented for research purposes with large digital computers rather than with technology suitable for packaging in head-worn hearing aids. However, considerable possibility exists as well to develop consonant enhancement algorithms with subminiature analog circuitry that are suitable for being included in head-worn and even in ITE hearing aids. Some of these approaches have already been utilized for many years in head-worn hearing aids. For example, a single-channel syllabic compressor hearing aid with a low-enough compression threshold and appropriate time constants significantly improves the CVR. Regardless of whether large digital or subminiature analog approaches are used, the goal is to accomplish this CVR increase without audible artifacts so that speech and background environmental sounds are not altered in an unnatural or unpleasant manner. Indeed, inappropriate manipulation of the speech signal can lead to a degradation in speech recognition (Plomp, 1988).

TECHNIQUES FOR SPEECH ENHANCEMENT

Overviews of speech-enhancement techniques are found in Lim (1983), Montgomery (1984), Revoille and Holden-Pitt (1990), and Williamson and Punch (1990). From those references, a simple categorization of speech-enhancement techniques might include (1) duration enhancement, (2) spectral sharpening or increasing spectral contrast, (3) temporal envelope expansion, and (4) consonant enhancement relative to vowels. Some of the techniques that involve alteration or exaggeration of specific speech cues or speech segments within these four categories will be reviewed herein. Many, but not all, of these techniques utilized DSP to achieve the desired speech enhancement, and several of the methods discussed may actually fall into more than one of the above categories for speech enhancement.

Many of the first ideas for speech enhancement resulted directly from investigations conducted to determine what speech cues are important for perception. For example, because of the findings of Picheny, Durlach, and Braida (1985), in which intelligibility of clearly spoken speech was superior to that for normally spoken speech, some of the very first acoustic alterations of speech attempted to duplicate the acoustic features of clearly spoken speech (Picheny, Durlach, and Braida, 1986). Experiments in manipulating the speech waveform have been conducted to alter such features as vowel duration and amplitude, consonant duration and amplitude, extent of formant transitions, voice onset time and burst amplitude of stop consonants, and the amount of frication noise for voiceless fricatives. Many efforts in speech enhancement have concentrated on improving the intelligibility of frequently confused unvoiced fricatives and plosive sounds. For example, in an early effort, Drucker (1968) suggested that improved intelligibility may result by first detecting the presence of these low-energy-level sounds and then adaptively high-pass filtering the fricatives and inserting short pauses before the plosives.

Duration Enhancement

To compensate for reduced temporal resolution of impaired auditory systems, several researchers have investigated varying the duration of speech components. This type of algorithm may also help to determine whether some hearing-impaired listeners can perceive temporal cues more easily than spectral cues (Revoille et al., 1982). Duration variation of vowels and consonants has provided substantial increases in consonant recognition for 25 moderately to profoundly hearing-impaired listeners (Revoille et al., 1986). For this investigation, the preceding vowel was lengthened for syllables with final /z/ or /v/ and shortened in syllables with final /s/ or /f/. However, in another study, 100% increases in consonant duration did not generally produce an increase in consonant recognition scores for elderly hearing-impaired listeners at two presentation levels (Gordon-Salant, 1987). Similarly, for consonant duration increases of up to 30 msec, Montgomery and Edge (1988) reported no increase in California Consonant Test scores at a 65 dB SPL presentation level, and only a 5% increase at 95 dB SPL.

Spectral Contrast Enhancement

Spectral sharpening or contrast enhancement has been advocated to help compensate for reduced frequency selectivity of impaired auditory systems (Boers, 1980). Several researchers have investigated spectral contrast enhancement with formant bandwidth reduction and with principal components compression. In order to study lateral suppression effects in the auditory system for vowels, van Veen and Houtgast (1985) evalu-

ated sharpening as well as smoothing the spectral envelopes of synthetic vowel-like sounds. The degree of smoothing or sharpening was quantified via a summation of sinusoidal spectral modulations or peak and valley ripples in the spectrum. It was found that perceptual differences were mainly associated with spectral sharpening via amplifying waveforms with ripple densities of two ripples per octave. Similarly, Sidwell and Summerfield (1985) found that enhancing spectral contrast for steady-state vowel-like maskers produced increased peak-to-valley intensity differences in masking patterns for both normal-hearing and hearing-impaired listeners up to 2.5 kHz.

Summerfield, Foster, and Tyler (1985) evaluated the effect on stop consonant recognition of narrowing and broadening the formant bandwidths in synthetic speech by 0.25 to 8 times normal. Examples of the speech spectra resulting are reproduced in Figure 12.10. Broadening the formant band-

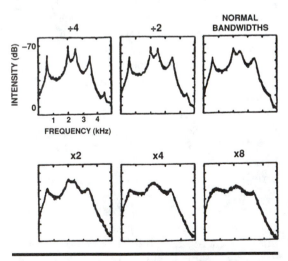

FIGURE 12.10. Long-term power spectra of the vowel /e/ from the syllables get, debt, and bet, showing the effects of varying formant bandwidths from 0.25 to 8.0 times nominally normal values. Reprinted with permission from Summerfield, Foster, and Tyler, 1985. Copyright © by Elsevier Science Publishers.

widths produced a definite decrease in percent correct stop consonant identification for both hearing-impaired and normal-hearing subjects. Although some persons in both groups benefited from one-half the normal formant bandwidths, the authors found that, in general, no benefit was provided by spectral sharpening.

Bustamante and Braida (1986a) reported on a principal components compression tech-

nique for reducing gross speech amplitude changes while maintaining spectral contrast. They advocated compressing only the first two principal components, corresponding to overall level (PC1) and spectral tilt (PC2), in order to preserve rapid fluctuations of speech while reducing overall level variation. Examples of the temporal waveforms of PC1 and PC2 are reproduced in Figure 12.11 before and after their compression. To compensate for the

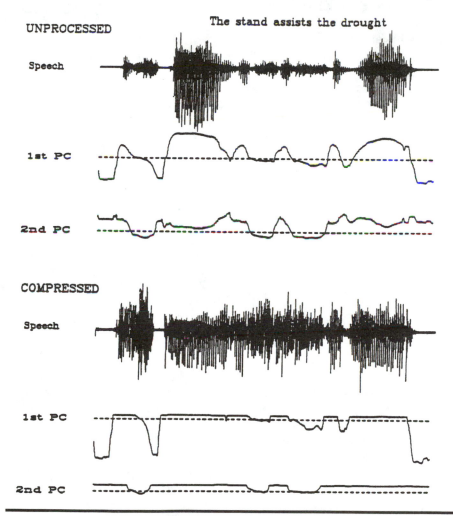

FIGURE 12.11. Example of principal components compression. Temporal waveforms of speech and first and second principal components unprocessed (top) and after compression of PC1 and PC2 (bottom) are shown. Reprinted with permission from Bustamante and Braida, 1986a.

combination of reduced dynamic range and reduced frequency selectivity, Bustamante and Braida (1986b) evaluated wideband compression with sharpening of short-term spectral shape. This was accomplished with an orthogonal decomposition of the critical band spectrum, a technique similar to principal components decomposition, and expanding the component weights responsible for peak-valley ratio. With a CVC nonsense syllable recognition task, a modest benefit over linear amplification for four hearing-impaired listeners resulted for a male speaker, but not for a female speaker. Wideband compression combined with expansion of higher-order principal components produced no change or reduced intelligibility for the four hearing-impaired listeners relative to wideband compression alone.

In a subsequent study (Bustamante and Braida, 1987), for four hearing-impaired listeners, wideband compression and compressing PC1 was found to produce improved intelligibility relative to linear processing. However, compressing both PC1 and PC2 reduced intelligibility relative to linear processing. In a related approach, to account for different frequency responses being preferred at different input levels, Levitt, Neumann, and Toraskar (1986) recommended compressing three orthogonal polynomial components from the short-time spectrum. The three components were a constant term representing RMS level, slope, and convex/concave curvature. Compression of the constant term, which is analogous to conventional wideband compression, improved the dynamic range for hearing-impaired subjects. The effect of compressing spectral tilt was evaluated by switching between flat and rising responses and has been studied by Haggard et al. (1987). They found a decrement in performance from selectively manipulating spectral tilt relative to a fixed spectral tilt. Trying to improve the results

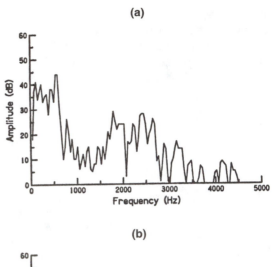

(a)

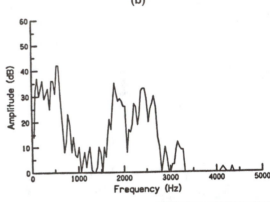

(b)

FIGURE 12.12. Example of unprocessed (a) and contrast-enhanced (b) spectra. The enhancement was applied differentially to midfrequency peaks. Reprinted with permission from Bunnell, 1990.

with the principal components compression procedure, Bunnell (1990) enhanced the spectral contrasts for F2 and F3 only, and not for F1. Examples of speech spectra prior to enhancement and after F2 and F3 enhancement are reproduced in Figure 12.12. With reduced spectral contrast, correct identifications of stop consonants were reduced for ten hearing-impaired persons; enhancing spectral contrast raised the number of correct identifications for /b/ and /g/, but not for /d/ (Figure 12.13).

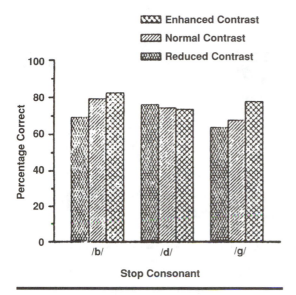

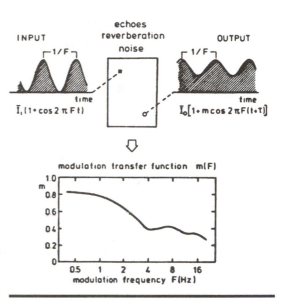

FIGURE 12.13. Percent correct identification of three stop consonants in three spectral contrast conditions. Reprinted with permission from Bunnell, 1990.

FIGURE 12.14. Top: Reduction in depth of sinusoidal modulation of a noise carrier caused by echoes, reverberation, and noise in an enclosure. Bottom: Using the modulation transfer function m(F) to quantify the degree of preservation of the original intensity modulations as a function of modulation frequency. The carrier is octave-band-filtered noise. Reprinted with permission from Houtgast and Steeneken, 1985.

Modulation Envelope Expansion

As opposed to *spectral* contrast enhancement, modulation envelope expansion increases the contrasts in the fine structure of *temporal* speech waveforms. As shown in the top portion of Figure 12.14, reverberation and noise decrease the temporal modulation depth of signals in auditoriums (Houtgast and Steeneken, 1985). This degradation is greater for higher modulation frequencies than for lower modulation frequencies as shown in the bottom of Figure 12.14, and it is thought that this reduces intelligibility in auditoriums.

Schroeder (1979) and Plomp (1988) have suggested that selective expansion or compression of the temporal modulation envelope under certain conditions may improve speech intelligibility for hearing-impaired persons. Langhans and Strube (1982) evaluated this approach by applying compression or expansion or linear processing after determining the modulation frequency from FFT-derived short-time spectra. Preprocessing was performed in 32 bands with competing noise added thereafter at SNRs of 0, 5, and 10 dB with the following algorithm: 20:1 compression if the modulation frequency was less than 2 Hz; 5 dB expansion if the modulation frequency was between 2 Hz and 5 Hz; and linear amplification if the modulation frequency was greater than 18 Hz. A 30% improvement in intelligibility was obtained for 240 monosyllables over the unprocessed condition. After determining the short-time spectrum in 20 uniformly wide bandpass filters, Clarkson and Bahgat (1991), using a similar algorithm to that of Langhans and Strube, obtained a 6% improvement in Modi-

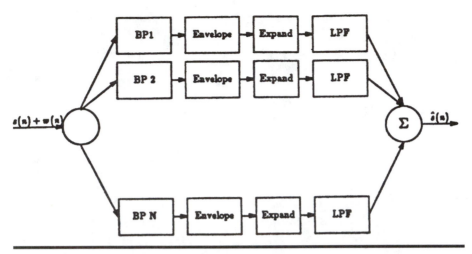

FIGURE 12.15.   Block diagram of system that enhances speech using envelope expansion. BPI is the bandpass filter for the ith band; LPF is low-pass filtering; x(n) is the measured input consisting of signal s(n) and noise w(n), and S(n) is the enhanced output. Reprinted with permission from Clarkson and Bahgat, 1991.

fied Rhyme Test scores for normal-hearing listeners in competing white noise presented at 0 dB SNR. A block diagram of their system is reproduced in Figure 12.15.

CVR Enhancement

Increasing the acoustic energy of consonants relative to vowels via consonant amplification shows promise for improved consonant recognition for hearing-impaired persons. This is the type of processing compression circuits perform and has been advocated for improving SNR as compared to linear processing for low-level signals (Villchur, 1973; Dillon, 1989). Compression has been studied for use in hearing aids for about 40 years (Walker and Dillon, 1982). Much of the research work on the effects of compression for the hearing impaired has been performed with analog compressors. For example, Niederjohn and Grotelueschen (1976) studied the effects of high-pass filtering followed by automatic amplitude normalization (syllabic compression) on speech intelligibility in

high levels of competing noise. They utilized rapid attack and release times (8 msec) in the compressor so as not to interfere with the transient characteristics of speech. It was noted that because of its quick response time, the compressor would produce an attenuation of high-level vowel energy that would tend to increase the CVR. Significant intelligibility advantages were found for high-pass filtering followed by amplitude normalization over that for unprocessed speech. Dreschler (1988a) indicated that syllabic compression equalizes levels between successive sounds, thus increasing consonant levels. Although syllabic compression has considerable intuitive face validity in compensating for the reduced dynamic range of hearing-impaired persons, up to this time it has not been employed in a high percentage of hearing aid fittings. Several researchers have shown little, if any, benefit of syllabic compression compared to linear amplification. Walker and Dillon (1982) and Dreschler (1988b) speculated that the benefits of recruitment compensation by the compressor may be negated by temporal distortions from the compressor attack and recovery times and its alterations of the normal intensity cues in speech.

Another type of compressor, the compression limiter, generally has a much higher compression threshold and a higher compression ratio than a syllabic compressor. Because compression limiting is only active at high signal levels, it may provide some CVR enhancement without significantly altering the dynamics of conversational speech signals compared to the effect of a syllabic compressor (Walker and Dillon, 1982).

A multiband compressor having independent compression circuits for each frequency band has been advocated to eliminate the problem of single-channel compressors in which gain across the entire frequency range is reduced by low-frequency noises. With multichannel compression, low-frequency noise would theoretically cause gain reduction only in the low-frequency band(s) and the weaker high-frequency components of speech, critical for good speech intelligibility, would continue to be maximally amplified (Kates, 1986). Bustamante and Braida (1987) concluded that multichannel compression provides an advantage over linear amplification for lower input-level signals but not for higher input-level signals. However, there are several studies that have failed to demonstrate significant improvements in speech intelligibility in noise using multichannel compression systems as compared to single-channel compression and linearly amplifying hearing aids having appropriate frequency shaping (e.g., Abramovitz, 1980; Barfod, 1976; Lippman, Braida, and Durlach, 1981). O'Connell et al. (1988) found no significant differences in NST scores or Hearing Aid Performance Inventory (HAPI) for six hearing-impaired persons between a body-worn, programmable digital hearing aid and the subjects' own hearing aids. The digital hearing aid was programmed to function as a

four-channel compression device, and the testing was conducted following a brief field trial with the digital instrument. NST scores were obtained at six speech levels (45 to 80 dBA) with two competing noise levels (42 and 57 dBA) and with a quiet background. In general, the subjects were quite satisfied with their own conventional hearing aids, which had been fitted at the Central Institute for the Deaf (CID). The gain in each of the four channels for the digital hearing aid was programmed to the approximate real-ear gain specified by a modified Pascoe fitting procedure, while the subjects own instruments were set as fitted originally by the CID clinic.

Some researchers have stated that high compression ratios with multichannel compression may degrade the relative intensity cues required to identify stops or fricatives (De Gennaro, Braida, and Durlach, 1986; Plomp, 1988). Interfering with the high-frequency components of the speech signal compressors may be even more of a problem with fast-acting multichannel syllabic compression hearing aids than with single-channel syllabic compressors (King and Martin, 1984). The optimal time constants for multichannel compression in hearing aids are still debatable in terms of whether the circuit should react to and alter the rapid level changes of speech—a kind of deliberate distortion of the speech signal itself—or whether the natural temporal cues of speech should be preserved. Plomp (1988) has criticized fast-acting multichannel compressors with many independent compression bands for reducing the natural amplitude contrasts in speech. Therefore, Plomp contends that longer compressor time constants should be used in multichannel compression hearing aids. However, Villchur (1989) reminds us that Licklider and Pollack in 1948 demonstrated that speech was perfectly intelligible after infinite amplitude clipping had produced a signal with no amplitude contrasts. Villchur maintains that although multichannel compression decreases the peak-to-valley level differences within speech, the audibility of weaker components of speech, such as consonants, are preserved after compression.

Whereas compression produces less change in output SPL for a given change in input SPL, expansion does the opposite, as shown by the input/output characteristic in the lower portion of Figure 12.16. This input/output characteristic was obtained with varying levels of a speech-shaped noise input to a

hearing aid with an expander. Note that the ratio of output SPL change to input SPL change is greater than 1 up to about a 70 dB input SPL. Use of expansion for increasing perception of low-level consonants has been suggested by Kates (1984). In his implementation, the level of high-frequency energy was sensed in a number of channels. After determining the presence of a consonant from the short-term spectral shape, if the speech level in a high-frequency band exceeded a preselected threshold, a 3:1 dynamic range expansion was applied in that band. Linear amplification was performed at frequencies below 500 Hz. Cummins, Hecox, and Williamson (1989) advocated an input/output function with three piecewise linear sections: Low-level signals up to the first compression kneepoint are expanded, signals having levels exceeding the first kneepoint but less than the second compression kneepoint are amplified linearly, and signals exceeding the level of the second compression knee point are compressed.

Several researchers have conducted behavioral evaluations to investigate the effectiveness of expansion for improving speech recognition. For example, Yanick and Drucker (1976), using modified dbX™ compressors in two channels, concluded that a combination of expansion and compression was superior both to compression alone and to linear amplification. With an SNR of +6 dB, they reported a 10% improvement in recognition scores for six hearing-impaired listeners with compression and expansion combined as compared to compression alone. However, Walker, Byrne, and Dillon (1984) evaluated speech intelligibility for a six-channel expander/compressor for a small group of hearing-impaired subjects. Their expander operated on low-level signals in the high-frequency channels, while the compressor was used for high-level signals. They concluded that expansion degraded speech intelligibil-

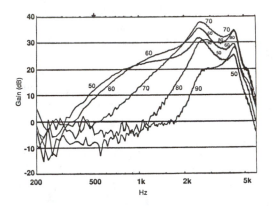

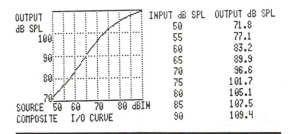

FIGURE 12.16. Example of a hearing aid that reduces low-frequency gain while expanding high-frequency gain. Top: Family of frequency response curves with speech-shaped noise input levels ranging from 50 dB to 90 dB SPL in 10 dB steps, per ANSI S3.42-1992. Bottom: Input/output characteristic with same noise with its input level ranging from 50 dB to 90 dB SPL in 5 dB steps. Reprinted with permission from Preves et al., 1991.

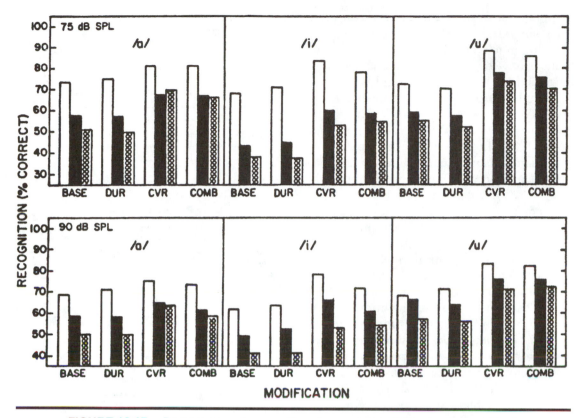

FIGURE 12.17.   Percent correct recognition of nonsense syllables by three subject groups (open bars = normal hearing, black bars = gradually sloping losses, transverse bars = sharply sloping losses), in four acoustic modifications (baseline, 100% consonant duration increase, 10 dB CVR increase, and combined 100% duration and 10 dB CVR increases), in three vowel contexts (/a,i,u/) and two presentation levels (75 and 90 dB SPL). Reprinted with permission from Gordon-Salant, 1987.

ity for low levels or, at best, did not change it as compared to six-channel linear frequency shaping. The outcome of this study might have been influenced by the degradation of the speech signal resulting from automatically manipulating the gain simultaneously in six bands. As a follow-up study, it may be worthwhile to evaluate an expander/compressor system with fewer channels.

Gordon-Salant (1987) found that a CVR increase of 10 dB resulted in an overall 14% increase in consonant recognition percent cor-

rect for elderly persons with gradually sloping and sharply sloping, mild to moderate high-frequency hearing loss. Her results are reproduced in Figure 12.17 and include the effects of duration increases discussed previously. For these tests, nineteen consonants, paired with three vowels, were presented at 75 dB and 90 dB SPL with competing twelve-talker babble at a +6 dB SNR. In the same study, increasing consonant duration by 100% and combining the amplitude and duration enhancements produced no improvement, and even a decrement in consonant recognition scores for some subjects.

Using much the same protocol, for consonants from the California Consonant Test amplified by 10–21 dB at 65 and 95 dB SPL presentation levels, an improvement in intelligibility of 10% was reported for the lower-level presentations only by Montgomery and Edge (1988). In that study, this amount of consonant enhancement resulted in the consonants and vowels having equal amplitude (CVR = 0 dB), which may have been too large an increase for some of the mild to moderately hearing-impaired subjects. In another study, Freyman et al. (1991) reported improved recognition with normal-hearing listeners for voiced stops in competing white noise as a result of amplifying consonants by 10 dB. They theorized that the improvement may have been the result of amplification of the burst release, which may have strengthened the modulation envelope cues.

Recognizing that the optimal CVR may vary on an individual basis, Kennedy and Levitt (1990) obtained an overall 15% improvement in NST scores for nine moderate to moderately severe hearing-impaired listeners with 3, 6, 9, and 12 dB increases in consonant level. As shown in Figure 12.18, too much consonant amplification for certain consonants for some subjects resulted in an intelligibility decrease from that obtained for the "ideal" amount of enhancement. Thus, the optimal CVR varied with the particular combination of consonants and vowels as they interacted with the characteristics of a particular auditory system. If a CVR optimization technique were to be used in hearing aids, one would first have to test for the set of optimal CVRs for a listener and then utilize automatic speech recognition algorithms in real time to determine which vowels and consonants were present, so as to apply the appropriate amount of consonant emphasis.

The combination of adaptive high-pass fil-

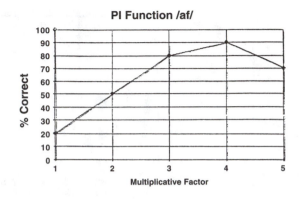

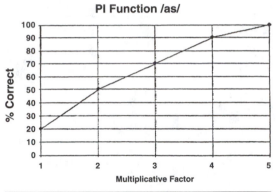

FIGURE 12.18.   Effect of amount of consonant level emphasis (CVR increase) on percent correct recognition of two nonsense syllables for the same subject. (1 = no enhancement; 2 = +3 dB; 3 = +6 dB; 4 = +9 dB; 5 = +12 dB consonant level enhancement.) Rollover between 4 and 5 for /af/ (top graph) demonstrates that the optimum CVR was not always found to be at the level of the most consonant emphasis. Reprinted with permission from Kennedy and Levitt, 1990.

tering and expansion of high-frequency gain, as shown in Figure 12.16, has been investigated for potentially increasing CVR with analog circuitry small enough to be packaged in ITE hearing aids (Preves et al., 1991; Ochs, Sammeth, and Tetzeli, 1992). The intent of this algorithm was first to attenuate high-energy vowels with adaptive high-pass filtering, leaving mainly low-energy consonants as the resultant. This residual signal was then expanded to further increase the CVR. Higher CVRs were reported with this combination algorithm, as compared to adaptive high-pass filtering alone, for some, but not all, consonants. Fortune and Preves (1991) and Tetzeli, Sammeth, and Ochs (1991) obtained higher CVRs and NST scores for some, but not all, consonants with adaptive high-pass filtering followed by expansion as compared to that for adaptive high-pass filtering alone for persons with sharply sloping high-frequency losses.

DIGITAL NOISE REDUCTION ALGORITHMS

Obtaining an improved SNR with hearing aids is challenging because of different types of speech degradation caused by changes in the spectral and temporal characteristics of background noise as the listening environment changes. These different types of speech degradation may be better addressed individually by different signal processing methods (Lim, 1982). For example, increased reverberation in some listening environments can diffuse an interfering noise signal so that it arrives at the hearing aid from many different directions and at many different arrival times. Because of the changing nature of background noise to which hearing aid wearers are exposed, many of the traditional techniques used for steady-state noise reduction are not applicable for hearing aid use without modification. The hearing aid designer must be aware of these problems and apply different solutions when appropriate. Then, a sophisticated hearing aid of the future could store different noise reduction algorithms so that the hearing aid wearer could select an algorithm suitable for a particular listening environment.

Unlike fixed filters that are employed in most conventional analog hearing aids, adaptive digital filters are able to modify their frequency response as well as other characteristics to achieve noise reduction. Techniques for noise reduction can be simply categorized into single-microphone approaches and multiple-microphone approaches.

Digital Noise Reduction Techniques with a Single Microphone

In one-microphone noise reduction approaches, the spectrum of the noisy speech signal is split up into bands with a bank of parallel bandpass filters or with an FFT so as to attenuate a particular spectral band. The amount of attenuation in each band depends on how much the measured speech power exceeds an estimate of the background noise. Included in single-microphone noise reduction approaches are spectral power subtraction and adaptive Wiener filtering. McAulay and Malpass (1980) found that these algorithms were equally effective for processing speech in a quiet background. However, their results showed that neither approach did an adequate job of suppressing noise when speech was absent. The following sections briefly explore these two approaches.

Spectral Power Subtraction. In this noise reduction approach, the short-time spectral magnitude of speech is estimated from a time slice of the speech mixed with noise and then combined with the phase of the speech and noise to produce enhanced speech (e.g., Berouti, Schwartz, and Makhail, 1979; Boll, 1979). This technique requires frequent spectral subtractions of samples of the noise signal from samples of the speech mixed with noise to obtain an estimate of the speech signal from moment to moment. Characteristics of the noise are estimated during silent intervals in the speech. Evaluation of this technique using nonsense sentences mixed with wideband random noise showed that, while intelligibility scores were not improved, the processed speech sounded less noisy and had improved quality as compared to the unprocessed speech (Lim, 1979). If the spectrum of the noise is similar to that of speech, as is the case for competing speech babble, algorithms that simply subtract the noise spectrum from the incoming signal will also subtract a significant amount of the speech itself (Lim, 1982; Tuzman, 1989). For high speech SNRs, the algorithm usually decides that it is most likely that speech is present and the speech envelope is comparatively easily extracted. However, for low speech SNRs, the model often assumes that noise alone is present, and in this case, some investigators have noted considerable distortion, resulting in a music-like residual noise (e.g., Ephraim and Malah, 1984). To work successfully, the algorithm needs to determine the average amount of noise power present and, therefore, whether speech is present or not. To aid in this decision, temporal differences between speech (which is more impulsive in nature) and noise (which is hopefully more steady state in nature) can be used.

Adaptive Wiener Filters. Adaptive hearing aids that utilize the long-term differences between speech and noise can be classified as Wiener filters with adaptation. A Wiener filter produces an estimate of the speech signal without any noise. An adaptive Wiener filter changes from moment to moment so as to approximate the ideal filter as the speech and competing noise change. Qualitatively, a multichannel Wiener filter does the following: In each channel, if the system decides there is predominately noise present, the gain in that channel is adaptively reduced. For this type of noise reduction system to work best, some knowledge is required beforehand of the speech and noise signals and the transfer characteristics of their transmission paths from the speech and noise sources to the

hearing aid microphone. The system can work particularly well when the noise does not change too much (quasi-steady-state noise). Frequently, as for the spectral subtraction approach, with adaptive Wiener filtering, an estimate is made of the noise during silent periods in the speech. Under digital control, the parameters of a digital filter are adaptively changed to estimate the noise. However, if the noise changes in character or if the long-time spectrum of the noise is similar to that of speech (e.g., for several competing talkers), performance degrades. One implementation of a multichannel adaptive Wiener filter reported a large improvement in the quality of processed speech by increasing the number of channels to 24 (Doblinger, 1982). It was reported that for signal-to-noise ratios greater than 6 dB, the device "nearly eliminated" disturbing noise while introducing negligible speech distortion, having achieved a 32 dB noise reduction. As is frequently the case with other single-microphone processors, this noise reduction system was not as effective in lower SNR listening conditions. The computer utilized in this implementation was an Intel 2920 DSP chip, one of the first off-the-shelf DSP chips. This remarkable device (for that era) included an analog-to-digital converter, a microprocessor, and a digital-to-analog converter all on one chip. Unfortunately, this particular DSP chip required two 9 V batteries to operate, one requiring about 100 milliamperes current drain to operate (Preves, 1986).

In a more marketable implementation of an adaptive Wiener filter, from the standpoint of size and cosmetics, a special-purpose digital computer packaged on a custom-designed (not off-the-shelf) CMOS integrated circuit adaptively reduced noise (Zeta Noise Blocker) (Graupe, Beex, and Causey, 1980). The Zeta Noise Blocker (ZNB) was small enough to be incorporated into BTE and even ITE hearing aids. In conjunction with switched capacitor

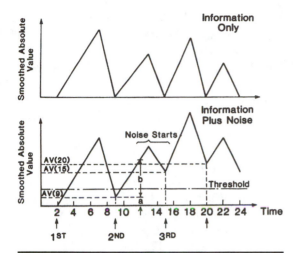

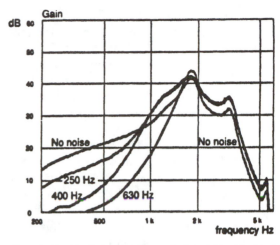

FIGURE 12.19. Illustration of temporal processing by the Zeta Noise Blocker. Top: Time representation of energy of smoothed speech pulses without additive noise. Bottom: Time representation of energy of smoothed speech pulses with additive noise. Sampling to identify noise occurs during the pauses in the speech pulses as indicated by the arrows. Reprinted with permission from Graupe, Beex, and Causey, 1980.

FIGURE 12.20. Change in frequency response for a hearing aid with Zeta Noise Blocker with pulsed speech-spectrum noise alone (no noise) and summed with steady-state narrow bands of noise at three frequencies. Reprinted with permission from Bareham, 1990.

analog filters, the digital computer in the ZNB essentially attempted to separate speech components from noise simultaneously in several frequency bands. To accomplish this, temporal differences between speech and quasi-steady-state noise were utilized as shown in Figure 12.19. Here the noise was sensed during the silent intervals between vocal cord pulses of speech at the bottom of the troughs of the speech waveform pulses. If noise was present, these troughs would "fill up" and the adaptive Wiener filter reduced the gain in the corresponding frequency band. Figure 12.20, reproduced from Bareham (1990) shows that the frequency response of a ZNB hearing aid did not change for a pulsing speech-shaped noise input (representing speech in quiet). However, for pulsing speech-shaped noise mixed with steady-state narrowband noise

centered at three different frequencies (to represent different frequency regions of steady-state noise), gain was attenuated in the frequency range of the narrowband noise. These tests indicated that the ZNB could distinguish between a steady noise (assumed undesirable) and speech represented by a pulsing broad-band noise. In spite of its evident performance benefits, cosmetic packaging, and availability from a number of hearing aid manufacturers in a variety of hearing aids, the ZNB was not a commercial success and has essentially disappeared from the market. Speculations on reasons for this lack of success generally point out too-noticeable, drastic changes in frequency response and in the resulting sound quality as listening environment changed, whether excessive noise was present or not.

Investigations into whether there is an improvement in speech intelligibility with competing noise utilizing the ZNB are equivocal. A study that used a nonintegrated circuit prototype of the ZNB in a body aid (Stein and Dempsey-Hart, 1984) and another investigation using an actual ZNB integrated circuit in a postauricular aid (Wolinsky, 1986) found significant improvement in intelligibility for the majority of subjects. Another study (Klein, 1989) found a trend for a wide-band linear hearing aid to be superior to the ZNB adapting condition and for both the linear aid and ZNB adapting condition to be superior to the ZNB nonadapting (linear) condition for five hearing-impaired subjects. Van Tasell, Larsen, and Fabry (1988) found no significant improvement for spondee words mixed with speech-spectrum noise with the ZNB using an SRT-in-noise test paradigm, and Larsen (1986) found no subjective preferences favoring the ZNB in adaptive mode over linear mode. Both of these investigations utilized in-the-ear modules and the first generation of the ZNB integrated circuit. It was concluded that the amount of improvement obtained depends on the amount of spectral similarity of the speech materials and interfering noise employed. It is more difficult to demonstrate an improved SNR if the speech and competing noise are spectrally similar than, for example, if high-frequency-weighted nonsense syllables and a low-frequency-weighted interfering noise such as speech-spectrum noise are used (Van Tasell, 1988).

Adaptive Noise Canceling and Beamforming with Two or More Microphones

Because the long-term spectral characteristics of speech and interfering noise signals are often similar, the effectiveness of many conventional DSP algorithms for SNR enhancement using one microphone is limited. This occurs because these algorithms generally are based on some form of subtraction of the noise from the speech, often reducing the speech energy significantly as well as the

noise energy. With two or more microphones, more-sophisticated algorithms can be utilized that somewhat avoid this problem. More than one microphone can provide superior noise cancellation because each microphone receives a different representation of the desired target signal and the undesired noise signal(s). A classic two-microphone noise reduction scheme exploits the correlation of the noise signal in two microphones and has been called adaptive noise canceling or ANC (Widrow et al., 1975). To date, many of the digital noise reduction laboratory evaluations have utilized this popular ANC approach. In Figure 12.21, the signal from the top microphone is the primary input, while the signal from the bottom microphone is used as the reference input. In practice, the reference microphone is placed at some distance away from the primary microphone and as close as possible to the interfering noise source. The object of this noise reduction scheme is to obtain a good estimate of the desired speech signal in the primary microphone.

The adaptive filter is updated periodically by trying to eliminate the difference between the noise signals in the primary microphone and reference microphone. This filtering algorithm has been termed least mean squares

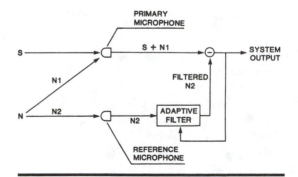

FIGURE 12.21.   Block diagram of basic adaptive noise canceler (ANC). Reprinted with permission from Weiss, 1987.

(LMS), referring to minimizing the error between the two inputs by adjusting the adaptive filter. Like many of the single-microphone noise reduction systems, many two-microphone schemes sense the noise during silent periods of the desired speech signal to adjust the adaptive noise canceler (Strube, 1981). However, unlike single-microphone noise reduction systems that perform Wiener filtering, ANC has the advantage that no knowledge of the desired speech and the undesired noise signals is required to adjust the adaptive filter. The ideal setup in order for the two-microphone adaptive noise canceler to work perfectly is to have the interfering noise signal correlated in both microphones, but to have only the desired speech signal in the primary microphone. Thus, ideally, the primary microphone senses speech and noise while the reference microphone senses correlated noise only. Also, ideally, the desired speech signal should be uncorrelated with the noise signals. Under these conditions, much of the noise will be canceled in the system output and up to 20 dB improvement in SNR is possible. Realizing these ideal requirements in practice necessitates a large spacing between the two microphones and requires having the reference microphone close to the interfering noise source—both unrealistic requirements for hearing aids. In real-world use of this two-microphone algorithm for hearing aids, the reference microphone output contains some desired speech signal as well as undesired noise, which causes part of the desired speech signal to be canceled. Additionally, room reverberation can invalidate the requirement mentioned previously that the desired speech signal and the undesired noise are uncorrelated (Peterson et al., 1987).

Many of the references cited herein for adaptive noise cancellation have used computer simulations and/or large, laboratory-grade components to test the effectiveness of the algorithm instead of actual hearing aids

worn by hearing-impaired listeners in real-world listening environments. For example, in one study, a microphone was used to pick up speech and noise for the primary channel, but the reference channel input was taken from the electrical output of a speech-noise generator passed through a low-pass filter rather than from a microphone (Brey et al., 1987). This experimental configuration formed an artificially perfect input to the reference channel—the speech signal was totally absent and only the noise signal was present. Another investigation of the two-microphone ANC technique reported an 18–22 dB reduction in speech babble or speech-weighted noise with a resulting 27% to 40% improvement in CID W-22 word recognition for hearing-impaired listeners (Harris et al., 1988). However, for this study, two loudspeakers separated by two meters were used, one for the speech with the primary microphone close by, and one for the noise with the reference microphone close by. This is hardly a practical simulation of the spacing between hearing aid microphones but was evidently done to ensure that the speech signal would be much stronger in the primary channel than in the reference channel. Thus, the excellent results of this study perhaps reflect the best improvements obtainable under idealized conditions. Although promising, perhaps test results from such experimental protocols should be regarded as having only academic interest until such algorithms and the required instrumentation can be made available and are evaluated with actual hearing aids in situ. Although real-world conditions prevent attaining the ideal microphone positions for hearing aids, the adaptive noise canceling technique still holds considerable promise for improved performance.

As another way of dealing with the effects of the physical environment on the input signals, some investigators of adaptive noise cancelers have utilized directional microphones to ensure that the reference microphone output contains only noise that is correlated to the noise in the primary microphone (Miller, 1986; Weiss, 1987). In these approaches, a directional microphone facing backwards was employed to help ensure that only noise was sensed for the reference channel. For the Weiss study, an omnidirectional microphone was used at the same ear of KEMAR for the primary channel to sense both the desired signal from the frontal azimuth and the noise. Laboratory-size components were employed for the microphones and the adaptive noise canceler, and the microphone output signals were tape recorded for offline presentation to the adaptive filter. Weiss concluded that in real-world, reverberant environments, the advantage provided by the relatively complicated system of directional microphone and omnidirectional microphone feeding an adaptive noise canceler would be minimal over that provided by a single directional microphone facing forward in a conventional hearing aid. This same approach was incorporated in a prototype noise canceling digital hearing aid (Staab, 1990).

As an extension of ANC, researchers have examined the possibility of using beamformers to compensate for the loss of directionally selective noise reduction capacity of hearing-impaired auditory systems. A beamformer is implemented with two or more microphones and an adaptive filter. It produces large attenuations or nulls at specific angles of incidence to cancel noises from several directions. If the number of microphones exceeds the number of disturbing noise sources, a null can be generated to attenuate the noise in the direction of each disturbance. Generally, the beamformer is constrained to provide maximum gain straight ahead at 0 degrees, or what is called the "look" direction.

In order to allow the use of two microphones as in an actual hearing aid fitting, a preprocessor, as shown in Figure 12.22, has been added to the adaptive noise canceler to

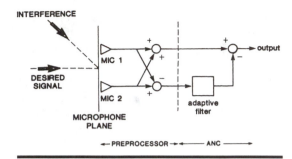

FIGURE 12.22. Basic adaptive noise canceler (ANC) with preprocessor to help cancel desired signal in reference channel for real-world hearing aid microphone positions.

help ensure that only noise correlated to the noise in the primary channel is present in the reference channel (Peterson et al., 1987). This configuration has been called the Griffiths-Jim beamformer. One of the cross-coupled

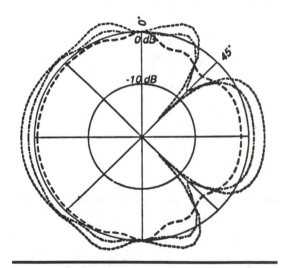

FIGURE 12.23. ANC attenuation, averaged from 0–4.3 kHz, as a function of arrival direction. Short dashes, dots and dashes, and long dashes indicate gain in simulated anechoic, living room, and conference room listening environments, respectively. Desired signal is at 0 degrees, and the interfering noise is at 45 degrees. Reprinted with permission from Peterson, 1987. Copyright © 1987 IEEE.

links and summing junctions in the preprocessor subtracts microphone 1 signal from microphone 2 signal for the purpose of canceling the desired signal to leave only noise in the reference input going to the adaptive filter. The other cross-coupled link and summing junction in the preprocessor adds microphone 1 signal to microphone 2 signal to produce the desired signal and correlated noise in the primary input of the adaptive noise canceler. In theory, two microphones implemented in this way can cancel one noise source adaptively by moving the null direction provided by the canceler automatically

to the direction of the undesired noise. The directivity patterns achieved in one such two-microphone approach (Peterson, 1987) are shown in Figure 12.23. These represent patterns similar to those of first-order gradient supercardioid directional microphones used in hearing aids during the 1970s. For comparison, the range of directivity patterns possible with first-order gradient directional microphones of the type used in hearing aids is reproduced from Marshall and Harry (1941) in Figure 12.24.

In another study, a two-microphone adaptive noise canceling beamformer of the type

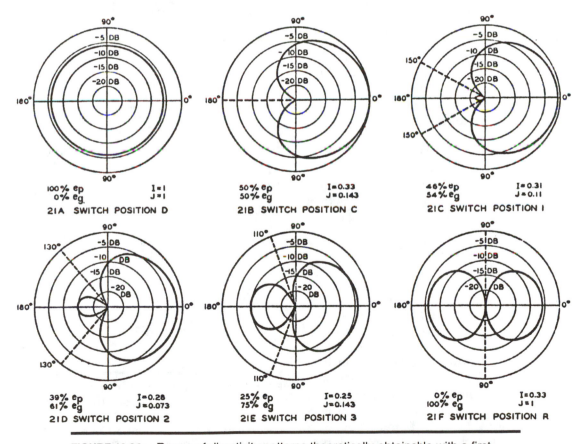

FIGURE 12.24. Range of directivity patterns theoretically obtainable with a first-order gradient directional microphone in free space. Reprinted with permission from Marshall and Harry, 1941.

suggested by Widrow was implemented with a plug-in board for a personal computer (Farassopoulos, 1989). With this system, an SNR improvement of 14–24 dB was reported for an anechoic chamber, depending on the direction of the uncorrelated pseudo-random, flat-spectrum noise source. In this implementation, the microphones were located on either side of KEMAR's head and near the ear canal entrance of each ear. With the speech incident at 0 degrees azimuth, because of the symmetrical microphone locations, little or no speech energy was present in the reference input of the adaptive noise canceler. Adding a second noise source resulted in less attenuation, particularly when the noise sources were from opposite sides of the head, until a third microphone was added at the front of head [Figure 12.25(a)]. This three-microphone beamformer produced a double-null directivity pattern as shown in Figure 12.25(b) for noise sources at +40 degrees and –60 degrees.

One important question that comes to mind is whether beamformers can produce more effective noise attenuation than directional microphones. A higher degree of directivity with directional microphones than that shown in Figure 12.24 would be possible with second-order gradient directional microphones, for which sample polar patterns are shown in Figure 12.26. However, hearing aids have not utilized higher-order gradient directional microphones because they are generally implemented with a bundle of parallel tubes having length in excess of one foot in order to provide good directionality at low frequencies. Such a packaging approach would not be cosmetically acceptable for head-worn hearing aids. The advantage of adaptive beamformers over directional hearing aid microphones is that the nulls in the directivity pattern provided by a beamformer move automatically to follow changes in direction of the noise

(a)

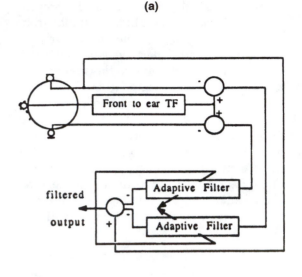

(b)

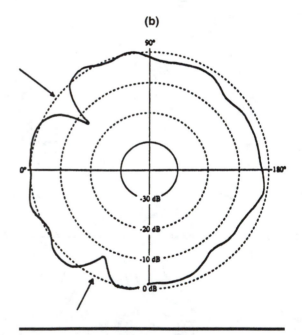

FIGURE 12.25. (a) Three-microphone beamformer configuration. (b) Directivity pattern produced by beamformer in (a) with two uncorrelated noise sources positioned at 40 degrees and at –60 degrees. Reprinted with permission from Farassopoulos, 1989. Copyright © 1989 IEEE.

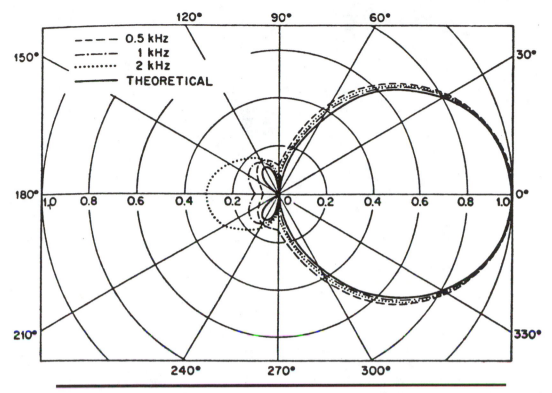

FIGURE 12.26.   Theoretical and measured directivity patterns at three frequencies obtainable with a second-order gradient directional microphone in free space. Reprinted with permission from Sessler and West, 1975.

sources. It is also possible to achieve polar patterns with more directivity using beamformers by using more microphones, as shown in Figure 12.27 for four microphones. In another example, Hoffman and Buckley (1990) evaluated a five-microphone array located symmetrically around the head at 45-degree intervals from –90 degrees to +90 degrees, as shown in Figure 12.28(a). The authors included the head shadow effects of a typical hearing aid wearer in their simulations. In their implementation, an adaptive digital spatial filter was formulated from the output of the microphone array and was advocated as a preprocessor for an ordinary analog hearing aid. With such a filter, the di-

rection of the nulls adapts to follow the locations of the interfering sources as they change direction and frequency [Figures 12.28(b) and 12.28(c)]. In one test of the beamformer, a 30 dB attenuation was reported of isotropic, speech-shaped noise in the presence of two 0 dB SNR interfering sources located at –60 degrees and +30 degrees.

Using white noise for both the desired signal and the undesired noise, Peterson et al. (1990) found improved speech reception threshold estimates for two- and four-microphone adaptive beamformers operating on one or two noises in simulated anechoic and living room environments for negative SNRs. The performance of their system degraded

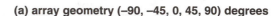

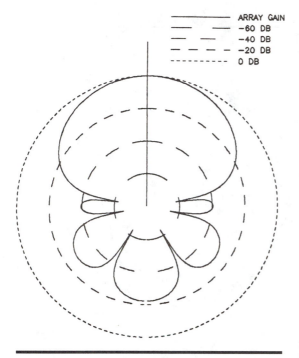

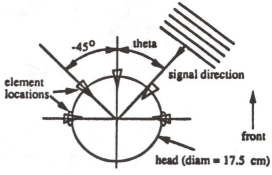

FIGURE 12.27. Directivity pattern attainable with a four-microphone nonadaptive array. Reprinted with permission from Beex and DeBrunner, 1990. Copyright © Elsevier Science Publishers.

for SNR greater than 0 dB and when the desired signals in the microphones were not equal due to reverberation, two conditions commonly found while wearing hearing aids. Both of these real-world difficulties caused a reduction in the desired signal due to the smearing into the noise(s) and to null misalignment. At high SNR, due to imperfect cancellation of the desired signal in the two microphones, the desired signal may be stronger than the noise in the reference channel, resulting in more desired signal than noise cancellation. This study did not include the effects of diffraction from a hearing aid wearer that would add to the null misalignment problem. The authors also have been testing the effectiveness of a portable, battery-powered, wearable version of the adaptive beamformer.

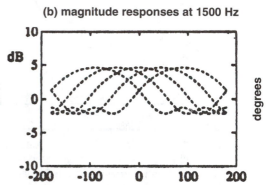

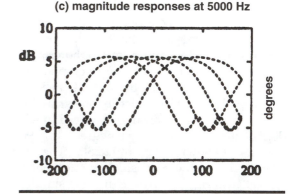

FIGURE 12.28. (a) Positions of five-microphone beamformer array around head. Sample nulls produced for each element overlaid at (b) 1500 Hz and (c) 5000 Hz. Reprinted with permission from Hoffman and Buckley, 1990. Copyright © 1990 IEEE.

Many of the signal processing techniques advocated for reducing noise and enhancing speech do not perform well when reverberation is present. A few of the studies cited herein have investigated the effects of simulated reverberation on the SNR improvement obtained with particular digital processing algorithms. Some investigators have evaluated the effectiveness of multimicrophone noise canceling techniques in reverberant surroundings. For example, the ability of a two-microphone adaptive digital system to remove echoes by exploiting the differences in the reverberated speech signal at the two ears has been studied (Bloom, 1982). His results show that although mean speech recognition scores were unchanged for both normal and hearing-impaired listeners, perceived and measured reverberation time was clearly reduced by processing.

To test the effect of various degrees of reverberation, Peterson et al. (1987) and Peterson (1987) presented processed sentences to normal-hearing listeners at 0 degrees azimuth and competing SPIN babble at 45 degrees azimuth in simulated anechoic, living room, and conference room environments. Test results were then compared to unprocessed sentences and babble presented in the same simulated test environments. In this study, simulated signals, rather than actual microphone-processed signals, were used. Although the simulated microphones were spaced 20 cm apart, no attempt was made to simulate the diffraction effects due to the wearer's head and torso that are encountered by actual hearing aid microphones. Results of this investigation showed SNR improvements, at 50% correct, of 30 dB for the anechoic (nonreverberant) environment, 14 dB for the living room, and 0 dB for the conference room, the most reverberant environment. As a follow-up study, an evaluation of a real-time system, as opposed to beamformer simulation, has been made using the same stimuli with a two-microphone adaptive array on KEMAR using an Ariel DSP

board plugged into a personal computer (Greenberg, 1989). In this study, the microphones were located for one test in an eyeglass frame and for another test in one eyeglass temple with the eyeglasses mounted on the KEMAR head. Tests were run with one and two SPIN babble noise sources from several directions.

As mentioned previously, the use of digital signal processing algorithms in hearing aids to improve SNR and to enhance speech can, if care is not taken, introduce other types of distortions that are unique to the digital processing algorithms themselves. For example, one time domain adaptive noise canceler technique (Sambur, 1978) reportedly results in an artificial enhancement of low-frequency content and attenuation of high-frequency content, causing the elimination of unvoiced speech sounds and an introduction of artificial reverberation (Chabries, et al., 1987). On a similar note, it has been pointed out that some digital processing algorithms actually reduce intelligibility relative to unprocessed signals (Lim and Oppenheim, 1984).

DIGITAL ALGORITHMS FOR REDUCING ACOUSTIC FEEDBACK OSCILLATION

Some of the approaches to feedback cancellation for hearing aids have been adopted from those used for public address systems. The most common technique is to decrease the gain in the frequency region of the acoustic feedback oscillation. This has been most commonly implemented by low-pass filtering, although recently notch filtering has been used to produce nulls in the frequency response at the feedback frequencies. Other approaches to feedback reduction for hearing aids include frequency shifting and phase shifting (Preves, 1988). To date, these techniques have been implemented in mass-produced hearing aids with analog technology. However, digital technology also lends itself to the important application of preventing oscillation in hearing aid fittings due to acoustic feedback. Feedback reduction can be thought of as a special case of noise reduction, and adaptive digital filtering techniques for cancellation have been investigated. The first step usually taken for digitally canceling the feedback path is to determine the open loop transfer function of the acoustic feedback path (e.g., Egolf et al., 1985; Egolf et al., 1989). Then, if an additional filter that is tuned to the inverse frequency response and inverse phase of the acoustic feedback path is inserted in the forward path of the hearing aid amplifier, cancellation results (e.g., Egolf, 1987; Levitt, Dugot, and Kopper, 1988). Similarly, an identical acoustic feedback network may also be synthesized by using a second microphone (Egolf et al., 1987). When the synthesized acoustic feedback network is subtracted from the actual acoustic path, feedback cancellation results.

One problem with any acoustic feedback cancellation scheme is that changes in proximity of objects to the hearing aid cause changes in the acoustic feedback characteristics. Several researchers have extended the capability of the nonadaptive synthesized acoustic feedback path approach by making it tunable or adaptive (e.g., Best, 1985; Graupe, 1988; Bustamante, Worrall, and Williamson, 1989; Kates, 1991; Dyrlund and Bisgaard, 1991). With this capability, the system could compensate for the effects of changes in the acoustic feedback path caused by movement of the hearing aid wearer. As an example, in the Kates approach, which was implemented via computer simulations rather than actual hearing aid instrumentation (Figure 12.29), the feedback path was broken by disconnecting the output amplifier and a 50 msec noise probe signal was injected to synthesize the open loop transfer function. A low duty cycle was employed for the probe mode so as not to introduce significant audible artifacts to the hearing aid wearer. The presence of acoustical feedback oscillation

was determined by comparing the power in the largest sinusoidal component in the microphone output signal to a predetermined threshold. In one approach employed by Kates [Figure 12.29(a)] the additional filter was updated periodically during the probe sequence via a Least Mean Squares (LMS) algorithm so as to null out the acoustic feedback signal. In a second approach [Figure 12.29(b)] a Wiener filter was used to adjust an additional filter at the end of the probe sequence. The acoustic feedback path was attenuated by 50 dB as a result. (Both the LMS algorithm and the Wiener filter have been mentioned previously in this chapter for noise attenuation.)

Bustamante, Worrall, and Williamson (1989) investigated three approaches to feedback suppression after estimating the transfer function of the acoustic feedback path with a series of clicks. Using a TMS32010 DSP system connected to a hearing aid microphone and receiver in a BTE hearing aid housing, first a time-varying delay was generated periodically. Maximum stable gain increased, but the accompanying distortion introduced a warbling quality to the processed signals. With this approach, a 1–2 dB maximum stable gain improvement was all that was possible with a reasonable amount of distortion. Next, notch filters were adaptively placed at the acoustic feedback oscillation frequencies. However, the notch filter bandwidths were too wide and they attenuated too much of the desired signal as well as the feedback frequencies. In a modification of this approach, no formant attenuation was observed when a fixed time delay was added in the reference signal path prior to the adaptive filter. The time delay was made roughly equal to the average group delay of the feedback path in a stable frequency region. The result was a 3–4 dB increase in maximum stable gain. The third approach attempted to cancel the feedback path by assuming that it could be represented by a fixed

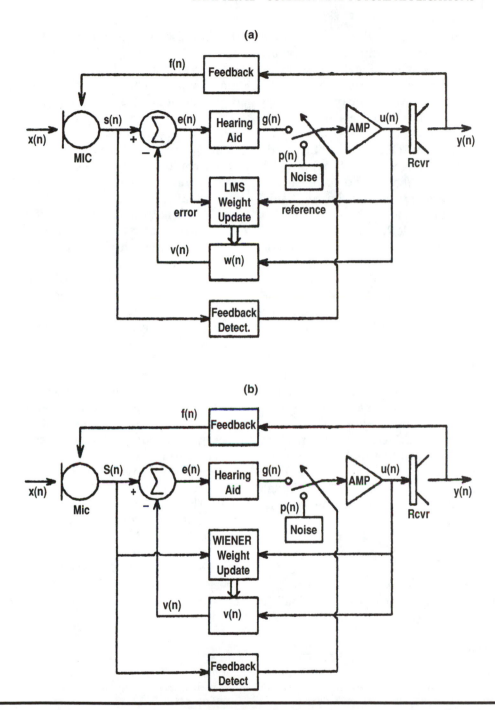

FIGURE 12.29.   Block diagram for hearing aid feedback cancellation system (a) using an adaptive procedure for estimating the filter coefficients during a probe sequence and (b) based on computing the Wiener filter coefficients. Reprinted with permission from Kates, 1991. Copyright © 1991 IEEE.

delay of about 0.85 msec (the average group delay of the feedback path) followed by an adaptive filter. Maximum stable gain measured on KEMAR was increased by up to 10 dB by this approach with little or no sacrifice in sound quality. For field trials, the third algorithm was implemented in a pocket processor coupled to a BTE earpiece with a cord. Users reported that feedback was suppressed in most situations that would have caused feedback with conventional hearing aids without such processing.

As another example, Dyrlund and Bisgaard (1991) evaluated a digital implementation of the feedback transfer function subtraction approach. As in the other adaptive approaches, the system was trained by re-estimating the acoustic feedback path transfer function with an injected noise signal. The processing device was body worn, connecting to high-gain BTE or ITE instruments with a cord. Ten to fifteen dB of improvement in feedback margin was achieved, which the authors believed would be achieved regardless of degree of earmold venting. This device has since been introduced into the marketplace for widespread distribution in a high-gain BTE hearing aid. This device thus represents one of the few uses of true digital processing available in production hearing aids at the time of this writing.

CONCLUSIONS

The technology of hearing aids is changing rapidly. Digital signal processing (DSP) holds the promise of significantly extending the signal processing capability and performance features of hearing aids beyond those of currently available analog and hybrid analog/digital devices. One advantage of DSP is incorporating several adaptive strategies for different applications simultaneously—for example, noise and feedback reduction programs could be operating concurrently with speech enhancement strategies geared to the individual hearing aid wearer. However, in spite of the advantages it could offer, for several reasons the use of DSP in hearing aids appears to be still in the infancy stage. Over the past fifteen years, many researchers have investigated the application of DSP to solve some of the performance problems in hearing aids. The outcomes of many of these studies do not show overwhelming evidence for putting DSP in hearing aids at this time. Some of the noise reduction algorithms evaluated cause considerable distortion in the processed signal, leading to plainly audible artifacts for the listener. Additionally, the results of some of these approaches are more practical from a packaging standpoint for incorporation into actual hearing aids than are others. Some of the approaches advocated are not compatible from a cosmetic view for hearing aid applications. These performance and packaging problems must be reconciled before DSP can be routinely utilized in hearing aids. The cost, performance features, and packaging must first become acceptable to the majority of prospective hearing aid wearers before true digital will be widely incorporated and marketed.

REFERENCES

Abramovitz, R. (1980). Frequency shaping and multiband compression in hearing aids. *Journal of Communication Disorders* 13:483–488.

Agnew, J. (1988). Hearing instrument distortion: What does it mean for the listener? *Hearing Instruments* 39(10):10–20.

Bareham, J. (1990). Hearing aid measurement using dual channel signal analysis. *Hearing Instruments* 41(3):34–36.

Barfod, J. (1976). Multi channel compression hearing aids, Report 11, The Acoustics Lab., Tech. Univ. of Denmark.

Beex, A., and DeBrunner, V. (1991). Restricted geometry acoustic arrays for highly directional patterns. *Applied Acoustics* 33:63–77.

Berouti, M., Schwartz, R., and Makhoul, J. (1979). Enhancement of speech corrupted by acoustic noise. International Conference on Acoustics, Speech and Signal Processing, Washington, DC.

Best, L. (1985). Digital suppression of acoustic feedback in hearing aids. Master's thesis, University of Wyoming, Laramie, WY.

Bloom, P. (1982). Evaluation of a dereverberation technique with normal and impaired listeners. *British Journal of Audiology* 16:167–176.

Boers, P. (1980). Formant enhancement of speech for listeners with sensorineural hearing loss. I.P.O. (Institut voor Perceptie Onderzoek, The Netherlands) Annual Progress Report 15:21–28.

Boll, S. (1979). Suppression of acoustic noise in speech using spectral subtraction. *IEEE Transactions on Acoustics, Speech and Signal Processing* 29:113–120.

Bratt, G., Peek, B., Bacon, S., and Logan, S. (1987). Variance from prescribed frequency response in custom ITE hearing aids. Presented at the American Speech-Language-Hearing Association Convention, New Orleans.

Brey, R., Robinette, M., Chabries, D., and Christiansen, R. (1987). Improvement in speech intelligibility in noise employing an adaptive filter with normal and hearing-impaired subjects. *Journal of Rehabilitation Research and Development* 24(4):75–86.

Bunnell, T. (1990). On enhancement of spectral contrast in speech for hearing-impaired listeners. *Journal of the Acoustical Society of America* 88(6):2546–2556.

Bustamante, D., and Braida, L. (1986a). Principal component amplitude compression. Presented at the 106th meeting of the Acoustical Society of America.

Bustamante, D., and Braida, L. (1986b). Wideband compression and spectral sharpening for hearing-impaired listeners. *Journal of the Acoustical Society of America* 80(suppl. 1):S12–S13.

Bustamante, D., and Braida, L. (1987). Principal-component amplitude compression for the hearing impaired. *Journal of the Acoustical Society of America* 82(4):1227–1242.

Bustamante, D., Worrall, T., and Williamson, M. (1989). Measurement and adaptive suppression of acoustic feedback in hearing aids. *Proceedings of IEEE ASSP*: 2017–2020.

Carlson, E. (1988). An output amplifier whose time has come. *Hearing Instruments* 39(10):30–32.

Chabries, D., Christiansen, R., Brey, R., Robinette, M., and Harris, R. (1987). Application of adaptive digital signal processing to speech enhancement for the hearing impaired. *Journal of Rehabilitation Research and Development* 24(4): 65–74.

Clarkson, P., and Bahgat, S.(1991). Envelope expansion methods for speech enhancement. *Journal of the Acoustical Society of America* 89(3):1378–1382.

Conger, C. (1987). A programmable gain response digital hearing aid. Master's thesis, University of Minnesota.

Cummins, K., Hecox, K., and Williamson, M. (1989). Adaptive, programmable signal processing hearing aid. U.S. Patent #4,887,299.

DeGennaro, S., Braida, L., and Durlach, N. (1986). Multiband syllabic compression for severely impaired listeners. *Journal of Rehabilitation Research and Development* 23:17–24.

Dillon, H. (1989). Hearing aid amplification method and apparatus. U.S. Patent #4,803,732.

Doblinger, G. (1982). "Optimum" filter for speech enhancement using integrated digital signal processors. International Conference on Acoustics, Speech and Signal Processing.

Dreschler, W. (1988a). The effect of specific compression settings on phoneme identification in hearing-impaired subjects. *Scandinavian Audiology* 17:35–43.

Dreschler, W. (1988b). Dynamic-range reduction by peak clipping or compression and its effects on phoneme perception in hearing-impaired listeners. *Scandanavian Audiology* 17:45–51.

Drucker, H. (1968). Speech processing in a high ambient noise environment. *IEEE Transactions on Audio and Electroacoustics* 16:165–168.

Dyrlund, O., and Bisgaard, N. (1991). Acoustic feedback margin improvements in hearing instruments using a prototype DFS (Digital Feedback Suppression) system. *Scandinavian Audiology* 20:49–53.

Egolf, D., Howell, H., Weaver, K., and Barker, S.

(1985). The hearing aid feedback path: Mathematical simulations and experimental verification. *Journal of the Acoustical Society of America* 78(5):1578–1587.

Egolf, D. (1987). Acoustic feedback suppression in hearing aids, final report: Vol. II, unpublished report to the Veterans Administration (Dept. of Elect. Eng., Univ. of Wyoming, Laramie, WY).

Egolf, D., Larson, V., Ahlstrom, C., Rainbolt, H., and McConnell (1987). The development and evaluation of a prototype acoustic feedback suppressor. Presented at the American Speech-Language-Hearing Convention, New Orleans, LA.

Egolf, D., Haley, B., Howell, H., Legowski, S., and Larson, V. (1989). Simulating the open-loop transfer function as a means for understanding acoustic feedback in hearing aids. *Journal of the Acoustical Society of America* 85(1):454–467.

Ephraim, Y., and Malah, D. (1984). Speech enhancement using a minimum mean-square error short-time spectral amplitude estimator. *IEEE Transactions on Acoustics, Speech and Signal Processing* 32(6):1109–1120.

Farassopoulos, A. (1989). Speech enhancement for hearing aids using adaptive beamformers. *Proceedings of IEEE ICASSP*, 1989:1322–1325.

Fortune, T., and Preves, D. (1991). Consonant perception and the modification of real ear consonant-to-vowel ratios produced by analog in-the-ear hearing aids. Presented at the American Speech-Language-Hearing Association Convention, Atlanta, GA.

French-St. George, M. (1992). CID Digital Hearing Aid Project. Presented at Amplification in the 90's, St Louis, MO.

Freyman, R., and Nerbonne, G. (1989). The importance of consonant-vowel intensity ratio in the intelligibility of voiceless consonants. *Journal of Speech and Hearing Research* 32:524–535.

Freyman, R., Nerbonne, G., and Cote, H. (1991). Effect of consonant-vowel ratio modification on amplitude envelope cues for consonant recognition. *Journal of Speech and Hearing Research* 34:415–426.

Gilman, S. (1986). Processor controlled ear responsive hearing aid and method. U.S. Patent #4,596,902.

Gordon-Salant, S. (1987). Effects of acoustic modification on consonant recognition by elderly hearing-impaired subjects. *Journal of the Acoustical Society of America* 81(4):1199–1202.

Graupe, D. (1988). Method of and means for adaptively filtering screeching noise caused by acoustic feedback. U.S. Patent #4,73,818.

Graupe, D., Beex, A., and Causey, D. (1980). ARMA filter and method for designing the same. U.S. Patent #4,188,667.

Greenberg, J. (1989). A real-time adaptive-beamforming hearing aid. Master's thesis, Massachusetts Institute of Technology.

Haggard, M., Trinder, J., Foster, J., and Lindblad, A. (1987). Two-state compression of spectral tilt: Individual differences and psychoacoustical limitations to the benefit from compression. *Journal of Rehabilitation Research and Development* 24(4):193–206.

Harris, R., Brey, R., Robinette, M., Chabries, D., Christiansen, R., and Jolley, R. (1988). Use of adaptive digital signal processing to improve speech communication for normally hearing and hearing-impaired subjects. *Journal of Speech and Hearing Research* 31:265–271.

Hecox, K., and Punch, J. (1988). The impact of digital technology on the selection and fitting of hearing aids. *American Journal of Otology* 9(Suppl):77–85.

Hoffman, M., and Buckley, K. (1990). Constrained optimum filtering for multi-microphone digital hearing aids. Presented at ASILOMAR'90.

Houtgast, T., and Steeneken, H. (1985). A review of the MTF concept in room acoustics and its use for estimating speech intelligibility in auditoria. *Journal of the Acoustical Society of America* 77(3):1069–1077.

Kates, J. (1984). Speech intelligibility enhancement. U.S. Patent #4,454,609.

Kates, J. (1986). Signal processing for hearing aids. *Hearing Instruments* 37(2):19–22.

Kates, J. (1991). Feedback cancellation in hearing aids: Results from a computer simulation. *IEEE Transactions on Signal Processing* 39(3):553–562.

Kennedy, E., and Levitt, H. (1990). Optimal C/V intensity ratio at MCL. Presented at ASHA Convention, Seattle.

King, A., and Martin, M. (1984). Is AGC beneficial in hearing aids? *British Journal of Audiology* 18:31–38.

Klein, A. (1989). Assessing speech recognition in

noise for listeners with a signal processor hearing aid. *Ear and Hearing* 10(1):50–57.

Knowles (1988). The Knowles amplified receiver. Knowles Report 10676–1.

Langhans, T., and Strube, H. (1982). Speech enhancement by nonlinear multiband envelope expansion. *Proceedings of IEEE ICASSP*:156–159.

Larsen, S. (1986). The effect of a self-adaptive filter on speech reception thresholds in noise for hearing impaired subjects. Master's thesis, University of Minnesota.

Lenk, J. (1974). *Handbook of Modern Solid-State Amplifiers* (pp. 28, 254). Englewood Cliffs, NJ: Prentice Hall.

Levitt, H., Neumann, A., Toraskar, J. (1986). Orthogonal polynomial compression amplification for the hearing impaired. *Journal of the Acoustical Society of America* 80(Suppl. 1):S12.

Levitt, H., Dugot, R., Kopper, K. (1988). Programmable digital hearing aid system. U.S. Patent #4,731,850.

Levitt, H. (1987). Digital hearing aids: A tutorial review. *Journal of Rehabilitation Research and Development* 24(4):7–20.

Licklider, J., and Pollack, I. (1948). Effects of differentiation, integration and infinite peak clipping upon the intelligibility of speech. *Journal of the Acoustical Society of America* 20:42–51.

Lim, J. (1983). *Speech Enhancement*. Englewood Cliffs, NJ: Prentice Hall.

Lim, J. (1979). Evaluation of a correlation subtraction method for enhancing speech degraded by additive white noise. *IEEE Transactions on Acoustics, Speech, and Signal Processing* 26:471–472.

Lim, J. (1982). Signal processing for speech enhancement. In: G. Studebaker and F. Bess (eds.), *The Vanderbilt Hearing-Aid Report* (pp. 124–130). Upper Darby, PA: Monographs in Contemporary Audiology.

Lim, J., and Oppenheim, A. (1984). Enhancement and bandwidth compression of noisy speech. Proceedings of the IEEE:1586–1604.

Lippmann, R., Braida, L., and Durlach, N. (1981). Study of multichannel amplitude compression and linear amplification for persons with sensorineural hearing loss. *Journal of the Acoustical Society of America* 69:524–531.

Marshall, R., and Harry, W. (1941). A new microphone providing uniform directivity over an extended frequency range. *Journal of the Acoustical Society of America* 12:481–498.

McAulay, R., and Malpass, M. (1980). Speech enhancement using a soft-decision noise suppression filter. *IEEE Transactions on Acoustics, Speech and Signal Processing* 29(2):137–145.

Miller, E. (1988). Digital signal processing in hearing aids: Implications and applications. *Hearing Journal* 41(4):22–26.

Miller, H. (1986). Electronic noise-reducing system. U.S. Patent #4,589,137.

Montgomery, A. (1984). A review of speech signal enhancement for the hearing impaired. Proceedings of Symposium on Hearing Technology, Gallaudet University.

Montgomery, A., and Edge, R. (1988). Evaluation of two speech enhancement techniques to improve intelligibility for hearing-impaired adults. *Journal of Speech and Hearing Research* 31:386–393.

Moorer, J., and Berger, M. (1986). Linear-phase bandsplitting: Theory and applications. *Journal of the Audio Engineering Society* 34(3):143–151.

Morely, R., Engel, G., Sullivan, T., and Natarajan, S. (1988). VLSI based design of a battery-operated digital hearing aid. *Proceedings of IEEE ICASSP*.

Niederjohn, R., and Grotelueschen, J. (1976). The enhancement of speech intelligibility in high noise levels by high-pass filtering followed by rapid amplitude compression. *IEEE Transactions on Acoustics, Speech and Signal Processing* 24:277–282.

Nielsen, B. (1986). Digital hearing aids: Where are they? *Hearing Instruments* 37(2):6.

Nielsen, L., Wu, E., Hoffman, M., Buckley, K., and Soli, S. (1990). Design and evaluation of FIR filters for digital hearing aids with arbitrary amplitude and phase response. *Journal of the Acoustical Society of America* 87(Suppl. 1):S24

Nunley, J., Staab, W., Steadman, J., Wechsler, P. and Spencer, B. (1983). A wearable digital hearing aid. *Hearing Journal* 36:10.

O'Connell, M., Skinner, M., Engebretson, M., Miller, J., and Pascoe, D. (1988). Evaluation of a digital hearing aid and fitting system. *Journal of the Acoustical Society of America* 84(Suppl. 1):S40.

Ochs, M., Sammeth, C., and Tetzeli, M. (1992). Acoustic analysis of syllables processed by linear and nonlinear hearing aid circuits. Presented at the American Academy of Audiology Meeting, Nashville, TN, April.

Pascoe, D. (1975). Frequency responses of hearing aids and their effects on speech perception of hearing-impaired subjects. *Annals of Otology, Rhinology and Laryngology* 23(Suppl.):84.

Peterson, P. (1987). Using linearly constrained adaptive beamforming to reduce interference in hearing aids from competing talkers in reverberant rooms. *Proceedings of IEEE ICASSP*: 2364–2367.

Peterson, P., Durlach, N., Rabinowitz, W., and Zurek, P. (1987). Multimicrophone adaptive beamforming for interference reduction in hearing aids. *Journal of Rehabilitation Research and Development* 24(4):103–110.

Peterson, P., Wei, S., Rabinowitz, W., and Zurek, P. (1990). Robustness of an adaptive beamforming method for hearing aids. *Acta Otolaryngologica* (Suppl. 469):85–90.

Picheny, M., Durlach, N., and Braida, L. (1985). Speaking clearly for the hard of hearing, I: Intelligibility differences between clear and conversational speech. *Journal of Speech and Hearing Research* 28:96–103.

Picheny, M., Durlach, N., and Braida, L. (1986). Speaking clearly for the hard of hearing, II: Acoustic characteristics of clear and conversational speech. *Journal of Speech and Hearing Research* 29:434–446.

Plomp, R. (1988). The negative effect of amplitude compression in multichannel hearing aids in the light of the modulation-transfer function. *Journal of the Acoustical Society of America* 83(6):2322–2327.

Preves, D. (1986). Future developments in hearing aid technology. In: W. Hodgsen (ed.), *Hearing Aid Assessment and Audiologic Habilitation* (pp. 317–320). Baltimore: Williams and Wilkins.

Preves, D. (1987). Digital hearing aids. *ASHA* 29:45–47.

Preves, D. (1988). Principles of signal processing. In: R. Sandlin (ed.), *Handbook of Hearing Aid Amplification, I: Technical and Theoretical Considerations* (pp. 87–94). Boston, MA: College Hill Press.

Preves, D., and Newton, J. (1989). The headroom problem and hearing aid performance. *Hearing Journal* 42(10):21.

Preves, D., Fortune, T., Woodruff, B., and Newton, J. (1991). Strategies for enhancing the consonant to vowel ratio with in the ear hearing aids. *Ear and Hearing* 6(Suppl. 12):1395–1535.

Revoile, S., Pickett, J., Holden, L., and Talkin, D. (1982). Acoustic cues to final stop voicing and impaired- and normal-hearing listeners. *Journal of the Acoustical Society of America* 72:1145–1154.

Revoile, S., Holden-Pitt, L., Edward, D., Pickett, J., and Brandt, F. (1987). Speech-cue enhancement for the hearing impaired: Amplification of burst/murmur cues for improved perception of final stop voicing. *Journal of Rehabilitation Research and Development* 24(4):207–216.

Revoile, S., Holden-Pitt, L., Edward, D., and Pickett, J. (1986). Some rehabilitative considerations for future speech-processing hearing aids. *Journal of Rehabilitation Research and Development* 23(1):89–94.

Revoile, S., and Holden-Pitt, L. (1990). Some acoustic enhancements of speech and their effect on consonant identification by the hearing impaired. Presented at Arrowhead, California, Conference.

Roeser, R., and Taylor, K. (1988). Audiometric and field testing with a digital hearing instrument. *Hearing Instruments* 39(4):14.

Sammeth, C. (1989). Hearing instruments: From vacuum tubes to digital microchips. *Hearing Instruments* 40(10):9–12. *Journal of Rehabilitation Research and Development*.

Sammeth, C., Preves, D., Bratt, G., Peek, B., and Bess, F. (1993). Achieving prescribed gain/frequency responses with advances in hearing aid technology. *Journal of Rahabilitation Research and Development*.

Sambur, M. (1978). Adaptive noise cancelling for speech signals. *IEEE Transactions on Acoustics, Speech, and Signal Processing* 26(5):419–423.

Schroeder, M. (1979). Acoustics in human communications. Plenary lecture, 97th Meeting of the Acoustical Society of America, Cambridge, MA.

Sessler, G.M., and West, J.E. (1975). Second order gradient unidirectional microphones. *Journal of the Acoustical Society of America* 58(1):278.

Sidwell, A., and Summerfield, Q. (1985). The effect of enhanced spectral contrast on the internal representation of vowel-shaped noise. *Journal of the Acoustical Society of America* 78(2):495–506.

Staab, W. (1987). Digital hearing instruments, *Hearing Instruments* 38(11):18–26.

Staab, W. (1985). Digital hearing aids. *Hearing Instruments* 36(11):14.

Staab, W. (1990). Digital/programmable hearing aids—an eye towards the future. *British Journal of Audiology* 24:243–256.

Stein, L., and Dempsey-Hart, D. (1984). Listener-assessed intelligibility of a hearing aid self-adaptive noise filter. *Ear and Hearing* 4:199–204.

Strube, H. (1981). Separation of several speakers recorded by two microphones (cocktail-party processing), Signal Processing, 3, 4, North-Holland Publishing Co.: 355–364.

Studebaker, G., Sherbecoe, R., and Matesich, J. (1987). Spectrum shaping with a hardware digital filter. *Journal of Rehabilitation Research and Development* 24(4):21–28.

Summerfield, Q., Foster, J., and Tyler, R. (1985). Influences of formant bandwidth and auditory frequency selectivity on identification of place of articulation in stop consonants. *Speech Communication* 4:213–229.

Tetzeli, M., Sammeth, C., and Ochs, M. (1991). Effects of nonlinear amplification on speech intelligibility and sound quality. Presented at the American Speech–Language–Hearing Association Meeting, Atlanta, GA.

Tuzman, A. (1989). Spatial filtering for hearing aids. Master's thesis, University of Minnesota.

Van Tasell, D. (1988). Noise reduction hearing aids. Presented at the American Speech and Hearing Association Workshop on Amplification: Evaluation, dispensing, and devices, Minneapolis, MN.

Van Tasell, D., Larsen, S., and Fabry, D. (1988). Effects of an adaptive filter hearing aid on speech recognition in noise by hearing-impaired subjects. *Ear and Hearing* 9(1):15–21.

van Veen, T., and Houtgast, T. (1985). Spectral sharpness and vowel dissimilarity. *Journal of the Acoustical Society of America* 77(2):628–634.

Villchur, E. (1973). Signal processing to improve speech intelligibility in perceptive deafness. *Journal of the Acoustical Society of America* 53(6):1646–1657.

Villchur, E. (1989). Comments on "The negative effect of amplitude compression in multichannel hearing aids in the light of the modulation-transfer function" [*Journal of the Acoustical Society of America* 83:2322–2327 (1988)]. *Journal of the Acoustical Society of America* 86(1):425–427.

Walker, G., Byrne, D., and Dillon, H. (1984). The effects of multichannel compression/expansion amplification on the intelligibility of nonsense syllables in noise. *Journal of the Acoustical Society of America* 73(3):746–757.

Walker, G., and Dillon, H. (1982). Compression in hearing aids: An analysis, a review and some recommendations. National Acoustics Laboratory Report No. 90. Canberra: Australian Government Publishing Service.

Weiss, M. (1987). Use of an adaptive noise canceler as an input preprocessor for a hearing aid. *Journal of Rehabilitation Research and Development* 24(4):93–102.

Widin, G. (1987). The meaning of digital technology. *Hearing Instruments* 38(11):28–33.

Widrow, B., Glover, J., McCool, J., et al. (1975). Adaptive noise cancelling: Principles and applications. *Proceedings of the IEEE* 63:1692–1716.

Williamson, M., and Punch, J. (1990). Speech enhancement in digital hearing aids. In: C. Sammeth (ed.), *Seminars in Hearing*. New York: Thieme Medical Publishers.

Wolinsky, S. (1986). Clinical assessment of a self-adaptive noise filtering system. *Hearing Journal* 39(10):29–32.

Yanick, P., and Drucker, D. (1976). Signal processing to improve intelligibility in the presence of noise for persons with ski-slope hearing impairment. *IEEE Transactions on Acoustics, Speech, and Signal Processing* 24:507–512.

Author Index